# EARLY INTERVENTION I
## Working with Infants and Toddlers

**Katharine G. Butler, PhD**
Editor, *Topics in Language Disorders*
Syracuse University
Syracuse, New York

## TOPICS IN LANGUAGE DISORDERS SERIES

AN ASPEN PUBLICATION®
Aspen Publishers, Inc.
Gaithersburg, Maryland
1994

Library of Congress Cataloging-in-Publication Data

Early intervention / Katharine G. Butler, editor.
p. cm.
Compilations from Topics in language disorders.
Includes bibliographical references and index.
Contents: 1. Working with infants and toddlers—2. Working with
families and parents.
ISBN: 0-8342-0584-x (v. 1)—ISBN: 0-8342-0585-8 (v. 2)
1. Communicative disorders in children—Treatment. 2. Communicative
disorders in infants—Treatment 3. Language disorders in children—Treatment.
I. Butler, Katharine G.
II. Topics in language disorders
RJ496.C67E38 1994
618.92'85506—dc20
93-36266
CIP

Editorial Resources: Ruth Bloom

Library of Congress Catalog Card Number: 93-36266
ISBN: 0-8342-0584-x
Series ISBN: 0-8342-0590-4

Printed in the United States

1 2 3 4 5

# Table of Contents

**Early Intervention I: Working with Infants and Toddlers**

v   Preface

1   **Part I—Identification of At-Risk and Disabled Infants and Toddlers**

3   **A collaborative approach to developmental care continuity with infants born at risk and their families**
Ginny Laadt-Bruno, Patricia K.Lilley, and Carol E. Westby

17   **Neonates and infants at risk for hearing and speech–language disorders**
David A. Clark

29   **Identifying expressive language delay at age two**
Leslie Rescorla

36   **Toward an integrated view of early language and communication development and socioemotional development**
Barry M. Prizant and Amy M. Wetherby

52   **Delivering communication-based services to infants, toddlers, and their families: Approaches and models**
M. Jeanne Wilcox

65   **Part II—Assessment Strategies: Implications from Practice and Research with Normal and Disordered Populations**

67   **Ins and outs of the acquisition of spatial terms**
Cheryl K. Messick

79   **Freeing talk from the here-and-now: The role of event knowledge and maternal scaffolds**
Joan Lucariello

95   **Language sampling for repeated measures with language-impaired preschoolers: Comparison of two procedures**
Barbara A. Bain, Lesley B. Olswang, and Glenn A. Johnson

110   **Normal and disordered phonology in two-year-olds**
Carol Stoel-Gammon

122 **Early assessment and intervention with emotional and behavioral disorders and communication disorders**
Geraldine Theadore, Suzanne R. Maher, and Barry M. Prizant

137 **Bringing context back into assessment**
Truman E. Coggins

149 **Part III–Intervention Strategies: Applications from Practice and Research with Normal and Disordered Populations**

151 **The role of world knowledge in language comprehension and language intervention**
Linda M. Milosky

164 **Intervention issues for toddlers with specific language impairments**
Lesley B. Olswang and Barbara A. Bain

182 **Providing services to children with autism (ages 0 to 2 years) and their families**
Barry M. Prizant and Amy M. Wetherby

205 **"Verb-alizing": Facilitating action word usage in young language-impaired children**
Kathy L. Chapman and Brenda Y. Terrell

219 **Index**

# Preface

*Topics in Language Disorders* is a transdisciplinary journal that is devoted to discussion of issues surrounding language acquisition and its disorders. *TLD* has the following major purposes: (1) providing relevant information to practicing professionals who provide services to those who are at-risk or have language disabilities; (2) clarifying the application of theory and research to practice; (3) bringing together professionals across disciplines, who are researchers and clinicians from the health education arenas both as authors and as readers; (4) clarifying the application of theory to practice among professionals and students-in-training; and (5) contributing to the scientific literature while making each issue accessible and relevant to an interdisciplinary readership.

Typically, each *TLD* journal is devoted to a single topic, although the constellation of articles may vary. A few may be wholly clinical in nature, while most blend practice and research. In the *TLD* book series, each book provides a critical but highly sensitive evaluation of current research and translates that analysis into a framework for service delivery. Hence, in this *TLD* book, the reader will find a distillation of the best of the journal's current offerings as well as some seminal articles that may enhance the readers' conceptual knowledge. Offerings are provided by professionals from a variety of disciplines: speech-language pathology, human development, psychology, and medicine (including pediatrics and neonatology).

The authors represented within the covers of *Early Intervention I: Working with Infants and Toddlers* were gathered together to provide a current perspective on the rapidly growing specialty area of early childhood services. An accompanying volume, *Early Intervention II: Working with Parents and Families*, provides additional information on this important topic. Both volumes stress a family systems approach. In reality, it is impossible to separate consider-

ation of infants and toddlers from consideration of their parents and families (Billeaud, 1993; Donahue-Kilburg, 1992). As many researchers and clinicians have advocated, professionals from a variety of disciplines must work together to provide services to very young children within a family-centered context. Given the twin goals of prevention and intervention, this book provides an overview of identification, assessment, and intervention with the zero to three population who are either at-risk or exhibit communication disorders.

## PART I. IDENTIFICATION OF AT-RISK AND DISABLED INFANTS AND TODDLERS

Part I provides readers with a glimpse of neonatal intensive care units and demonstrates the potential for language specialists to work within the medical setting to provide continuity of care from hospital to home. Secondly, a variety of medical problems whose sequelae are known to involve disorders of communication are presented. Thirdly, identification of expressive language difficulties in toddlerhood provides a framework for considering the fourth item, dealing with the socioemotional aspects of language development—an oft-ignored area of concern. Finally, a number of approaches and models for the delivery of communication-based services are provided.

In "A Collaborative Approach to Developmental Care Continuity with Infants Born At-Risk and Their Families," Laadt-Bruno, Lilley, and Westby provide an exciting exemplar of a program that is currently in place at the University of New Mexico (UNM) School of Medicine within the Division of Neonatology, Department of Pediatrics. The team approach utilized in this setting includes occupational and physical therapy, child development, family therapy, and speech-language pathology. While this array of professionals is not unusual, the two-tiered team structure developed by the authors and their colleagues from other disciplines suggests that team membership that is flexible and that can be modified as infant and family needs change is responsive to the realities of service provision and cost effectiveness. As the authors conclude, "no single professional can address the diverse needs of infants born at-risk and their families....Professionals and families must collaborate...[in order to] support and encourage infants to maintain their developmental trajectory to the greatest degree possible during hospitalization and beyond."

Clark, in "Neonates and Infants At Risk for Hearing and Speech-Language Disorders," reminds readers of the multiple factors that may cause hearing and speech-language disorders. He focuses on prenatal, perinatal, and early childhood risks of later developmental delay. Noting that "the earlier an infection occurs in the pregnancy, the more profound are the physical and neurological abnormalities in the newborn." He elaborates on a number of aspects of in utero fetal infections, chromosomal abnormalities, environmental toxin, perinatal and postnatal acquired infections, as well as a number of syndromes, asphyxia, prematurity, intracranial hemorrhage, bilirubin, ototoxic drugs, and environmental noise in the NICU. In support of a team approach, he notes that "physicians must ensure that the newborn with any identifiable risk is evaluated by competent developmentalists, speech-language pathologists, and educators in order to limit the adverse impact of any impairment."

Rescorla, in "Identifying Expressive Language Delay at Age Two," joins other researchers in noting that language delay is a major risk factor for later educational and mental health problems. When identified in the preschool, she maintains such language delay has a strong predictive correlation with later learning disabilities. She also cites the extant evidence that young children with language delay also have higher rates of behavioral and psychiatric disorders than do children with normal lan-

guage. This latter statement is sometimes rejected by language clinicians in various settings where mental health problems are treated exclusively by professionals in other fields. Noting that language delay identified at age two is likely to continue, she provides a review of pediatric screening instruments and parent report inventories but points out that "the gold standard" has not yet been met for most assessment instruments. She continues by discussing the MacArthur Communicative Development Inventory (CDI), as constructed by Bates and her colleagues, and is now published commercially. She follows her review of the CDI with a discussion of the Language Development Survey (LDS) that she developed in 1981. She concludes that LDS is a highly efficient instrument with data collected on more than 900 children. This screening tool might well be used as a first cut at initial identification, with the CDI being used as a more comprehensive parental report followed by a language evaluation, as necessary.

The theme of early communication development and socioemotional status is picked up again in Prizant and Wetherby's offering, "Toward an Integrated View of Early Language and Communication Development and Socioemotional Development." Although it has been noted that approximately 50% to 60% of the children and adolescents who have emotional and behavioral disorders also have communication disorders, the co-occurrence of these disorders within the same child requires an integrative approach among professionals in assessment and intervention. Thus, the need for social workers, child psychiatrists, psychologists, and language specialists to share perspectives is obvious. Nevertheless, the collaboration across disciplines is far from a reality in many settings. The authors note that infancy researchers are beginning to "demonstrate interest in exploring continuities between early affective or behavioral state communication and later emerging intentional and propositional communication." Readers will be interested in the very early (prior to 12 months of age) signals that infants provide as affective and referential communication systems meld together. Stressing the need for speech-language pathologists and other language specialists to integrate a mental health perspective, the authors note that early appropriate communication and language intervention utilizing family strengths may prevent the development of emotional and behavioral difficulty in very young children. As the authors trace the development of language and communication across the preschool years, they provide a series of guideposts that underscore the important role played by communication not only with and between infants and toddlers and their parents, but also with their siblings and other peers. Appropriate and collaborative intervention may well increase young language-disordered children's ability to interact and establish positive relationships in day care centers and early intervention and preschool programs. Finally, Prizant and Wetherby cite the evidence that children who experience early communicative impairments may be at "double risk, because of the effects of emotionally stressful environments (i.e., abusive or neglectful environments) on young children may include secondary language and communication delays." Very recently this finding has been supported by new evidence reported in *Topics in Language Disorders* 13:4, August 1993 ("Child Abuse: Cognitive, Linguistic, and Developmental Considerations," L.S. Snyder and K.J. Saywitz, co-Issue Editors).

Wilcox, a leader in the field of early intervention and communication disorders, presents a cohesive discussion of "Delivering Communication-Based Services to Infants, Toddlers and Their Families: Approaches and Models." Noting that there are multiple approaches and models, Wilcox establishes the view that most often approaches are combined rather than used singly. These approaches include remediation, prevention, and compensation. All of these approaches share the goal of improving developmental outcomes. Obviously, prevention is the controlling factor unless or until a language disorder is identified. When a communication disorder is identified, either compensation or remediation, one (or a combination of the two) is in order. Wilcox also comments upon the necessity for some formal mechanism for interprofessional collaboration. Readers new to the field may be interested in Wilcox's discussion of multidisciplinary, transdisciplinary, and interdisciplinary models. Role release as a component of the transdiciplinary model has been a subject of intense interest among professionals who feel strongly about a profession's scope of practice as detailed in licensing laws in various states. Wilcox concludes that communication has a central role in early intervention planning, and that the most appropriate model "includes a programming team....Early intervention personnel should be well versed in each of the approaches and make decisions in accordance with the needs of individual infants, toddlers, and families." Who could disagree?

In the next section, six carefully selected articles provide a bird's eye view of assessment strategies based upon recent research with normal and language-disordered populations. Focusing on semantic, lexical, and phonological acquisition, maternal scaffolding in the service of the infant's emerging event knowledge, the use of language sampling procedures, and concluding with the assessment of communicative intentions within a variety of contexts, this section provides a wealth of information for very early assessment techniques.

## PART II. ASSESSMENT STRATEGIES: IMPLICATIONS FROM PRACTICE AND RESEARCH WITH NORMAL AND DISORDERED POPULATIONS

This section begins with a presentation by Messick, "Ins and Outs of the Acquisition of Spatial Terms," that may provide language clinicians with a new perspective on "teaching prepositions," for example. In many preschool classrooms, the teaching of spatial terms is thought to be a simple, easily learned activity. Messick dispels this notion as she provides the theoretical constructs that underlie the acquisition of spatial prepositions, nouns, and adjectives in the child's lexicon. She urges professionals to begin by examining the child's conceptualization of these words, as well as the toddler's comprehension and production of them. She provides the reader with the available information regarding the developmental progression of spatial term acquisition, but emphasizes that children as young as 18 months use context to make decisions regarding such words as *in*, *on*, and *under*. Thus, children *appear* to understand and produce spatial terms when they have not yet actually comprehended the words' meanings. Messick suggests a number of assessment strategies using objects rather than pictures and concludes with an equal number of intervention strategies, also using objects in naturalistic as well as direct instruction. Language specialists will appreciate Messick's efforts to provide readers "direct instruction" on the topic of spatial terms.

We begin with a question, What does TD mean? What does it mean on a beautiful Fall day standing outside a college football stadium? In that context one could only assume TOUCHDOWN. But what does TD mean when the reader encounters it within the covers of this volume? The context of the book's title and Lucariello's article "Freeing Talk from the Here-and-Now: The Role of Event Knowledge and Maternal Scaffolds," provides a comprehension clue, and the author's first sentences dispel the mystery: "At least two sources of language acquisition, the cognitive and the social-interactive relate to the acquisition of temporally displaced (TD) speech, defined as talk about objects and events displaced in time from the present situation. The ability to talk about the nonpresent, that is, past and future

happenings and persons and things not in the perceptual field is one of the most important characteristics of linguistic communication, indeed setting it apart from other forms of communication." TD, or displaced reference, may be found in children's language between 20 and 24 months and is highly related to the mother's or caretaker's scaffolding. Lucariello's own research leads her to suggest that it is the interactive nature of parental scaffolding and the child's increasing event knowledge through conversational routines that assists children in the acquisition of TD speech. Mothers who provide infants and toddlers with highly scripted contexts, i.e., a commonly occurring routine activity that is highly familiar and predictable to both adult and child, contribute to both past talk and future talk. The author provides a number of suggestions for both assessment and intervention; readers will not be surprised to find that she suggests that the language specialist use multiple means over multiple observational contexts, with multiple tests or scales, and multiple methods. By using a variety of dynamic measures of the child's ability to produce TD speech, the clinician assesses the child's cognitive functioning while identifying intervention goals and objectives. The author concludes with specific suggestions for intervention and training.

Continuing with the theme that standardized assessment procedures are limited in their scope and depth, Bain, Olswang, and Johnson discuss "Language Sampling for Repeated Measures with Language-Impaired Preschoolers: Comparison of Two Procedures." The authors propose that sampling early semantic production also requires adult input, or scaffolding, and familiarity of tasks and materials, which the authors identify as "predictability." The authors discuss their recent research and conclude that free-play situations that were structured were sufficient to provide opportunities for two-word utterances. They conclude that "clinicians need not focus on creating special events and episodes, but rather on providing enough interesting materials to ensure opportunities will arise for language behaviors of interest."

"Normal and Disordered Phonology in Two-Year Olds" is discussed by Stoel-Gammon who cites the tremendous individual variation which may be found among infants and toddlers, as she urges an emphasis on broad assessment of the entire communicative system. She contrasts normal and atypical phonological development and assists readers in ascertaining the limits of normal variation. Stoel-Gammon asserts that the range of variability declines between age two and age three, thus making the diagnosis of phonological disorders easier following the toddler's second birthday. She concludes with a discussion of atypical error patterns and the lexicon-phonology interface, and the suggestion that a "late talker" may be the child with less than 50 words or a phonetic inventory of only 4 or 5 consonants. Stoel Gammon makes a final appeal: "...normal phonological development cannot be determined by comparing the child's performance with a set of speech-sound norms like those used to evaluate older children. Examination of the subparts of the phonological system is not enough...."

Prizant returns with his colleagues, Theadore, and Maher, in Part II to confront issues related to "Early Assessment and Intervention with Emotional and Behavioral Disorders." Such issues include the infant's or toddler's behavioral difficulties, including overactivity, impulsivity, aggression, and low tolerance for frustration as well as behavioral control and regulation of emotional arousal. Other symptoms of emotional difficulties may be seen in severe separation anxiety, fearfulness of new situations and avoidance or withdrawal from interactions. Having absorbed the earlier articles in this text, readers will not be surprised to find that these authors recommend observation of predictable routines between parent or caregiver and child, and less predictable or familiar routines, including free play and other interactional activities. They strongly suggest a transactional approach to early intervention, returning to the theme expressed in Part I of this volume, whereby the family context is paramount in providing the social and emotional interaction required for normalizing language development. Once again, the authors note that, "When disturbed interactional patterns appear to be deeply rooted in dysfunctional caregiver behavior related to extremely stressful life circumstances, speech-language pathologist must work closely with mental health professionals to ensure that other emotional and social supports are addressed." The authors conclude by providing a number of valuable service delivery options.

Coggins, in "Bringing Context Back into Assessment," brings closure to Part II with his review of past and present approaches to early language assessment. He specifies that since "communicative intents are acquired in context-dependent situations, communication and context stand as essential variables to manipulate during the assessments of developmentally young children. Clearly, the only way in which speech-language clinicians will ultimately attain a complete and satisfying understanding of a handicapped child's social use of language is to bring context back into the assessment process. He, too, addresses the importance of communicative intentions, followed by a discussion of the patterns of performance one might find in clinical populations. Readers will find his suggestions for manipulating contextual variables for assessment purposes to be consonant with earlier discussions in this section and to summarize the importance of dynamic approach to the assessment process.

Part III, which follows, assists readers in pulling together assessment and intervention principles. As most experienced clinicians have long known, it is difficult to separate assessment and intervention, since ongoing assessment embeds itself within every intervention procedure of consequence.

## PART III. INTERVENTION STRATEGIES: APPLICATIONS FROM PRACTICE AND RESEARCH WITH NORMAL AND DISORDERED POPULATIONS

Miloskey begins Part III with a discussion of "The Role of World Knowledge in Language Comprehension and Language Intervention," in which she describes how *world knowledge* is closely aligned with *word knowledge*. She notes that "the implications of "a world-knowledge-driven model are considerable for the clinician. Therapy stimuli or targets cannot be considered as merely words or language, but must be considered as packets of information about the world." Thus, the goals of therapy are to assist children in using relevant knowledge about the world and about language to add to that language knowledge "store" from which they may comprehend and integrate new knowledge. Miloskey continues with a discussion of later language learning, describing how words come to have a "history" and how interventionists must establish goals which take into account the child, the context, and world and word history.

Olswang and Bain pick up from their earlier commentary on assessment to provide readers with an insightful discussion of "Intervention Issues for Toddlers with Specific Language Impairments." Specific Language Impairment (SLI) is reflected in children's performance at age level in all aspects other than language development (in which they perform at least 6 months below their chronological age or minus one standard deviation on standardized texts). Treatment of SLI children is seen as involving (1) changing or alleviating the underlying language deficit; (2) making the child more proficient in certain discrete aspects of linguistic comprehension and production, without

suggesting that the child is "cured"; and/or (3) providing a number of compensatory strategies to assist the child in gaining a higher level of language sophistication. They illustrate service delivery options by suggesting teaching strategies, such as milieu teaching, inductive teaching, and joint action routines, followed by a dissection of the clinical decision-making process.

Prizant and Wetherby also return to provide insight on intervention in "Providing Services to Children with Autism (Ages 0 to 2 Years) and Their Families." Stressing that early diagnosis of autism is a difficult task, the authors, nevertheless, provide a description of early symptomatology and early identification. Acknowledging that we know little about very early intervention (ages 2 and below), they note that intervention prior to age 5 rather than after age 5 would lead language specialists to opt for the earliest possible moment to use developmental strategies with very young autistic children. They note a number of approaches to early assessment of cognition, language, and symbolic behavior, followed by a helpful discussion of approaches to early intervention, including home- vs. center-based approaches. They conclude with a set of well defined expectations for appropriate intervention specifically with adult-child interactions involving caregivers, noting that progress is then realized for both child and family.

Part III of this volume concludes with Chapman and Terrell's apt description of "'Verbalizing': Facilitating Action Word Usage in Young Language Impaired Children." While their work is applicable to autistic children, it is also applicable to children with lesser degrees of language impairment. When facilitating the use of action-related terms, they suggest focused stimulation and the use of scripts. They conclude that intervention undertaken in this manner will provide language-impaired children with the opportunity to increase single word utterances which then may facilitate transition to later stages of language.

In closing, this volume brings to readers a progress report on research and practice in language acquisition and disorders. We have increased reason to hope that *early* intervention will increase infants' and toddlers' ability to communicate. Milne (1927) captured the essence of "zero to three" when he wrote:

When I was One I had just begun,
When I was Two I was almost new,
When I was Three I was nearly me.

The authors in this volume have captured the essence of what it means to work with an infant or toddler in the years that lead to becoming "me."

## REFERENCES

Billeaud, F.P. (1993). *Communication disorders in infants and toddlers: Assessment and intervention*. Boston, MA: Andover Medical Publishers.

Butler, K.G. (1993). (Ed). Child abuse: Cognitive, linguistic, and developmental considerations. *Topics in Language Disorders, 13*(4); L.S. Snyder & K.J. Saywitz, Issue Co-editors.

Donahue-Kilburg, G. (1992). *Family-centered early intervention for communication disorders: Prevention and treatment*. Gaithersburg, MD: Aspen Publishers.

Milne, A.A. (1927). *Now we are six*. Toronto, Canada: McClelland & Stewart, LTD.

—*Katharine G. Butler, PhD*
Editor, *Topics in Language Disorders*

# Part I
# Identification of At-Risk and Disabled Infants and Toddlers

# A collaborative approach to developmental care continuity with infants born at risk and their families

**Ginny Laadt-Bruno, MA**
*Occupational Therapist*
*Department of Pediatrics, Neonatology*
*    Division*
*University of New Mexico School of*
*    Medicine*
*Albuquerque, New Mexico*

**Patricia K. Lilley, MS**
*Speech-Language Pathologist*
*Department of Pediatrics, Neonatology*
*    Division*
*University of New Mexico School of*
*    Medicine*
*Albuquerque, New Mexico*

**Carol E. Westby, PhD**
*Speech-Language Pathologist*
*University of New Mexico*
*University Affiliated Program*
*Albuquerque, New Mexico*

## CHANGING ISSUES IN EARLY INTERVENTION

The complexity and magic of early childhood development have been described in great detail during the past 20 years. Research on early attachment, social/emotional development, parent-child interaction, and development of sensorimotor skills has provided an understanding of issues that must be considered when working with infants and families. Infant development is currently viewed within the context of family structure and cultural heritage. This view influences the manner in which professionals provide services to infants and toddlers who are at risk for developmental concerns or in which developmental concerns have been identified (Krehbiel, Munsick-Bruno, & Lowe, 1991).

Service delivery models for infants born at risk or with identified developmental disorders must take into account (1) the changing nature of at-risk infant populations and family environments; (2) changes in atti-

*Acknowledgments to Roberta Krehbiel, PhD, LuAnn Papile, MD, Julia Stephens, MEP, Developmental Care Staff.*

*Top Lang Disord* 1993;14(1):15–28

tudes regarding collaboration with families and changes among agencies in determining families' and children's needs and how best to provide services; (3) legislative changes mandating services; and (4) development of interdisciplinary and transdisciplinary professional teams.

The number of infants and toddlers requiring early intervention services is increasing. This is related in part to broadened definitions of who is eligible for and who may benefit from services. In addition, improved medical technology has affected infant survival. The number of infants with chronic illness who survive has increased. More than 50% of infants weighing less than 750 grams are surviving (Bauchner, Brown, & Peskin, 1988). The increasing prevalence of infants exposed to environmental teratogens that prolong hospitalization and affect maternal-infant relationships has been described by the American Academy of Pediatrics as the "new morbidity." Examples include infants who were exposed to drugs or alcohol during the prenatal period or who are born to mothers with the human immunodeficiency virus (HIV) or the acquired immunodeficiency syndrome (AIDS) (Spiegel & Mayers, 1991; Zuckerman & Bresnahan, 1991).

Appropriate services for infants born at developmental risk and their families require collaboration among professionals and families within a family context (Gorski, 1991). The identification of the family's key role in any intervention program leads to recognition of the unique characteristics of families. Legislation has mandated services to younger populations and changed the ways in which assessment and intervention are provided. The 1986 Public Law 99-457 (Part H), an amendment to the Individuals with Disabilities Educa-

tion Act, mandated services to children with developmental disabilities from birth through two years of age.

Changing populations and legislation have resulted in changes in assessment and intervention paradigms. There is a stronger emphasis on coordination of services among families and professionals. A major shift toward recognizing the importance of service coordination is underscored through funding of the service coordinator position. The law has facilitated team decision making by encouraging collaboration with families and other professionals (Briggs, 1991; Gilbert, Sciarillo, & Van Rembrow, 1992). The shift to interventions with children who are younger and more fragile medically has promoted development of collaborative consultation models that focus on prevention and integration of medical, educational, and therapeutic services for young children and their families (Krehbiel, Munsick-Bruno, & Lowe, 1991; McGonigel & Garland, 1988).

Developmental assessment and intervention services for infants and toddlers who are considered to be at risk may begin within the hospital setting and assist infants and families through the transition to their homes and communities. This article describes a collaborative consultation process developed by the University of New Mexico (UNM) Developmental Care team of University Hospital to address the needs of newborns at risk and their families.

## TEAM STRUCTURE

The Developmental Care (DC) clinical team within the Division of Neonatology, Department of Pediatrics, reflects multiple disciplines, including occupational therapy, physical therapy, child development, speech-language pathology, and family therapy. The program also employs translators and family liaisons who are parents of children who have "graduated" from the Newborn Intensive Care Unit (NICU). The DC team structure and function must be flexible yet consistent to fit the unique features of the acute care setting. The most difficult issue is allocating staff time and effort and matching the person with the appropriate skills for the problem area with the selected infant-family so as to facilitate continuity of care over time, including transition into the community and follow-up through repeated hospitalizations. Staff assignment is especially difficult during the newborn period and early infancy, a period characterized by rapidly changing developmental needs. Unlike the infant, who has ever-changing needs, parents and family members often seek consistency in staff, searching for stability in a time of uncertainty.

The DC team uses a two-tiered team structure to address infant and family needs in hospital special care nursery settings. Other staff groups, including social services, nursing, and medical care, also tend to be organized in two tiers. Figure 1 depicts the team structure and organization.

The major difference between the DC team and the other staff groups is that it is comprised of professionals from multiple disciplines, whereas other staff groups are comprised of service providers from the same discipline. The inner tier team is infant-family specific. Its composition is determined by the needs of a particular infant and family. Its members function in an interdisciplinary manner, as they collaborate in the development of a unified service plan. Typically, team composition builds over time as infant-family needs unfold and as it becomes clear that an infant will be hospi-

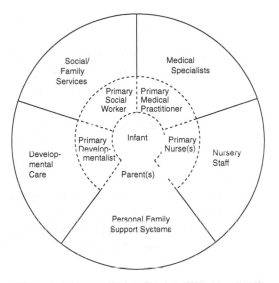

**Figure 1.** UNM Children's Hospital two-tiered team structure to address infant family needs. Source: Copyright © 1993 Laadt-Bruno, G., Lilley, P., & Westby, C. All rights reserved.

talized for a long period. On admission, the initial team consists of the physician, nurse, and family. As needs change, a member of the DC team, social worker, nutritionist, or others are added.

Each infant's team is drawn from a larger pool of resources in the outer tier. For example, the primary developmentalist for a specific infant team may be any person from the DC clinical group. The primary developmentalist is typically designated within two weeks of hospital admission. The members of the DC team in the outer tier function as a transdisciplinary team and provide backup to the developmentalist for a specific infant-family. All members are referred to as "developmentalists." Information, knowledge, and skills are transferred across discipline boundaries, as members teach and learn from one another and assume interchangeable roles and responsibilities. For example, the speech-language pathologist (SLP) may be the developmental specialist on the inner tier team serving a child with cleft palate, but he or she also is expected to provide information regarding sensori-motor issues that in a multidisciplinary team would be the province of the occupational therapist.

The structure and function of the developmental care team is unique within the hospital setting. Typically, each discipline is set up as a department, division, or service unit that functions in relative isolation as illustrated around the second tier. The functional style around the second tier is best described as multidisciplinary, with each group working independently. Individuals among disciplines collaborate around specific questions or issues. For example, an SLP from the DC team may be the representative member on a multidisciplinary team that addresses care coordination issues for the pediatric subacute care unit; or, an occupational therapist from DC may participate in an orientation for new nurses.

Within the DC program, this two-tiered team structure allows for consistency for individual infants-families, plus backup support and flexibility for sharing skills and addressing the diverse demands of providing developmentally oriented services, education, and research. The developmental staff work in conjunction with all strata of medical personnel (the second tier) in the hospital to identify infants who will need developmental assessment, care coordination, intervention, or follow-up services. For about 40% of families seen, a developmental care clinician is assigned as the primary care coordinator and service provider during weekly developmental clinical case review meetings. This system serves to minimize the number of caregivers and provide consistency in care. The primary developmentalist, as well as the primary nurse,

serve as the coordinator for the infant and family. This system integrates developmental care with medical routines and creates continuity links between the hospital and home community. The triple foci of developmental intervention in the hospital is first to support normal development through individualizing each infant's social and physical environment; second, to promote and maintain systems for care continuity throughout the hospital experience and through transition into the community; and third, to attend to specific problems as they are identified. This approach means that medical staff must be developmentally oriented, and nonmedical staff must become well informed about medical conditions and procedures. Cross training between disciplines is necessary. Coordination and collaboration are of prime importance.

## COLLABORATIVE SERVICE DELIVERY APPROACHES

Collaboration operates in several areas at multiple levels along the care continuum for the clinician based within the DC program. In this model, every service encounter is viewed as a teaching opportunity. In this way, developmental interventions are integrated into nursery and hospital routines by other staff and the family during daily caretaking routines and procedures in timely and meaningful ways throughout the infant's 24-hour day. Also, it gives the best chance for developmental programs to be carried out in a manner that is consistent with and relevant to the infant's needs, considering state of arousal, diurnal rhythms, medical condition, and social and physical setting. Therefore, integration of individualized developmental care into hospital routines supports the infant's development and may prevent some of the iatrogenic effects of NICU care and long-term hospitalization (Als, 1983; Als, Lawhon, & Brown, 1986).

This integrated medical/developmental approach to developmental intervention underscores the interactive nature between medical and developmental processes ongoing within the infant. Research emphasizes the importance of encouraging development of central nervous system organization during illness. The alternative orientation is to wait until the infant is "medically stable" before focusing on developmental processes. DC staff believe that addressing medical and developmental needs simultaneously by integrating developmental care within daily routines offers a more holistic and individualized approach. The infant's developmental age and medical status, and the physical and social environment, are recognized as important interactive contextual variables for the infant, family, and staff. This orientation is basic to the DC approach throughout the child's care continuum, from nursery admission at birth through discharge and transition into the community. Figure 2 displays the components of continuity care for infants and their families.

As depicted in the graph, newborns and young infants at UNM Children's Hospital are cared for in one of four nurseries. These nurseries include the maximum care NICU, the extended care nursery (ECN) for infants who remain critically ill for an extended period, the intermediate care nursery (ICN) for infants who are relatively stable, and the newborn nursery (NBN) for normal newborns, drug-exposed infants, and infants who may have conditions such as Down syndrome or cleft lip and palate.

In addition to the newborn nurseries, the DC team also consults with the Pediatric In-tensive Care Unit (PICU), Pediatric Sub-acute Care (PSAC), and the General Pediatric Unit. All clinical staff wear pagers and rotate call or are assigned to specific areas for consistent coverage. For NICU, a standing order for initial assessment or triage within the DC team occurs based on risk criteria drawn from the literature and staff experience. The DC orientation requires constant vigilance, creativity, and patience to seek out ways of integrating developmental principles into hospital staff attitudes, beliefs, routines, and skills.

When an infant's hospitalization is prolonged, collaboration becomes even more important. With continued medical fragility and increasing age of the infant, more people interface with the infant and family in an effort to maintain the infant's developmental trajectory and to get the infant well enough for discharge home. Families need staff consistency to be able to maintain a sense of relationship with their infant, who is not under their care and, in spite of all efforts, may still die.

The DC staff, in conjunction with other neonatology, pediatric, and nursery staff, use three approaches alone or in combination to address the developmental needs of infants born ill or premature:

1. The developmentally shaped environment, to promote developmentally supportive care (Als, 1983, 1984);
2. Developmental care continuity (Krehbiel, Munsick-Bruno, & Lowe, 1991; Lawhon & Melzar, 1988), and
3. Problem-focused therapy.

Based on averages from the past three years, all infants receive the developmentally shaped environment service, 54% of infants receive developmental care continuity services, and 5% of infants receive problem-focused therapy.

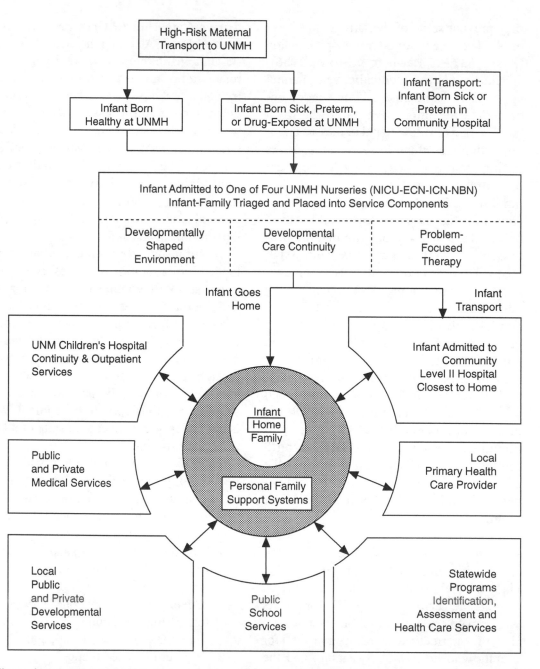

**Figure 2.** Infant-family care continuum between hospital and home/community. *Source:* Copyright © 1993 Laadt-Bruno, G. All rights reserved.

## Developmentally shaped environment

The developmentally shaped environment service component is provided for all infants in the special care nurseries. Developmentally shaped environment is primarily provided by bedside nursing staff in collaboration with family members, usually the mother, with backup from DC staff. This service component is considered as baseline nursery care. Based on infant behavioral observations (Als, 1984), each infant's immediate and ambient environment is shaped to encourage infant organization and self-regulation to the greatest degree possible. For example, a concerted effort by medical staff is made to decrease excessive ambient light and noise. Nursing routines are clustered or spaced to match the infant's normal sleep/wake cycles and stamina. Developmental, medical, and nursing staff observe, along with the family, for developmental differences (e.g., feeding problems, temperament or sleep difficulties, or subtle neuromuscular alterations) that warrant further examination. Developmental assessment, consultation, and intervention are provided as needed on a referral basis during the infant's hospital stay and through discharge with selected families.

Infants receiving only this developmental service approach typically are in the nursery for less than two weeks and are not assigned a developmental primary.

## Developmental care continuity

Developmental care continuity is the primary service model carried out by the DC program staff in collaboration with others. Infants and families receiving this service approach are assigned a DC team primary developmentalist when it becomes clear that the infant will remain in the hospital for at least 30 days or that the infant and family will need help in making the transition from the hospital to home community. In this approach, developmental assessments are combined with intervention strategies from admission through discharge or transition to another hospital closer to home or to home (see Figure 2). The program provides coordinated DC continuity for infants whose potential for developmental problems is considered to be greater than that of the general population. Approximately half of the infants cared for in the special care nurseries and a select population of infants from the regular nursery who experienced prenatal exposure to illicit drugs are followed in this manner. Criteria for increased risk of developmental concern include factors such as birth weight below 1,250 g, central nervous system–related problems (e.g., seizures, birth asphyxia, meningitis, periventricular/intraventricular hemorrhage, gastrointestinal problems requiring surgery; ventilatory assistance required for more than 10 days, and prenatal alcohol or drug exposure).

Individual infants seen through other inpatient or outpatient services who qualify as "at risk" are also followed in this manner. The care continuity approach uses a culturally sensitive, family-centered approach. It is integrated within the hospital's medical systems. Collaboration with other hospital services and community, university, and statewide resources occurs in the least restrictive and least intrusive manner for the family. Focusing on prevention, it provides anticipatory guidance and integration of medical and developmental issues to generate plans of care that support optimal developmental outcomes for infants and their families. Standard procedures include, but are not limited to, individualized neuro-developmental assessment with collaboration among medical caregivers, family, and DC staff to integrate recommendations from all members of the team. The developmental primary for an infant in the care continuity component routinely anticipates discharge from the time of admission and helps the family participate in the hospital discharge process along with other inner-tier infant-family team members. Once infants are medically stable, they are ready to go to the community hospital or home. By this time, most infants are nippling all their feedings and are able to remain in a crib or open bassinet. Parents have been able to hold and feed their infant and are doing most of the routine caretaking during visits. Family collaboration with the DC team may include recommended parent-infant activities and assistance in planning for continued follow-up at UNM or other community programs.

The developmentalist's role focuses on increased intra- and interagency collaboration for service coordination at the outpatient level. The primary focus of developmental care services after discharge from the hospital is to provide encouragement to establish normal family routines and mechanisms to promote health, family-infant well-being, and integration into community services and systems, as needed, in a timely manner. Major efforts must be made early to help the parents recognize and attend to those aspects of the infant's development and the family structure that are healthy and normal. Extended telephone consultation to families or telephone collaboration with physicians, early childhood service providers, or other agencies is also available. A toll-free telephone number for families and professionals is maintained by DC to help families coordinate trips and appointments and provide access to developmental consultation. This is especially important in a rural state such as New Mexico. Amy's case is an example of care continuity services:

Amy was born at 28 weeks gestation weighing 590 grams (approximately 1 lb., 5 oz.). She was vigorous at birth with Apgars of 7 and 8. Amy initially required only supplemental oxygen, although she was eventually intubated for increased apnea episodes. Amy's extremely low birth weight, guarded medical prognosis, and results of a behavioral observational assessment by a member of the DC team, indicated she was to be followed under the developmental care continuity service component. Approximately two weeks later in the DC weekly clinical meeting, the SLP was designated as Amy's "primary developmentalist." This decision was based on the knowledge that Amy probably would require prolonged ventilatory support and that feeding concerns were likely. Support from OT and PT staff on the DC team, as needed, was assured based on the two-tiered structure of the team.

Table 1 summarizes the significant events that followed which illustrate the SLP's function on the Developmental Care team and her collaboration with Amy's family and the NICU interdisciplinary team.

**Problem-focused therapy**

Problem-focused therapy, the third service component, is most typical of services offered through hospital-based departments such as speech, occupational therapy, physical therapy, or rehabilitation departments. The therapist carries out hands-on treatment

**Table 1.** Collaborative Consultation Services for Amy

| Time | Problem | Recommendations | Outcomes |
|------|---------|-----------------|----------|
| An estimated date of birth (40 weeks post conception) | Had been intubated for over 60 days<br>Oral hypersensitivity to touch | Neonatologists recommended tracheostomy<br>Regular oral program to maintain oral function while intubated; minimize intrusive procedures such as suctioning | Family refused; respiratory status improved; extubated 3 weeks later<br>Hypersensitivity continued |
| Following extubation nipple feedings initiated | Poor coordination of suck-swallow-breathe pattern<br>Developed less tolerance of gavage feedings | Medical staff decided to use nasogastric tube for gavage feedings | Nippling skills did not improve |
| | Mother questioned if NG causing nippling problems | Nutritionist and SLP decided to try nipple feedings without NG tube<br>Used formula with increased calories to reduce volume of feedings | Increased successful nipple feedings<br>Reduced need for gavage feeding<br>Good weight gain for home discharge after one month<br>SLP reviewed feeding suggestions with mother<br>Follow-up to continue in outpatient pulmonary clinic |
| 5 weeks after discharge from NICU Amy rehospitalized with pneumonia | Orally intubated on ventilator; after 2 weeks extubated<br>Refused nipple feeding and required NG tube again | SLP reinstituted activities to encourage nipple feeding | Little progress with feeding; medical staff discussed surgery for gastrostomy tube; family agreed to surgery; Amy discharged one week after surgery |
| 2 weeks following rehospitalization discharge | Mother wanted to begin oral feeding | SLP provided home treatment activities to support oral function<br>Health insurance paid for pediatric rehabilitation nurse to assist family with feeding Amy at home<br>Bi-monthly consultation with Developmental Care team and nurse | Greater tolerance of oral program<br>Maintained oral skills for suck/swallow<br>Beginning acceptance of varied tastes |

with the infant at regular intervals, often daily. At UNM Children's Hospital, this approach is used when the therapeutic emphasis has shifted from one of encouraging normal developmental processes and trajectories to one in which an abnormality has been identified and training others to provide treatment would be difficult. This approach often, but not always, is delivered simultaneously with the care continuity approach discussed earlier. Often other staff or family members are present during treatment and learn to carry out aspects of the treatment program under the direction of the therapist. Therapists who deliver direct therapy services in this mode still need to be sensitive to infant, family, and staff routines and environments. This sometimes is difficult for therapists who operate within departments that keep tight schedules so that service and billing opportunities are maximized. Infants who receive problem-focused therapy at UNM Children's Hospital tend to be those with syndromes and congenital physical anomalies or associations present at birth that are known to be associated with developmental alterations (e.g., Down syndrome, fetal alcohol syndrome, cleft palate, clubbed foot, myelomeningocele, congenital amputee) or severe sensory loss (e.g., deafness, blindness).

The basic configuration of service needs for these children can be anticipated at birth or within the newborn period. The starting point and future course are relatively evident. Interventions consist of neurodevelopmental assessment plus individual program planning and implementation soon after the child is identified. Periodic assessment is determined on a case-by-case basis. Referral to in-hospital therapy services such as physical therapy may also occur. Coordinated transition to needed community services is initiated in the hospital when the child is being prepared for home. Carlos is a child who received all three service approaches over time.

Carlos was born at 38 weeks gestation. The pregnancy was uncomplicated with prenatal care begun during the second trimester. Delivery was vaginal without complications with Apgar scores of 1 at one minute, 3 at five minutes, and 6 at ten minutes. Resuscitation included use of supplemental oxygen that progressed to intubation and ventilatory support. Initial chest X-ray studies showed obvious vertebral and rib anomalies. The attending pediatrician arranged for Carlos to be transported by ambulance to the UNM NICU approximately 60 miles away. Carlos' admitting diagnosis included respiratory distress and rib and spine anomalies of upper thoracic rib and spine anomalies.

Carlos' 14-month hospital stay was within the NICU acute care and extended care units. The initial assessment by Developmental Care indicated he would require services under the Developmental Care Continuity and problem-focused service components in addition to a developmentally shaped environment. The SLP became his primary developmentalist. Early medical diagnostic procedures focused more on his respiratory problems with the anticipation that his overall development would be within normal limits. Carlos' skeletal and thoracic anomalies were later identified as requiring more intervention. Table 2 summarizes Carlos' needs during his hospitalization and the types of services he received.

A major challenge for Carlos' family and medical caregivers was to transition him to his home. The uniqueness of Carlos' medical status and his dependence on a mechanical ventilator prompted referral to the New Mexico Medically Fragile Children's Program. This program provides comprehensive services for children with complex medical needs. Transition plans were initi-

**Table 2.** Service Delivery Approaches for Carlos

| Time | Problems and strengths | Type of service |
|---|---|---|
| Beginning at admission | Difficulty regulating arousal levels; easily stressed with movement, handling, and social interactions resulting in gaze aversion and dropping oxygen saturation levels<br>Age appropriate self-calming ability by maintaining flexed body posture, keeping hands near his face and mouth, and sucking on endotracheal tube | **Developmentally shaped environment** (SLP completed Neonatal Individualized Developmental and Assessment Program)<br>SLP gave parents information so they could identify and respond to Carlos' stress cues and would time their interactions when he was most physiologically stable<br>Respecting baby's rhythms when arranging routine care |
| Beginning at two months | Tracheostomy performed due to prolonged ventilator dependence<br>Problems maintaining weight gain due to increased work of breathing and feeding intolerance<br>Vomiting of bottle feedings; difficulty tolerating full strength formula | **Developmental care continuity**<br>Instituted nipple feeding after tracheostomy<br>Instituted gavage feedings to maintain weight<br>Introduced solids at 4 months<br>Continued strategies to facilitate oral feeding throughout hospitalization |
| Beginning at 4 ½ months | Assessment by Development Care SLP and PT indicated age appropriate cognitive development and delayed motor development at approximately 2-month level<br>CT scans showed anterior spinal defect in upper thoracic region with possible herniation of neural contents into an anterior meningocele | **Problem-focused therapy**<br>Formal referral for physical therapy |
| Beginning at 8 months | Age appropriate cognitive skills with delayed communication abilities | **Developmental care continuity**<br>SLP recommended Passy-Muir valve for Carlos' trach so he could vocalize; not initially available, so trach was downsized to allow air leak that would permit vocalization<br>SLP gave instructions to medical staff and family on how to reinforce Carlos' attempts to vocalize<br>SLP discussed use of sign language and reinforcement of communicative gestures with medical staff and family<br>After Passy-Muir valve became available, SLP taught staff and family how to care for it and gave further suggestions to encourage vocal imitation |

ated by hospital medical specialists, social services, and DC and were continued with active collaboration between these teams and the Medically Fragile Program. For example, the SLP, as coordinator, ensured developmental continuity with home-based early intervention services, including speech and language consultation. Primary discharge coordination was assumed by the Medically Fragile Program.

## SPECIALIZED COMPETENCIES OF THE SLP

### Discipline-specific competencies

Collaborative consultation in a hospital neonatal setting requires unique competencies of professional staff. The speech-language pathologist on the DC team provides specific knowledge on oral-motor and feeding issues, which tend to be particularly critical for many infants.

In the neonatal settings, SLPs must possess knowledge of normal and atypical infant development. They must be familiar with:

- prenatal conditions and complications of pregnancy that can affect development;
- perinatal concerns such as fetal distress, birth trauma, and prematurity; and
- postnatal conditions that affect development, such as genetic syndromes or cardiovascular, respiratory, or gastrointestinal problems.

The impact of these various conditions should be understood in terms of their potential effect on developmental and neurologic outcome. Infant behaviors that communicate significant information to their families and medical/developmental staff are invaluable for helping to support basic physiologic stability and recovery. They also provide a foundation for appropriate and individualized developmental support. Knowledge of infant behavioral arousal states, state regulation capacities, and general neurobehavioral organization including the infant's ability to self-organize provide the therapist with a useful tool in the development of appropriate individualized care (Gorga, Anzalone, Holloway, Hunter, Munsick-Bruno, 1993; Gorski, 1991).

Training in the development of feeding or prespeech capacity must include knowledge of feeding problems resulting from medical factors such as gastrointestinal surgery, prolonged oral intubation, or craniofacial anomalies. Nipple feeding is a complex activity that can be influenced positively or negatively by such factors as environmental stimuli, neurobehavioral organization, gestational age, various medical conditions, and neuromotor development (Morris & Klein, 1987; Vandenberg, 1990). Interventions for feeding difficulties require assessment of oral motor skills for sucking and swallowing and coordination of these with respiration. Children who are nonoral feeders and are being fed via gavage or gastrostomy feeding tubes will require intervention to reinstitute oral feedings or to maintain oral feeding skills until they can discontinue reliance on alternative feeding methods.

The SLP's skills in assessing swallowing problems and collaborating with physicians can result in more appropriate referral for videofluoroscopy. The ability to interpret videofluoroscopic swallow studies is essential. Other professionals will require the specialized support the SLP can provide in this area. Other specialty areas to be addressed by the SLP can include (Jacobsen & Shubat, 1991)

- treatment of oral aversion,
- feeding disorders related to failure to thrive,
- extended continuum of oral feeding development,
- prelinguistic/early language communication development,
- communication development and support for tracheotomized infants/toddlers (i.e., use of Passy-Muir speech valve, alternative methods of communication), and
- strategies for normalization of communication development in children with hearing impairment.

**Competencies for collaboration**

Collaborative consultation in the hospital neonatal setting requires unique competencies for relating to medical staff and families under stress. Knowledge of families and family systems theory is key to working with neonates. The SLP must develop a supportive and collaborative relationship with parents, as families of infants in the intensive care unit can be fragile themselves. For parents, the environment of the NICU and the acute care needed by their fragile newborn in an NICU are extremely stressful (Goldson, 1992). These families will be best served by SLPs who are knowledgeable about infants but also sensitive to their families' concerns. Treatment programs that enhance caregiver-infant interactions are more effective than those that focus on only the infant's behavior (Donahue-Kilburg, 1992).

Collaboration also extends to medical staff who work directly with the infant and family. SLPs need to provide information regarding their role in oral motor/feeding skills and communication versus the actual development of words or speech. Emphasis should be placed on the unique skills SLPs have in supporting early communication, enhancing parent-infant interaction, improving feeding skills, normalizing and supporting communication for infants with tracheostomies, and identifying infants at risk for hearing impairment.

Individual interpersonal skills for successful collaboration with families and medical staff include

- self-confidence in a high-stress environment working with other highly trained professionals,
- ability to provide mutual support to professionals and to avoid "turf" issues,
- flexibility and patience, and
- ability to balance the roles of learner and expert.

For the SLP who is providing service coordination for an infant moving toward hospital discharge, there is a shift in the type of support that will be needed by the infant, family, and hospital staff. The SLP should be knowledgeable about local community resources. Communication with medical staff and the family during hospitalization will allow for planning of needed community supports (informal and formal) in a timely manner. Working with the family to follow their identified needs can lead to formal collaboration with community-based physicians, public and private nursing services, developmental follow-up resources, early intervention programs, therapy providers, or other resources. Effective collaboration at this juncture results in a smooth transition to the home and community for both infant and family.

•  •  •

The roles of occupational and physical therapists, SLPs, nurses, medical specialists, and early childhood specialists/special educators are broadening to fill gaps between in- and outpatient services. Advances in medical care, resulting in survival of infants who are born prematurely or ill, increasing awareness of the sequelae of prenatal exposure to environmental teratogens such as maternal drug or alcohol use, increasing sensitivity regarding cultural and socioeconomic diversity, and legislation mandating family-centered service options for young children and their families are changing. Increasingly complex problems require innovative solutions. No single professional can address the diverse needs of infants born at risk and their families. Professionals must work collaboratively with one another and with families if they are to effectively address the complex needs of infants at developmental risk and facilitate the adjustment and coping of the families.

## REFERENCES

Als, H. (1983). Infant individuality: Assessing patterns of very early development. In J. Call, E. Galenson, & R. Tyso (Eds.), *Frontiers of infant psychiatry.* New York, NY: Basic Books.

Als, H. (1984). Manual for the naturalistic observation of newborn behavior (preterm and fullterm infants). Unpublished manuscript. The Children's Hospital, Boston, MA.

Als, H., Lawhon, G., & Brown, E. (1986). Individualized behavioral and environmental care for the very low birthweight preterm infant at high risk for bronchopulmonary dysplasia: Neonatal intensive care unit and developmental outcome. *Pediatric Clinics of North America, 35,* 1,207–1,226.

Bauchner, H., Brown, E., & Peskin, J. (1988). Premature graduates of the newborn intensive care unit: A guide to follow-up. *Pediatric Clinics of North America, 35,* 1,207–1,226.

Briggs, M.H. (1991). Team development: Decision making for early intervention. *Infant Toddler Intervention: A Transdisciplinary Journal, 1,* 1–9.

Donahue-Kilburg, G. (1992). *Family-centered early intervention for communication disorders.* Gaithersburg, MD: Aspen Publishers.

Gilbert, M., Sciarillo, W.G., & Van Rembrow, D.L. (1992). Service coordination through case management. In M. Bender & C.A. Baglin (Eds.), *Infants and toddlers: A resource guide for practitioners.* San Diego, CA: Singular.

Goldson, E. (1992). The neonatal intensive care unit: Premature infants and parents. *Infants and Young Children, 4* (3), 31–42.

Gorga, D., Anzalone, M., Holloway, E., Hunter, J., Munsick-Bruno, G. (1993). Knowledge and skills for occupational therapy in the neonatal intensive care unit. Unpublished manuscript. American Occupational Therapy Association, Rockville, MD.

Gorski, P.A. (1991). Developmental intervention during neonatal hospitalization: Critiquing the state of the science. *Pediatric Clinics of North America, 38,* 1,469–1,479.

Jacobsen, C.H., & Shubat, S.J. (1991). Hospital-based communication intervention with the at-risk newborn. *Infant Toddler Intervention: A Transdisciplinary Journal, 1,* 27–35.

Krehbiel, R., Munsick-Bruno, G., & Lowe, J.R. (1991). NICU infants born at developmental risk and the individualized family service plan/process (IFSP). *Children's Health Care, 20,* 28–33.

Lawhon, G., & Melzar, A. (1988). Developmental care of the very low birth weight infant. *Journal of Perinatal and Neonatal Nursing, 2* (1), 56–65.

McGonigel, M.J., & Garland, C.W. (1988). The individualized family service plan and early intervention team: Team and family issues and recommended practices. *Infants and Young Children, 1* (1), 10–21.

Morris, S., & Klein, M. (1987). *Pre-feeding skills.* Tucson, AZ: Therapy Skill Builders.

Spiegel, L., & Mayers, A. (1991). Psychosocial aspects of AIDS in children and adolescents. *Pediatric Clinics of North America, 38,* 153–167.

Vandenberg, K.A. (1990). Nippling management of the sick neonate in the NICU: The disorganized feeder. *Neonatal Network, 9,* 9–16.

Zuckerman, B., & Bresnahan, K. (1991). Developmental and behavioral consequences of prenatal drug and alcohol exposure. *Pediatric Clinics of North America, 38,* 1,387–1,496.

# Neonates and infants at risk for hearing and speech–language disorders

*David A. Clark, MD*
*Professor of Pediatrics*
*Louisiana State University School of*
*   Medicine*
*New Orleans, Louisiana*

APPROXIMATELY one child per thousand is born deaf. An additional two to three per thousand develop profound hearing loss in early childhood. Apart from craniofacial malformations, it is very difficult to identify neonates who will eventually manifest speech–language problems. This article will focus on prenatal, perinatal, and early childhood risks of later developmental delay, with a major emphasis on hearing impairment (Coplan, 1987; Fria, Paradise, Sabo, & Elster, 1987).

## PRENATAL RISK FACTORS

Children who have chromosomal abnormalities associated with hearing loss often have physical malformations involving the face or external ear. Because early craniofacial development is intimately related to the formation of the brain (Konigsmark, 1969), these obvious external signs suggest the possibility of central nervous system anomalies.

*Top Lang Disord,* 1989,10(1),1–12
© 1989 Aspen Publishers, Inc.

In the 18q— syndrome, the long arm of the number 18 chromosome is absent; these infants are growth retarded, with microcephaly, midfacial hypoplasia, and hypotonia. The pinnae are coarse and redundant, and the external canal is narrow or atretic. Occasionally there is atresia of the middle ear. In addition, numerous other malformations, especially of the eyes, limbs, and palate are found (Jones, 1988; Wertelecki & Gerard, 1971).

Turner syndrome (XO syndrome) occurs when the developing fetus has one less sex chromosome than normal, with a total of only 45 chromosomes. Most common among the physical abnormalities are growth retardation; small stature; short, webbed neck; broad chest with widely spaced nipples; and cupped, prominent ears. More than 50% of affected individuals have hearing impairment. Those not afflicted with congenital heart disease commonly survive into adulthood, usually with mild mental retardation, sexual immaturity, and infertility (Brook, Mursat, Zachmann, & Prader, 1974; Jones, 1988).

Down syndrome (trisomy 21) has an infant incidence of approximately one in 700 live births, making this condition one of the most common genetic malformations. In addition to mental retardation, these children frequently have hypoplasia of the frontal sinuses, small noses, and malformed ears, often with an angulated upper helix and small or absent ear lobes. The relatively low placement of the ears has been associated with chronic otitis media in 10% of these infants due to poor drainage of the middle ear into the posterior pharynx.

Many less common syndromes have been associated with the early onset of hearing impairment, subsequently leading to speech and language delay. Table 1 briefly outlines some of the more commonly recognized syndromes that have been associated with a nonchromosomal genetic basis for predisposition to hearing loss (Jones, 1988; Konigsmark, 1969).

Inborn errors of metabolism may result in progressive retardation, hearing loss, and developmental delay by accumulation of a toxic metabolite in the neuron. The mucopolysaccharidoses, a group of disorders of mucopolysaccharide metabolism, are prime examples.

Hurler syndrome (mucopolysaccharidosis, type I) is inherited as an autosomal recessive condition. In addition to growth retardation, these infants have progressive mental retardation, joint stiffness, visual impairment from clouding of the cornea, and coarse facial features. Similarly, Hunter syndrome (mucopolysaccharidosis, type II) is characterized by growth retardation, coarse facial features, and joint stiffness. By 3 to 4 years of age (juvenile type) such children display severe mental deficiency with hyperactivity and spasticity. Most youngsters have profound neuronal hearing loss before the age of 5. This enzymatic defect is inherited in an X-linked manner similar to hemophilia; therefore, there are no affected females.

Finally, Morquio syndrome (mucopolysaccharidosis, type IV) is inherited as an autosomal recessive deficiency of the enzyme 6-sulfo-N-acetylhexosominide sulfatase. Typically, children show severe growth retardation, corneal clouding, flaring of the rib cage, and a kyphotic spinal deformity. They usually do not have mental retardation but do develop profound sensorineural hearing loss (Mata-

**Table 1.** Syndromes with hearing impairment

| Syndrome | Etiology | Major features | Type of hearing loss |
|---|---|---|---|
| Cockayne | Autosomal recessive | Early senility<br>Retinopathy<br>Dermatitis | Sensorineural |
| Goldenhar | Unknown | Facial hypoplasia<br>Preauricular tags<br>Vertebral defects<br>Mental retardation<br>Microtia | Conductive, sensor-ineural |
| Kartagener | Autosomal recessive<br>(probable) | Situs inversus<br>Bronchiectasis<br>Sinusitis | Conductive |
| Melnick-Fraser | Autosomal dominant | Preauricular pits<br>Branchial cysts<br>Renal dysplasia | Conductive, sensor-ineural |
| Mohr | Autosomal recessive<br>(probable) | Reduplication of foot<br>bones<br>Cleft tongue | Conductive (defect of incus) |
| Multiple synostosis | Autosomal dominant | Fusion of finger joints<br>Nasal hypoplasia<br>Vertebral defects | Conductive (fusion of middle ear bones) |
| Oto-palato-digital | X-linked, semidomi-nant | Cleft palate<br>Broad digits<br>Short nails<br>Small stature<br>Mild retardation | Conductive |
| Velo-cardio-facial | Autosomal dominant<br>(probable) | Cleft palate<br>Prominent nose<br>Hypotonia<br>Small stature<br>Mental retardation | Conductive |
| Treacher Collins | Autosomal dominant<br>mutations | Malar hypoplasia<br>Small mandible<br>Cleft palate<br>Antimongoloid pal-pebral fissure<br>Coloboma<br>Malformed auricles<br>Sparse lower eyelashes | Conductive |
| Waardenburg, types I & II | Autosomal dominant | Broad nasal bridge<br>Partial albinism<br>(white forelock)<br>Medial flare of eye-brows<br>Wide-set eyes | Sensorineural (defec-tive organ of Corti, atrophic spiral ganglion) |

lon, Arbogast, Justice, Brandt, & Dorfman, 1974).

## ENVIRONMENTAL TOXINS

Several environmental toxins may have adverse effects on the developing fetus. In particular, a genetically normal fetus is dependent on his or her mother for both nutrition and elimination of the waste products of metabolism. If the mother is deficient in a crucial nutrient or has been exposed to a toxin, the fetus' early intrauterine development may be dramatically altered.

When a pregnant woman is exposed to a heavy metal, the effect on the fetus is often severe as well. Mercury contamination of food sources in Japan has caused severe impairment in infants, including microcephaly, growth and mental retardation, deafness, and blindness (Beckman & Brent, 1986). Other heavy metals such as lead and cadmium are probable ototoxins that have been firmly linked to fetal growth retardation and early identifiable neurobehavioral deficits (Bellinger, Levitson, Waternaux, Needleman, & Rabinowitz, 1987; Dietrich, Krafft, Bornschein, Hammond, Berger, Succop, & Bier, 1987).

Intrauterine exposure to maternal alcohol consumption has obvious adverse consequences for the fetus, resulting in the prenatal onset of growth deficiency, an underdeveloped brain, and mental retardation. Such effects vary from infant to infant, with the most easily identified children born to alcoholic women. Although hearing deficits have been identified in some affected children, the speech and language delays secondary to mental

retardation are much more prevalent (Jones, 1986; Jones, 1988).

## INFECTIONS

### In utero fetal infections

The transplacental passage of a virus, a parasite, or a spirochete (syphilis), especially during the first trimester, may compromise the fetus, causing congenital hearing deficits, mental retardation, and associated speech and language delays. Typically infected mothers have relatively few signs and symptoms of illness (Stagno & Reynolds, 1977). The earlier an infection occurs in the pregnancy, the more profound are the physical and neurologic abnormalities in the newborn. In general, the early transplacental viral infections interfere with normal formation of tissues, whereas the parasitic infections and syphilis usually destroy tissue that was forming normally.

The commonly known prototype of viral infections associated with hearing loss is rubella. Although the fetal rubella syndrome was first identified in 1941, the 1964 epidemic in the United States affected many neonates and clarified the subtleties of the disease process. The virus produces virtually no malformation if it crosses the placenta after the second trimester of pregnancy, in contrast with its impact during the first trimester: an inci-

*The earlier an infection occurs in the pregnancy, the more profound are the physical and neurologic abnormalities in the newborn.*

dence of 50% among newborns delivered by infected mothers. These infants have a deficiency of clotting and tend to bruise easily. In addition, infants afflicted with rubella syndrome typically have multiple organ system involvement; about 60% have moderate to severe mental retardation; approximately 50% have malformations or inflammation of the heart; and nearly 40% have serious eye disease (i.e., cataracts, glaucoma, corneal opacity, strabismus, or retinitis). More than 30% of the confirmed cases of fetal rubella syndrome show profound sensorineural hearing loss. The probable combination of congenital heart disease, mental retardation, blindness, and severe hearing impairment often requires a life-long commitment of special educational and health-related services for such children. Fortunately, in the 1970s an effective immunization program minimized the congenital rubella syndrome in the western world. However, the recent failure to immunize infants and young children has led to a resurgence of the disease, especially in inner cities (Bergstrom, 1980; Fraser, 1964; Jones, 1988).

Congenital cytomegalovirus (CMV) is another infection, much more subtle than rubella. The virus is prevalent in the general population, and no effective immunization is available. CMV, a member of the herpes virus group, is similar to varicella (chickenpox) and herpes; once the virus affects an individual, it remains for life. An infant born to a mother who had first-trimester CMV infection may be born apparently healthy, then develop progressive multiple organ system disease with pneumonia, hepatitis, myocarditis, and central nervous system involvement. The child may also be born with severe anoma-

lies, including microcephaly, cataracts, retinitis, intracerebral calcifications, anemia, jaundice, and limb deformities. Virtually all of these children have a very poor prognosis as a result of growth failure and severe mental retardation. Sensorineural hearing loss is a prominent feature of intrauterine infection and, more importantly, may be its only manifestation (Kumar, Nankervis, Jacobs, Ernhart, Glasson, McMillan, & Gold, 1984; Stagno & Reynolds, 1977).

Toxoplasmosis is a parasitic infection that the mother acquires from exposure to cat feces or poorly cooked meat, especially wild game. The parasite crosses the placenta and forms cysts anywhere in the fetus. When these cysts form within a developing brain, they can damage crucial neuronal relationships. In addition to hepatic disease, the central nervous system manifestations of toxoplasmosis are micro- or macrocephaly, hydrocephaly, seizures, mental retardation, and sensorineural deafness. Although there are antibiotics available to treat the infection, the damage caused by the cysts is irreversible (Stagno & Reynolds, 1977).

Most women are tested for syphilis during pregnancy and promptly treated if it is detected. A fetal infection seldom causes a congenital malformation; however, multiple organ systems may be acutely involved. The infected newborn may have no symptoms at birth or may exhibit jaundice, respiratory distress, an enlarged liver and spleen, and lethargy. Syphilis does not have a specific predilection for causing hearing loss but is often responsible for sensorineural hearing deafness as a consequence of a generalized central nervous system infection. Fortunately syphilis, if identified early, can be readily treated, and few newborns have permanent sequelae.

Numerous other maternal infections may be transmitted from the mother to the fetus. The epidemiology and the effect of these less common infections on the developing fetus are not nearly as well understood as are the preceding examples. Viruses that may have little overt neonatal impact but can produce long-term, progressively disabling diseases include hepatitis B, Epstein-Barr (mononucleosis), varicella, and the human immunodeficiency virus (HTLV III), the causative agent of AIDS.

### Perinatally or postnatally acquired infections

Any bacterial or viral infection that invades the central nervous system is capable of promoting hearing loss by damage to the auditory cortex, the eighth nerve and its nucleus, or the cochlea.

Herpes is one of the most virulent neonatal infections. It is usually acquired as an ascending infection from the mother's vagina, once the membranes have been ruptured, or from direct contact with lesions during delivery. There are several strains of the virus, classified as types I and II, either of which may infect the newborn. The most common presenting symptom is lethargy, suggesting central nervous system involvement. The typical rash is seen in only 50% of the cases at presentation. These infants may have respiratory distress, temperature instability, enlarged livers, jaundice, and poor clotting of the blood. The virus is aggressive, and that which may initially appear to be localized infection can rapidly extend to the central

nervous system. Despite intensive care and newer antiviral agents, the mortality rate remains high, and as many as 40% of the survivors have such serious long-term effects as seizures, mental retardation, and both central and sensorineural deafness (Beckman & Brent, 1986).

The newborn's defenses—especially those of the preterm infant—are extremely limited. Any bacteria within the vagina may gain access to the infant after the mother's membranes rupture, causing a generalized sepsis or meningitis. Group B streptococcus and listeria are two bacteria that seldom infect the older child or adult but are major neonatal pathogens. Thirty percent to fifty percent of women are colonized with group B streptococcus, and one per 250 of their newborns are infected. Group B streptococcus and listeria produce similar clinical courses. Each can cause an early onset of respiratory distress that can mimic the respiratory distress syndrome of surfactant deficiency seen in premature newborns. Each can also cause a delayed-onset infection, usually after 1 week of age, which primarily attacks the central nervous system as meningitis. Although both types of bacterial infection can be treated with antibiotics and the bacteria destroyed, permanent neurologic disability with mental retardation, speech–language disability, and especially hearing impairment may remain (Kaplan, Catlin, Weaver, & Feigin, 1984).

Although it is one of the most common infections in the first year of life, otitis media (middle ear infection) is not commonly diagnosed in the newborn. The eustachian tube, which should drain the middle ear to the posterior pharynx, has a small caliber, and the angle of drainage is less steep than that of adults. As a result, fluid accumulates in the middle ear and provides a medium in which bacterial or viral infections become established. The inflammatory process may cause conductive hearing loss from scarring and fixation of the tympanic membrane and from limitation of the motion of the ossicular chain.

## PREMATURITY, ASPHYXIA, AND INTRACRANIAL HEMORRHAGE

### Preterm and small-for-gestational age infants

Infants delivered at less than 37 weeks of gestation are designated as prematurely born. To date, the incidence of prematurity in the United States has remained fairly constant at approximately 7% to 8% of all newborns. Although prematurity alone, especially birth weight >2,500 g, is not the cause of mental retardation or learning impairment, preterm infants are much more likely to contract diseases that produce a wide range of developmental disabilities (Bergman, Hirsch, Fria, Shapiro, Holzman, & Painter, 1985; Cox, Hack, & Metz, 1981). In essence, the risk of neurologic sequelae and (by association) hearing, speech, and language delay in preterm infants is related to the number and severity of their problems.

Moreover, many of the conditions described earlier (e.g., transplacental infections, syndromes, chromosomal abnormalities, and environmental toxins) do produce infants who are small for their gestational age and who have neurologic dysfunctions. In fact, although no specific etiology may be identified for growth retardation,

such infants still have a three-to-tenfold increased risk of delayed development (American Academy of Pediatrics, 1982).

### Birth asphyxia

Prior to birth and during the process of delivery, an infant may receive insufficient oxygen across the placenta from the mother. Furthermore, asphyxia usually includes not only oxygen deprivation but also acidosis and hypercarbia (i.e., increased blood carbon dioxide). The combination of these metabolic insults may, in turn, affect any portion of the brain (Simmons, 1984).

The Apgar scoring system was devised in 1953 as a means of identifying the infant with asphyxia who was severely stressed and in need of prompt resuscitation. Although there is much debate over interpretation, there is little evidence to suggest that the 1-minute Apgar score is prognostic. The 5-minute Apgar score is more useful; yet in a large multicenter study, 95% of the surviving infants with an Apgar score of 3 or less did not have cerebral palsy, mental retardation, or other neurologic dysfunction (Duara, Suter, Bessard, & Gutberlet, 1986; Rowe, 1985).

### Intracranial hemorrhage

Intracranial hemorrhage seldom occurs in full-term infants; however, a preterm infant weighing less than 1,500 g and born at less than 32 weeks of gestational age is particularly susceptible to bleeding. The vascular bed of the developing brain in the region of the germinal matrix is not fully developed and is thus particularly prone to hemorrhage, which can be detected by ultrasonography or computerized axial tomography (CAT) scanning. This condition is found more commonly if an infant has suffered asphyxia, hypotension, acidosis, or respiratory distress requiring mechanical ventilation. In such instances, the blood itself is not the primary concern, since it will eventually be absorbed; damage results from insufficient blood flow and oxygen deprivation, particularly in areas of the brain near the site of hemorrhage. Unfortunately, tissue oxygen deprivation cannot be precisely determined clinically, and the detection of hemorrhage thus becomes a best estimate. Although a few infants with advanced intracranial hemorrhage (i.e., grade IV bleeds) develop normally, many infants with normal cranial ultrasounds are mentally retarded, with associated problems of hearing impairment and speech–language delays (Hendricks-Munoz & Walton, 1988; Marshall, Reichert, Kerley, & Davis, 1980).

## BILIRUBIN

Jaundice occurs as a result of the deposition of bilirubin in the skin. Bilirubin is a compound primarily formed from the normal destruction of red blood cells. To be excreted from the body, this substance must be transported to the liver, processed, and released into bile. Prior to birth, much of the bilirubin load has been passed across the placenta to the mother's liver and excreted. After birth, however, the newborn has to cope with the bilirubin burden and subsequently develops jaundice by the second to third day of life. Premature infants, with less well-developed hepatic function, have higher blood levels of bilirubin during their first week of life.

Bilirubin is toxic to the central nervous system, and it has a specific predilection for the basal ganglia and hippocampus. The toxicity of bilirubin results from its ability to interfere with crucial enzymes in the cell that release energy, causing the cell to die (Bergman et al., 1985; Nakamura, Takada, Shimabuka, Matsuo, Matsuo, & Negishi, 1985). The neurologic presentation features a high-pitched cry, lethargy, poor feeding, and hypotonia. In later stages, irritability, opisthotonos (i.e., arching of the body), and seizures may occur. Spasticity, athetosis, sensorineural hearing loss, and subsequent speech and language delay are long-term disabilities. In terms of treatment, jaundice is managed by adequate hydration, phototherapy, and, in a few extreme cases, an exchange transfusion of the blood.

## OTOTOXIC DRUGS

Medications taken during pregnancy that have been associated with neonatal deafness are primarily antibiotics, such as streptomycin, kanamycin, gentamicin, amikacin, tobramycin, and neomycin. Hearing loss with streptomycin is most thoroughly documented and involves high-frequency loss that is unrelated to fetal age or to total dose (Beckman & Brent, 1986; Davidson, Brish, Rein, & Rubinstein, 1980).

Diuretics may also have a direct effect

*Medications taken during pregnancy that have been associated with neonatal deafness are primarily antibiotics.*

on hearing loss. More importantly, if used in combination with a known ototoxic substance, these drugs are thought to increase ototoxicity by multiplying its concentration in the inner ear endolymph. Ethacrynic acid and furosemide (Lasix) are the diuretics of primary concern.

The precise risk of hearing loss with the use of ototoxic antibiotics in the newborn is difficult to establish, in large part because most neonates receiving such drugs have multiple other risk factors for auditory impairment. Animal studies and limited human data suggest that deficits as a result of asphyxia, infection, respiratory distress, and intracranial hemorrhage include a symmetrical high-frequency sensorineural loss with vestibular dysfunction. The maturity, birth weight, and hepatic and renal functioning of the infant, as well as the total dose of medication and the duration of therapy, are important factors. In order to minimize risk, antibiotics are given for a brief period, and serial blood levels are monitored in order to prevent excessive drug exposure.

Finally, because illicit drugs are widely used, many fetuses have been exposed to them. No specific association between neonatal hearing deficit and the use of narcotics, cocaine, crack, amphetamines, or marijuana has been found to date.

## ENVIRONMENTAL NOISE

Critically ill neonates require intensive monitoring of vital functions and continuous nursing observation. Environmental noise generated by machinery necessary to accomplish this care may intermittently reach potentially damaging thresholds. An infant incubator, for example, may produce noise levels of 60 decibels to 85 decibels, and additional noise can be added by cardiorespiratory monitors or ventilators. Such noise interferes with sleep and likely contributes to the higher incidence of hearing loss among premature and high-risk infants via cochlear damage (Kellman, 1982).

## SCREENING FOR HEARING IMPAIRMENT

Table 2 briefly summarizes the prenatal, perinatal, and neonatal factors that warrant early testing for hearing impairment (American Academy of Pediatrics, 1982; Poland, Wells, & Ferlauto, 1980). Most intensive care nurseries have established a screening program for the majority of their infants. In-hospital techniques are primarily behavioral; arousal, the startle reflex, and the auropalpebral reflex (APR) are the primary responses examined in response to generated sound of specific frequency and intensity (Eviator, 1984; Grimes, 1985).

The two most important factors resulting in speech and language delay are hearing impairment and altered development of, or damage to, the central nervous system. As has been indicated, there is clinical evidence that preterm infants more commonly have language delay, but there is little empirical information substantiating specific causes (Hubatch, Johnson, Kistler, Burns, & Moneka, 1985). The problems often seem to be elusive. For example, preterm infants with no overt neurologic impairment frequently show mild delay in early language development, and they also show more articulation defects at age

**Table 2.** Indications for audiological evaluation

| Source | Manifestations/indications |
|---|---|
| Family history of hearing disability | Relatives of immediate family with hearing impairment of genetic origin |
| Anomalies | |
| First or second brachial arch anomalies | Auricular dysplasia, micrognathia, microtia |
| Neural tube/neural crest/ectoderm anomalies | Defects of pigmentation, meningomyelocele, widely spaced eyes |
| Craniofacial syndromes | Cleft palate |
| Asphyxia | Low Apgar scores, acidosis, hypoxia, hypercardia |
| Infections | |
| Transplacental infection | Syphilis, rubella, cytomegalovirus, toxoplasmosis |
| Perinatally acquired sepsis or meningitis | Herpes, group B streptococcus, listeria |
| Infant infections | Middle ear infections, meningitis, rubeola |
| Neurologic abnormality | Autism, blindness, mental retardation, cerebral palsy, seizures, intracranial hemorrhage |
| Prematurity and growth retardation | Birth weight less than 2,500 g |
| Toxins | Elevated bilirubin levels<br>Exposure to ototoxic drugs<br>Exposure to heavy metals<br>Prenatal exposure to alcohol |

5, compared to the term population. Even when allowances are made for the degree of prematurity, delays appear to persist. Moreover, preterm infants with respiratory distress, when compared to control infants, often continue to display decreased receptive language skills at 18 to 24 months of age (Largo, Molinari, Pinto, Weber, & Duc, 1986). In addition, many syndromes have been reported with anatomical malformation of the palate, tongue, or lips as a component. Even with surgical correction, many of these children will manifest disorders of articulation (Avery & First, 1989).

As is the case in other areas of infant screening and assessment, to date there are few language screening tools for the practicing pediatrician. The Early Language Milestone (ELM) Scale is a brief, standardized instrument that allows professionals to screen receptive and expressive language development (Coplan, 1983, 1987) prior to full evaluation by a language specialist.

• • •

In summary, high-risk infants exhibit a myriad of problems of which interactions may impede speech and language develop

ment. Life-saving technology is advancing more rapidly than is the development of quality early assessment tools to identify and quantify the subtly affected infant. Thus physicians must ensure that the newborn with any identifiable risk is evaluated by competent developmentalists, speech-language pathologists, and educators in order to limit the adverse impact of any impairment.

## REFERENCES

American Academy of Pediatrics. (1982). Joint Committee on Infant Hearing position statement. *Pediatrics, 70,* 496–497.

Avery, M.E., & First, L.R. (1989). *Pediatric medicine.* Baltimore: Williams & Wilkins.

Beckman, D.A., & Brent, R.L. (1986). Mechanism of known environmental teratogens: Drugs and chemicals. *Clinics in Perinatology, 13,* 649–687.

Bellinger, D., Levitson, A., Waternaux, C., Needleman, H., & Rabinowitz, M. (1987). Longitudinal analyses and postnatal lead exposure and early cognitive development. *New England Journal of Medicine, 316,* 1037–1043.

Bergman, I., Hirsch, R.P., Fria, T.J., Shapiro, S.M., Holzman, I., & Painter, M.J. (1985). Cause of hearing loss in the high-risk premature infant. *Journal of Pediatrics, 106,* 95–101.

Bergstrom, L. (1980). Causes of severe hearing loss in early childhood. *Pediatric Annals, 9,* 23–30.

Brook, C.G.D., Mursat, G., Zachmann, M., & Prader, A. (1974). Growth in children with 45, XO Turner syndrome. *Archives of Diseases of Childhood, 49,* 789–794.

Coplan, J. (1983). *The Early Language Milestone Scale.* Tulsa, OK: Modern Education Corporation.

Coplan, J. (1987). Deafness: Ever heard of it? Delayed recognition of permanent hearing loss. *Pediatrics, 79,* 206–213.

Cox, C., Hack, M., & Metz, D. (1981). Brain stem–evoked response audiometry: Normative data from the preterm infant. *Audiology, 20,* 53–64.

Davidson, S., Brish, M., Rein, N., & Rubinstein, M. (1980). Ototoxicity in premature infants treated with kanamycin. *Pediatrics, 66,* 479–480.

Dietrich, K.N., Krafft, K.M., Bornschein, R.L., Hammond,

P.B., Berger, O., Succop, P.A., & Bier, M. (1987). Low-level fetal lead exposure effect on neurobehavioral development in early infancy. *Pediatrics, 80,* 721–730.

Duara, S., Suter, C.M., Bessard, K.K., & Gutberlet, R.L. (1986). Neonatal screening with auditory brainstem responses: Results of follow-up audiometry and risk factor evaluation. *Journal of Pediatrics, 108,* 276–281.

Eviator, L. (1984). Evaluation of hearing in the high risk infant. *Clinics in Perinatology, 11,* 153–173.

Fraser, G.R. (1964). Profound childhood deafness. *Journal of Medical Genetics, 1,* 118–151.

Fria, T.J., Paradise, J.L., Sabo, D.L., & Elster, B.A. (1987). Conductive hearing loss in infants and young children with cleft palate. *Journal of Pediatrics, 111,* 84–87.

Grimes, C.T. (1985). Audiologic evaluation in infancy and childhood. *Pediatric Annals, 14,* 211–219.

Hendricks-Munoz, K.D., & Walton, J.P. (1988). Hearing loss in infants with persistent fetal circulation. *Pediatrics, 81,* 650–656.

Hubatch, L.M., Johnson, C.J., Kistler, D.J., Burns, W.J., & Moneka, W. (1985). Early language abilities of high-risk infants. *Journal of Speech and Hearing Disorders, 50,* 195–207.

Jones, K.L. (1986). Fetal alcohol syndrome. *Pediatric Review, 8,* 122.

Jones, K.L. (1988). *Smith's recognizable patterns of human malformation* (4th ed.). Philadelphia: W.B. Saunders.

Kaplan, S.L., Catlin, F.S., Weaver, T., & Feigin, R.D. (1984). Onset of hearing loss in children with bacterial meningitis. *Pediatrics, 73,* 575–578.

Kellman, N. (1982, August). Noise in the intensive care nursery. *Neonatal Network,* pp. 8–17.

Konigsmark, B.W. (1969). Hereditary deafness in man.

*New England Journal of Medicine, 281,* 713–720, 774–778.

Kumar, M.L., Nankervis, G.A., Jacobs, I.B., Ernhart, C.B., Glasson, C.E., McMillan, P.M., & Gold, E. (1984). Congenitally and postnatally acquired cytomegalovirus infection: Long-term follow-up. *Journal of Pediatrics, 104,* 674–679.

Largo, R.H., Molinari, L., Pinto, L.C., Weber, M., & Duc, G. (1986). Language development of term and preterm children during the first five years of life. *Developmental Medicine and Child Neurology, 28,* 333–350.

Marshall, R.E., Reichert, T.J., Kerley, S.M., & Davis, H. (1980). Auditory function in newborn intensive care unit patients revealed by auditory brain-stem potentials. *Journal of Pediatrics, 96,* 731–735.

Matalon, R., Arbogast, B., Justice, P., Brandt, J.M., & Dorfman, A. (1974). Morquio's syndrome: Deficiency of a chondroitin sulfate N-acetylhexosamine sulfatase. *Biochemical and Biophysical Research Communications, 61,* 759–763.

Nakamura, H., Takada, S., Shimabuka, R., Matsuo, M., Matsuo, T., & Negishi, H. (1985). Auditory nerve and brainstem responses in newborn infants with hyperbilirubinemia. *Pediatrics, 75,* 703–708.

Poland, R.M., Wells, D.H., & Ferlauto, J.J. (1980). Methods for detecting hearing impairment in infancy. *Pediatric Annals, 9,* 31–44.

Rowe, L.D. (1985). Hearing loss: The profound benefits of early diagnosis. *Contemporary Pediatrics, 2,* 77–85.

Simmons, F.B. (1984). Auditory brain-stem responses in high-risk neonates. *Perinatology Neonatology, 8*(2), 17–21.

Stagno, S., & Reynolds, A. (1977). Auditory and visual defects result from symptomatic and subclinical congenital cytomegalovirus and toxoplasma infections. *Pediatrics, 59,* 669–678.

Wertelecki, W., & Gerard, P.S. (1971). Clinical and chromosomal studies of the 18q − syndrome. *Journal of Pediatrics, 78,* 44–47.

# Identifying expressive language delay at age two

*Leslie Rescorla, PhD*
*Assistant Professor*
*Department of Human Development*
*Bryn Mawr College*
*Bryn Mawr, Pennsylvania*

LANGUAGE DELAY in young children is a major risk factor for later educational and mental health problems. Language delay identified in the preschool years has a strong predictive relationship to later learning disabilities (Silva, Williams, & McGee, 1987; Tallal, 1988). Furthermore, children with language problems have higher rates of psychiatric and behavioral disorders than children with normal language (Beitchman, Nair, Clegg, & Patel 1986; Cantwell & Baker, 1987; Richman, Stevenson, & Graham, 1975). Recent studies investigating expressive language delay in 2-year-olds (Fischel, Whitehurst, Caulfield, & DeBarysche, 1988; Paul, 1989; Rescorla & Schwartz, 1990; Thal & Bates, 1988) suggest that approximately 50% of language-delayed toddlers continue to show lags in language skills at least up until age 3, even when their nonverbal ability and receptive language are normal.

With the recent passage of PL 99-457 mandating services for handicapped tod-

*Top Lang Disord*, 1991,11(4),14–20
© 1991 Aspen Publishers, Inc.

dlers, an efficient method for identifying language-delayed 2-year-olds is going to become increasingly useful. The need will be especially great for feasible ways to identify youngsters who are not already known to health or educational authorities because of mental retardation, neurological dysfunction, hearing impairment, or autism. However, the identification of language-delayed toddlers is hindered by a paucity of well-standardized language tests appropriate for very young children, as well as by the difficulties inherent in obtaining reliable test performance from 2-year-olds.

Several pediatric screening instruments aimed at the identification of language-delayed children have been developed in the last decade, most notably the Early Language Milestone Scale (ELM; Coplan, Gleason, Ryan, Burke, & Williams, 1982) and the Clinical Linguistic and Auditory Milestone Scale (CLAMS; Capute et al., 1986). Both the ELM and the CLAMS tap a wide range of communicative skills (gestural, receptive, and expressive), designed as they are to detect language deficits in infants as well as toddlers. Although these tools have been effective in pediatric practices for identifying infants and toddlers with severe developmental disorders, they have not been widely used in the general population to detect children with language delay.

Over the past 10 years, two parent report inventories geared at assessing language skills in toddlers in the general population have been developed and extensively researched: (1) the MacArthur Communicative Development Inventory: Toddlers (CDI), developed by Bates and her colleagues (Dale, 1990; Fenson et al.,

1989) and (2) the Language Development Survey (LDS), developed by Rescorla (1989). In contrast to the ELM and the CLAMS, the CDI and the LDS are designed for use with children from the age of 18 months, and they concentrate on expressive language. Both instruments are based on the premise that parental report is a practical, reliable, and valid method for assessing a toddler's progress in language acquisition, if such report is detailed and explicit. They are also predicated on the idea that the two most important areas of expressive language to assess in toddlers are vocabulary size and the development of syntax. Although the instruments differ in a number of respects, they both seem to be promising tools for speech-language pathologists to use in the identification of toddlers who are slow to talk. In this article, the CDI and the LDS will be described, and some of the pertinent literature about their reliability, validity, and application will be reviewed.

## THE CDI

About a decade ago, Bates and her colleagues (Bates, Bretherton, & Snyder, 1988; Bretherton, McNew, Snyder, & Bates, 1983) began to develop a comprehensive set of parent report instruments to assess communicative development from 8 to 36 months of age. They made the important decision to use a recognition-format vocabulary checklist, rather than to rely on global estimates of vocabulary size or recall of vocabulary items. Among the advantages of parent report that Bates et al. cite are that it is cost-effective and quick, and that it is based on experience with the child over an extended period of time and in multiple settings.

Research over the last decade on the CDI: Toddlers (in previous versions, called the Early Language Inventory, ELI) has demonstrated that this parent report instrument provides an accurate picture of the toddler's early language development. For example, Bates, Bretherton, and Snyder (1988) found a correlation of .83 between vocabulary size reported by the mother on the language checklist and total number of different words used by the child in 2 to 3 hours of naturalistic speech. Similarly, Dale, Bates, Reznick, and Morisset (1989) reported significant correlations between ELI vocabulary and performance on the receptive and expressive language items on the Bayley Scales (Bayley, 1969). In a study by Beeghly, Jernberg, and Burrows (1989) with 25-month-old children, total ELI vocabulary was correlated significantly with Bayley expressive and receptive language items, as well as with the number of different ELI words actually produced by the child during about 40 minutes of videotaped activity.

The most recent version of the inventory developed by Bates and her colleagues—the CDI: Toddlers—was examined in a large norming study in 1989 to 1990. Part I of the toddler inventory contains 680 vocabulary words arranged into 22 categories (e.g., animals, food and drink, outside things, body parts, places to go, descriptive words, question words, connecting words). Part II consists of 125 items pertaining to grammatical development. Some items ask about the frequency of use of various morphological inflections (e.g., "ing" for progressive tense, plural or possessive /s/, regular and irregular past

tense). Others employ a forced choice format in which the parent is asked to indicate which of two forms sounds most like his or her child (e.g., "doggie table" or "doggie on table"). In addition, the parent is asked to give examples of three of the child's longest sentences; this latter item was adopted from a similar item on the LDS. Preliminary data reported on 545 toddlers indicate mean vocabulary on the CDI: Toddlers to be about 300 words at 24 months, rising to about 500 words at 30 months. This mean vocabulary size is quite similar to reported vocabulary sizes on earlier versions of the CDI.

The most recently completed research with the CDI: Toddlers is a validity study with 24-months-olds by Dale (1990). Mean reported vocabulary on the CDI at 24 months was 372 words ($SD = 175.9$ words). Reported vocabulary was correlated .73 with the child's Expressive One-Word Picture Vocabulary score (Gardner, 1979). Similarly, the child's mean length of utterance (MLU) from a speech sample was correlated at .77 with the child's grammatical complexity score on the CDI and at .75 with the mean length of the three sample sentences listed by the mother.

The CDI: Toddlers is a parent report instrument whose validity has been demonstrated in many different research studies. Involvement of a large number of senior researchers and access to substantial amounts of funding have given the CDI a research base that is unparalleled in its geographical diversity and sample size. High and low socioeconomic status (SES) subjects; pre-terms and full-terms; and language-delayed, normal, and precocious children have all been successfully studied with the CDI. Because of its comprehensive nature, the CDI provides a vast amount of data. It is especially useful for providing an in-depth picture of the child's vocabulary by form class or a detailed profile of his or her mastery of specific syntactic features. On the other hand, the CDI has not been widely used for identifying toddlers with delayed language development (Thal & Bates, 1988). Therefore, the issue of what CDI criteria for language delay should be used at which ages, and the question of how these various criteria perform in terms of sensitivity and specificity against different "gold standards" of language delay, will be fruitful areas for future studies.

## THE LDS

The LDS was designed by Rescorla to be used as a quick and efficient epidemiological screening tool for the identification of language delay in 2-year-old children. Since its development in 1981, the LDS has been used with more than 900 children (Rescorla, 1989). Although the LDS has gone through several minor revisions, it has remained a one-page, double-sided survey form consisting of a checklist of about 300 vocabulary words arranged alphabetically by semantic category (e.g., animals, foods, vehicles, people, body parts, toys, action words, modifiers). The parent is asked to check off each word the child uses spontaneously. The parent also is asked whether or not the child uses word combinations and is asked to give three examples of the child's best sentences. Thus, like the CDI, the LDS differs from such pediatric language screening tools as the ELM or the CLAMS in that it requires the parent to supply details about what

words the child actually uses and to give examples of the child's sentences. Finally, the parent completes a set of items about demographic, health, and family information.

The first LDS studies were carried out in pediatric practices. In six different samples containing about 500 children ranging widely in SES, the overall reported prevalence of language delay using the criterion of "fewer than 50 words OR no word combinations at 2" ranged from 13% to 20%. In a reliability and validity study of the LDS carried out with 81 language-delayed and normal toddlers, the correlation between total LDS-reported vocabulary and children's naming of pictures and objects on the Bayley Scale and on the Reynell Expressive Language Scale (Reynell, 1977) was .87. Test–retest reliability of the LDS was .99 for total LDS words and ranged from .86 to .99 for the various semantic domains. Using the LDS criterion of "fewer than 50 words OR no word combinations at 2" against the "gold standard" of at least a 6-month delay in Reynell Expressive Language age, the LDS was able to identify 87% of the children concurrently found to be delayed on the Reynell, with a specificity of 86%. A second validity study carried out with 58 inner-city toddlers yielded a correlation of .79 between total words reported on the LDS and total number of Bayley objects and Preschool Language Scale (Zimmerman, Steiner, & Evatt, 1969) pictures named.

In a recent LDS study of 108 children from community recreation and day-care programs (Rescorla, Escarce, & Hadicke-Wiley, 1990; Escarce & Rescorla, 1991), mean vocabulary reported was 193 words, with 10% of the children 22 months or older having vocabularies under 50 words. Total LDS vocabulary correlated .78 with the child's score on naming Bayley objects and Stanford-Binet: Fourth Edition pictures (Thorndike, Hagen, & Sattler, 1986). Sixteen percent of the sample met the criterion of "fewer than 50 words OR no word combinations at 2." Using this criterion against a "gold standard" of "no Bayley objects named," the LDS had a sensitivity of 90% and a specificity of 95%.

The latest research using the LDS is an epidemiological survey of 92 children obtained through the census lists of a suburban school district (Rescorla, Escarce, & Hadicke-Wiley, 1990). Mean vocabulary was 183.71 words (*SD* of 97). More than half of the sample (58%) had vocabularies of more than 200 words, and 15% were reported to have fewer than 50 words. LDS vocabulary was correlated at .82 with total number of Bayley objects and Stanford-Binet pictures named. Eighteen percent of the sample had "fewer than 50 words OR no word combinations." Using this criterion, sensitivity was 100% and specificity was 91% against the "gold standard" of "no Bayley pictures named" and 100% and 93% for "no Binet pictures named."

The LDS has proven to be a highly efficient instrument for the identification of toddlers who are slow to talk. Data collected from more than 900 children have produced a number of stable and robust findings. Mean vocabulary on the LDS consistently has been about 150 words or more at age 2; the typical standard deviation of 80 to 90 reflects the wide variability in vocabulary size in normal toddlers. The CDI, which is double the

length of the LDS, generally yields vocabulary estimates exceeding 300 words at age 2. These findings suggest that neither the LDS nor the CDI yields a "complete" inventory of all the words in a given child's vocabulary, particularly when that vocabulary is large.

In LDS studies, the proportion of children with reported vocabularies of fewer than 50 words at age 2 consistently has been about 15%. Data from several studies have demonstrated high internal consistency reliability and test–retest reliability of the LDS. Maternal report of vocabulary has been highly correlated with the child's performance on a variety of picture-and object-naming tasks. Sensitivity of the LDS has been about 90% or higher using the criterion of "fewer than 50 words OR no word combinations," with a corresponding specificity of 90% or better.

•  •  •

Over the next decade, in response to the mandate of PL 99-457, speech-language clinicians are likely to be called on to screen large numbers of toddlers for possible language delay. Given the importance of early language delay as a risk factor for later learning disability, even in children with normal intelligence quotients (IQs) and good receptive language, it will be highly desirable to have language screening tools that are sufficiently sensitive to identify children who have delayed language in the absence of other major disabilities. The two parent report inventories reviewed in this article may prove useful for this purpose.

Speech-language clinicians may find it productive to identify language-delayed toddlers by employing a multistep screening process using these two parent report inventories followed by direct assessment of the child. First, the LDS might be used as a quick screening for the purpose of targeting 2-year-olds with very limited vocabularies and little or no emerging syntax. Because it takes only about 10 minutes for a parent to complete, is compact and inexpensive (a single sheet costs 25¢), and is easily "scored" (words are counted and the presence or absence of word combinations is determined), the LDS provides an excellent, quick screening for the purpose of initial identification. Children who appear to be language delayed on the basis of the LDS can then be looked at more intensively by obtaining parental report on the CDI.

Because of its comprehensive nature, the CDI is much longer than the LDS, takes approximately 30 minutes to complete, and is more expensive to purchase (50¢). Computer scoring is available for the CDI, but it can also be inspected by eye. Finally, children who appear to be delayed in vocabulary, word combinations, or morphological development on the CDI can then be examined by a speech-language clinician. Having already obtained detailed information about the child's expressive language skills from the LDS and the CDI, the clinician can be more selective and focused in choosing which instruments to administer directly to the child.

## REFERENCES

Bates, E., Bretherton, I., & Snyder, L. (1988). *From first words to grammar: Individual differences and dissociable mechanisms.* New York, NY: Cambridge University Press.

Bayley, N. (1969). *Bayley Scales of Infant Development.* New York, NY: The Psychological Corporation.

Beeghly, M., Jernberg, E., & Burrows, E. (1989). *Validity of the Early Language Inventory (ELI) for use with 25-month-olds.* Poster presented at the biennial meeting of the Society for Research in Child Development.

Beitchman, J.H., Nair, R., Clegg, M., & Patel, P.G. (1986). Prevalence of speech and language disorders in 5-year-old kindergarten children in the Ottowa-Carleton region. *Journal of Speech and Hearing Research, 51,* 98–110.

Bretherton, I., McNew, S., Snyder, L., & Bates, E. (1983). Individual differences at 20 months: Analytic and holistic strategies in language acquisition. *Journal of Child Language, 10,* 293–320.

Cantwell, D., & Baker, L. (1987). *Developmental speech and language disorders.* New York, NY: Guilford.

Capute, A.J., Palmer, F.B., Shapiro, B.K., Wachtel, R.C., Schmidt, S., & Ross, A. (1986). Clinical Linguistic and Auditory Milestone Scale: Prediction of cognition in infancy. *Developmental Medicine and Child Neurology, 28,* 762–771.

Coplan, J., Gleason, J.R., Ryan, R., Burke, M.G., &

Williams, M.L. (1982). Validation of an early language milestone scale in a high-risk population. *Pediatrics, 70,* 677–683.

Dale, P.S. (1990, July). *The validity of a parent report measure of vocabulary and syntax at 24 months.* Poster presented at the Fifth International Congress for the Study of Child Language, Budapest, Hungary.

Dale, P.S., Bates, E., Reznick, J.S., & Morisset, C. (1989). The validity of a parent report instrument of child language at 20 months. *Journal of Child Language, 16,* 239–249.

Escarce, E. & Rescorla, L. (1991). The Language Development Survey: A new tool for assessing expressive language development and delay in pediatric settings. Paper presented at the 12th Annual National Association of Pediatric Nurse Associates and Practitioners Conference, Philadelphia, PA, April 1991.

Fenson, L., Flynn, D., Vella, D., Omens, J., Burgess, S., & Hartung, J. (1989). *Tools for the assessment of language in infants and toddlers by parental report.* Poster presented at the Biennial Meeting of the Society for Research in Child Development.

Fischel, J., Whitehurst, G., Caulfield, M., & DeBaryshe, B. (1988). Language growth in children with expressive language delay. *Pediatrics, 82,* 218–227.

Gardner, M.F. (1979). *The Expressive One-Word Picture*

*Vocabulary Test.* Novato, CA: Academy Therapy Publishing Co.

Paul, R. (1989). *Outcomes of expressive language delay in toddlers.* Paper presented at the Biennial Meeting of the Society for Research in Child Development.

Rescorla, L., Escarce, E., & Hadicke-Wiley, M. (1990, July). *Epidemiology of expressive language delay at 2.* Paper presented at the Fifth International Congress for the Study of Child Language, Budapest, Hungary.

Rescorla, L. & Schwartz, E. (1990). Outcome of specific expressive language delay (SELD). *Applied Psycholinguistics, 11,* 393–408.

Rescorla, L. (1989). The language development survey: A screening tool for delayed language in toddlers. *Journal of Speech and Hearing Disorders, 54,* 587–599.

Reynell, J. (1977). *Reynell Developmental Language Scales.* Windsor: NFER.

Richman, N., Stevenson, J., & Graham, P.J. (1975). Prevalence of behaviour problems in 3-year-old children: An epidemiological study in a London borough. *Journal of Child Psychology and Psychiatry, 16,* 277–287.

Silva, P.A., Williams, S.M., & McGee, R. (1987). A longitudinal study of children with developmental language delay at age three: Later intelligence, reading, and behavior problems. *Developmental Medicine and Child Neurology, 29,* 630–640.

Tallal, P. (1988). Developmental language disorders. In J.F. Kavanagh & T.J. Truss, Jr. (Eds.). *Learning disabilities: Proceedings of the national conference.* Parkton, MD: York Press.

Thal, D. & Bates, E. (1988). Language and gesture in late talkers. *Journal of Speech and Hearing Research, 31,* 115–123.

Thorndike, R.L., Hagen, E.P. & Sattler, J.M. (1986). *Stanford-Binet Intelligence Scale: Fourth Edition.* Chicago, IL: Riverside Press.

Zimmerman, I., Steiner, V., & Evatt, R. (1969). *Preschool Language Scale.* Columbus, OH: Charles E. Merrill.

# Toward an integrated view of early language and communication development and socioemotional development

**Barry M. Prizant, PhD**
*Director, Communication Disorders
    Department*
*Bradley Hospital*
*Associate Professor of Psychiatry and
    Human Behavior*
*Division of Child and Adolescent
    Psychiatry*
*Brown University Program in Medicine*
*East Providence, Rhode Island*

**Amy M. Wetherby, PhD**
*Associate Professor*
*Department of Communication
    Disorders*
*Florida State University*
*Tallahassee, Florida*

OVER THE LAST 15 years, relationships among the development of communicative and linguistic abilities and of cognitive and social abilities in young children have received much interest (Bates, O'Connell, & Shore, 1987). However, interest in possible relationships among communication and language development and socioemotional development in young children has been far more limited. *Socioemotional development* refers to a young child's development of capacities to experience and express a variety of emotional states, to regulate emotional arousal, to establish secure and positive relationships, and to develop a sense of self as distinct from others and as capable of achieving goals in interactions with the social and nonsocial world. Howlin and Rutter (1987) noted that "the nature of the relationship between language, cognitive, behavioral and emotional development is poorly understood" (p. 290). Specific to emotional development, Cicchetti (1989) stated that "only if

*Top Lang Disord*, 1990,10(4),1–16
© 1990 Aspen Publishers, Inc.

we know how emotions relate to other aspects of knowledge we have about people's development will we be able to specify the necessary and/or sufficient conditions necessary to bring about change in the emotional domain" (pp. 400–401).

Recent literature in child psychiatry and communication disorders has documented a high cooccurrence of communication disorders and emotional and behavioral disorders in children (see Prizant et al., 1990, for a review). In clinical practice, frameworks for understanding communication disorders and emotional and behavioral disorders have been derived from research on early language and communication development and early socioemotional development. Researchers who study early childhood disorders have discussed the recent emergence of the field of developmental psychopathology, a multidisciplinary approach based on the premise that impairments in development should be understood in reference to normal developmental processes, and that knowledge of impaired development, in turn, provides insights into normal developmental processes (Cicchetti, 1984).

This approach recognizes that developmental perspectives that focus only on isolated domains of development without considering interrelationships among different aspects of development may be of limited value and not true to developmental realities (Sroufe & Rutter, 1984). Cicchetti (1989) stated that "the field of developmental psychopathology requires that multiple domains of development be studied, including cognitive, socioemotional, linguistic and biological processes. . . . Variables at many levels of analysis are viewed as being in dynamic

transaction with one another" (pp. 378–379). In a discussion of normal developmental processes, Blount (1982) noted that "emotional development includes the ties between affect and social and cognitive domains, and the mutual influences of those systems" (p. 140).

In this article, a more integrated perspective on early communication and socioemotional development in children is espoused. Given the enormous size of the separate literatures in language and communication development and in socioemotional development the most salient and interrelated aspects in each of these developmental domains will be the focus of inquiry. When relevant, examples from the literature on at-risk children will be given. It is beyond the scope of this article to review the research literature on at-risk or developmentally disabled children (see Dunst, Lowe, & Bartholomew, 1990; Vohr & Garcia-Coll, 1988), or approaches to assessment and intervention (see Greenspan, 1988; Theadore, Maher, & Prizant, "Early assessment and intervention with emotional and behavioral disorders and communication disorders," this issue). However, it is hoped that this discussion will stimulate speech–language pathologists and other professionals to develop greater clinical sensitivity to socioemotional issues in serving communicatively disordered children.

Achieving a more integrated perspective on communication and language development and socioemotional development has been hindered, in part, by the lack of clarity in uses of common terminology by professionals in different disciplines. For example, infancy researchers have used the term *communicative sig-*

*nals* in reference to signals that inform the receiver of an infant's physiological or emotional state (Brazelton, 1982; Tronick, 1980). Dunst and Lowe (1986) have referred to early communication (0–3 months) as *behavioral state communication*. Researchers studying later communication development, while acknowledging the continuity of development from early in the first year of life, have tended to focus attention on language development. More recently, greater attention has been given to patterns of nonverbal communication development, which typically appear at approximately 8 to 10 months, when normally developing children signal intentionally to achieve specific goals (Bates et al., 1987).

Infancy researchers are beginning to demonstrate interest in exploring continuities between early affective or behavioral state communication and later emerging intentional and propositional communication. For example, Adamson and Bakeman (1985) studied affective signaling in infants during the first and second year of life. They observed that affective displays provide infants with a means to comment on themes in play and serve as an early form of greeting. By 12 months of age, affective and referential communication systems become integrated. Recently, language development researchers have begun to integrate affective variables into their research paradigms. For example, Bloom (1987) demonstrated that in play interactions, normally developing children classified as early word learners tended to spend more time in neutral affect expression and, thus, demonstrated fewer expressions of positive and negative affect when compared to those classified as

late word learners who were more expressive affectively in early development (i.e., at 13 and 17 months of age). She interpreted these findings as indicating that stability in emotionality, as reflected in neutral affect expression, may allow for a reflective learning style, which is required for early word learning.

In relation to at-risk populations, Cicchetti (1989) and his colleagues have been investigating language and communication in maltreated children. At 31 months they found differences in language and communication between maltreated and nonmaltreated controls matched for low socioeconomic status, with the latter group demonstrating significantly greater abilities. Cicchetti noted that "these investigations provide compelling support . . . that social and emotional factors play important roles in the development of language" (p. 412). Research on low birth weight infants has found limitations in affective signaling as well as delays in communication development (Vohr & Garcia-Coll, 1988). This research represents some recent attempts to integrate aspects of socioemotional development and affective communication with aspects of language and communication development.

For practicing speech–language pathologists, integrating these perspectives is important for a variety of reasons. Although conclusive data are not yet available, it is likely that early appropriate communication and language intervention with at-risk or delayed children and their families may serve as a significant preventive measure against the development or exacerbation of emotional and behavioral problems in very young children (Baker & Cantwell, 1987). For clinicians working in early intervention, Public Law 99-457, the Early Intervention Program for Infants and Toddlers with Handicaps (1989), states specifically that professionals from different disciplines must work closely in an integrated and coordinated manner in planning appropriate programs for infants and their families. Infants or toddlers with communication delays or disorders may have, or be at risk for, the development of emotional and behavioral disorders (Baker & Cantwell, 1987). Finally, in the authors' clinical practice, they have found that consideration of socioemotional perspectives has a significant positive impact on both assessment and intervention efforts with children and their families.

## INTEGRATING KNOWLEDGE OF DEVELOPMENTAL ASPECTS

In-depth considerations of the interdependencies and mutual influences of early socioemotional and communication development are few. However, two models of development have been proposed that may provide a starting point for attempts at integration. The first model, proposed by Tronick (1989), addresses the role of the development of mutual (interactive) and self-regulatory capacities in young children's socioemotional development. The

*Infants or toddlers with communication delays or disorders may have, or be at risk for, the development of emotional and behavioral disorders.*

authors discuss the model as it pertains to communication and language development. The second model, the transactional model (Sameroff, 1987; Sameroff & Chandler, 1975; Sameroff & Fiese, 1990), is a more general attempt to conceptualize the complex developmental interdependencies among children, caregivers, and social contexts.

### Language, communication, and mutual and self-regulatory capacities

In the most general sense, the primary functions served by a child's growing communicative and linguistic competence involve the regulation of others' behavior and the regulation of his or her own behavior. Nonverbal communicative signals and communicative use of language allow a child to influence the behavior, attitudes, and beliefs of others and to regulate ongoing exchanges whether they be social exchanges, where the means and end are social-affective attunement, or exchanges undertaken to solve problems or to achieve specific goals.

A second important function of communication and language abilities relates to internal regulation, or self-regulation. Self-regulatory and other noncommunicative functions of language have been discussed for a number of years (Kuczaj & Bean, 1982; Vygotsky, 1976). The acquisition of a symbolic system to internally represent experiences enables a growing child to use internalized language to reflect, solve problems, anticipate, and plan. Thus, future actions can be based on prior experience. Additionally, inner language may serve a more specific directive function, enabling children to tell themselves what to do rather than simply being under the control of external agents (Luria, 1961).

Tronick (1989) recently considered the importance of an infant's developing mutual and self-regulatory capacities for his or her emotional well-being and emotional growth. Tronick hypothesized that an infant's early affective expressions may serve as communicative signals that function to help regulate emotional arousal. These may take the form of mutual (other-directed) regulatory behaviors as well as self-regulatory (self-soothing) behaviors. This conceptualization represents an important analog to communicative and non-communicative functions of language discussed above and provides a premise for conceptualizing the interface between emotional and communication development early in life.

**Transactional nature of development**

Sameroff and Chandler (1975) proposed a model for conceptualizing development that revolutionized the way developmental researchers consider relationships among child characteristics, caregiver characteristics, and environmental influences over time. These authors rejected linear, unidirectional models of causality in psychological and biological development (e.g., a particular child characteristic could be directly attributable to a biological factor, a caregiver characteristic, or an environmental variable). In the transactional model, developmental outcomes at any point in time are seen as a result of the dynamic interrelationships among child behavior, caregiver responses to the child's behavior, and environmental variables that may influence both the child and the caregiver. Transactional processes are op-

erative in moment-to-moment aspects of social exchange where caregiver–child influences are bidirectional, as well as over extensive periods of time where the cumulative experience of these bidirectional influences has a significant impact on child development and caregiver style (Sameroff & Fiese, 1990).

From the perspective of at-risk children, Dunst et al. (1990) recently presented a model of the development of communicative competence that is transactional in nature and is based on Goldberg's (1977) model of mutual efficacy in caregiver-child interaction. The model emphasizes the importance of bidirectional, contingent social responsiveness on the part of a caregiver and young child. Thus, over time, when a young child's social behavior can be accurately interpreted or read by a caregiver, and when the caregiver is able to respond in such a way as to meet the child's needs or to support social exchange, both caregiver and child develop a sense of efficacy. A cumulative effect of positive contingent exchange is that interactions become more predictable as expectancies and contingencies increase. Development is therefore influenced by a child's ability to produce readable signals, a caregiver's ability to respond appropriately to the child's signals, and the habitualization of such patterns. This highly simplified description of an extremely complex process must be viewed in the context of innumerable exchanges between a caregiver and child over time and under different circumstances. Furthermore, factors affecting a caregiver (e.g., psychological well-being, social support) will influence his or her availability and responsivity to the young child (Dunst et al., 1990).

Sameroff (1987) considered how premature birth, a significant biological risk factor, may result in a language delay within a transactional model. Sameroff noted that the fragile condition of a very low birth weight infant may cause anxiety in an otherwise composed caregiver, which may then lead to cautious and possibly less than optimal caregiving practices (e.g., overstimulation or understimulation). These practices may result in the development of irritability or difficult temperament or exacerbate any problems caused by biological factors. A caregiver may avoid an irritable child who is difficult to soothe or calm or who has limited self-soothing capacities, resulting in too few reciprocal interactive experiences and thus interfering with normal communication and language development. In this example, a hypothesized language delay may be determined partially by biological factors associated with prematurity (e.g., irritability, limited ability to self-soothe) and partly by the less direct, maladaptive transactional process that develops between caregiver and child. Following this model, it also is conceivable that caregivers of premature infants who demonstrate extreme sensitivity to their child's fragile state by providing appropriate levels of contingent sensory and social stimulation may mitigate or overcome the biological risk.

The transactional model is seen as a critical underlying premise in the attempt to integrate aspects of communication and language development with socioemotional development, as developmental processes in both domains are thought to be highly influenced by biological factors and by transactions between the child, his or her caregivers, and the environment (Cicchetti, 1989; Sameroff, 1987; Sameroff & Fiese, 1990).

### Stage-specific considerations

The achievements attained by children as they pass from infancy to early childhood change according to their stage in the continuum of development. Thus, relationships between communication, language, and socioemotional factors will be qualitatively different at different stages of development. While acknowledging the danger of oversimplifying the complexities and continuities of early development (Rutter, 1987a), the authors' attempt at integration is organized according to developmental stages of communication and language development and socioemotional development (Table 1). Using this framework, it is possible not only to present an overview of major milestones in these aspects of development, but also to consider both mutual influences and interdependencies when development proceeds normally and the effects of distortions or delays in the developmental process.

This developmental continuum is divided into three periods: infancy (approximately birth to 12 months of age), toddlerhood (approximately 12 through 24 months), and early childhood (approximately 24 through 48 months). Consideration beyond 48 months of age is beyond the scope of this article, but significant linguistic, communicative, and socioemotional achievements continue to occur into later childhood, adolescence, and throughout the life span (Maccoby & Martin, 1983; Owens, 1988).

**Table 1.** The relationship between communication and language development and socioemotional development in children aged 0–48 months

| Age (mos) | Achievements in communication and language development | Achievements in socioemotional development |
|---|---|---|
| 0–12 | Establishment of joint attention and social engagement with caregivers<br>Increased participation in joint activity routines<br>Early vocal and gestural intentional signaling for behavioral regulation, social interaction and joint attention<br>Comprehension of words in routinized interactions | Preintentional affective signaling of emotional states<br>Self-regulation of emotional arousal<br>Sharing of affect with caregivers<br>Establishment of attachment relationship<br>Ability to respond to soothing, comfort given by caregivers |
| 12–24 | Increased frequency, persistence, and intentionality in preverbal communication signaling<br>Acquisition of symbolic language for communication about immediate context and own actions<br>Internal symbolic representation of past events<br>Greater anticipation | Consolidation of attachment relationships<br>Greater awareness and assertiveness relative to own motives and goals and conflict with those of others (autonomy)<br>Establishment of internal representations of relationships and interactions |
| 24–48 | Increased communication about other's actions and about observed events<br>Increased distancing—symbolic communication about past and future events<br>Comprehension of conditional, causal, and other complex event relations<br>Early conversational competence | Ability to plan and to delay gratification to greater extent<br>Internal state communication and language<br>Development of self-image<br>Elaboration of internal representations of relationships<br>Stabilization of mood<br>Capacity for empathy<br>Development of peer relationships |

*Source:* Bates, O'Connell & Shore, 1987; Greenspan, 1988; Greenspan & Porges, 1984; Cicchetti, 1989.

## Infancy

In contrast to earlier theories of infancy as a time of reactivity and passivity, current theories acknowledge that from very early in development, infants are actively driven to achieve goals, including physiological and emotional regulation (Greenspan, 1988; Tronick, 1989). Greenspan (1988) noted that when infants' internal states are regulated, they are able to focus energy on the external animate and inanimate world, paving the way, according to Greenspan, for the establishment of emotional attachments. Internal goals include maintaining physiological homeostasis, establishing a feeling of security, experiencing positive emotions, and controlling negative emotions. External goals involve engaging the social and inanimate world, including interacting with others, maintaining proximity to caregivers, engaging in positive reciprocal interactions, and exploring objects (Tronick, 1989).

Prior to acquiring first words, children learn to communicate intentionally with preverbal gestures and sounds, to reference objects and events with indicative gestures (e.g., pointing), and to use conventional signals that have shared meanings (Bates et al., 1987). These preverbal communicative achievements provide the foundation for the emergence of language. From birth, a child's behavior systematically affects the caregiver, thus serving a communicative function. The caregiver's interpretation of such preintentional communicative behavior plays an important role in the development of intentional communication. Dore (1986) suggested that the caregiver induces in-

---

*At about 9 to 10 months of age, the child begins to use gestures and sounds to communicate intentionally — that is, the child deliberately uses a particular signal to have a preplanned effect on another person.*

---

tent in the infant by engaging in preverbal dialogues in which affective states are shared. These early social interactions involving shared affective experiences lead to the infant's awareness of the effect that his or her behavior can have on others (Bruner, 1981; Dore, 1986).

At about 9 to 10 months of age, the child begins to use gestures and sounds to communicate intentionally—that is, the child deliberately uses a particular signal to have a preplanned effect on another person (Bates, 1979). Bruner (1981) suggested that three innate communicative intentions emerge during the first year of life:

1. Behavioral regulation, which includes signals used to regulate another's behavior for purposes of obtaining or restricting an environmental goal;
2. Social interaction, which includes signals used to attract and maintain another's attention to oneself for affiliative purposes; and
3. Joint attention, which includes acts used to direct another's attention for purposes of sharing the focus on an entity or event.

Research has demonstrated that normal children express these three communicative intentions before the emergence of words (Wetherby, Cain, Yonclas, & Walker, 1988).

The sophistication of communicative means used to express these intentions increases with advancing cognitive, social, and language development. Bates (1979) found that giving and showing gestures are necessary precursors to the use of pointing to reference joint attention, and she concluded that these gestures are highly correlated with the subsequent emergence of naming. In other words, children learn to reference first with gestures and then with words. There is a gradual transition from preverbal sounds and gestures to first words. From about 9 to 12 months, children begin to use conventional sounds to signify a specific communicative function, such as *mama* as a general purpose request for objects, and to mark a predictable point in an episode, such as *bye bye* when closing a book.

In his discussion of the development of mutual and self-regulatory capacities in infancy, Tronick (1989) noted that the early affective expressions and displays of infants, which may be in reaction to internal or external stimuli, serve as other-directed mutual regulatory behaviors that may result in a caregiver helping to soothe the infant (if the infant is upset) or to aid the infant in reaching a goal (e.g., obtaining an object, reducing the amount of stimulation). This affective communication results in transforming an infant's experience of negative emotion to positive emotion.

Tronick added that infants also develop self-directed regulatory behaviors, including such coping strategies as gaze aversion, thumb sucking, and other behaviors that serve to either reduce the level of disruptive stimulation or enable a child to self-soothe. Tronick (1989) noted that

the distinction between self-directed and other-directed behaviors is not hard and fast. Self-directed behavior can function as communication, conveying the infant's evaluation of success and failure and his or her emotional state to a caregiver. The caregiver may then act on this communication to aid the infant's accomplishment of internal and external goals (p. 114).

After the first 6 to 8 months of life, infants develop greater cognitive capacities for observing and understanding the outcomes of their own behavior and are thus able to engage in more specific other-directed communicative efforts involving more intentional and purposeful communication with others. It is conceivable that, toward the end of the first year, the infant's growing experience of coping with internally or externally induced stressors, along with growing social and cognitive competence, results in a broader array of self-regulatory capacities of a more cognitive nature; the child is able to reflect and

to actively interpret affective communicative cues from others to make decisions in stressful circumstances. For example, Campos, Barrett, Lamb, Goldsmith, and Sternberg (1983) demonstrated in their research that infants as young as 10 months of age use the facial expressions of caregivers (e.g., joyful, fearful) to make decisions about crawling across a visual cliff, which presents an apparent, but not real, danger of falling. When parents look joyful, infants crawl across. When parents look fearful, infants use these facial cues to regulate their own behavior and will not cross.

Stern (1985) identified achievements in socioemotional development that appear to relate closely to a child's early development of intentional communication. He discussed the appearance of intersubjective relatedness at 7 to 9 months of age in normally developing infants. *Intersubjective relatedness* refers to the infant's deliberate attempts to share experiences with caregivers and the expectation that caregivers will share experiences with them. The three mental states that allow for intersubjectivity discussed by Stern include sharing affective states, or interaffectivity; sharing joint attention, or interattentionality; and sharing intentions, or interintentionality. Stern noted that "early in life affects are both the primary *medium* and the primary *subject* of communication" (p. 133). Responsive caregivers help infants to realize the instrumental communicative impact of their affective communication.

Toward the end of the first year, infants gain the capacity to actively signal either to achieve shared attention with others or to express their own intentions. However,

Stern believes that the affective exchange still predominates in communicative interactions with a primary caregiver at this time. Increasingly, however, communicative signals become more directed to the experiential world rather than simply communicating the child's own experience in an interaction with another person (Adamson & Bakeman, 1985). Stern (1985) noted that "most protolinguistic exchanges involving intentions and objects are at the same time affective changes . . . the two go on simultaneously" (p. 133). However, according to Stern, infants are far more adept at communicating emotions than specific intentions at the end of the first year.

Thus, this period of infancy represents a period of primarily emotional and affective and behavioral-state signaling in the first 6 to 8 months, with a fusion of affective signaling and later appearing intentional communicative signaling toward the end of the first year (Adamson & Bakeman, 1985).

It is interesting to note that children who have been maltreated in the first year of life (Cicchetti, 1989) or who were raised by depressed caregivers (Tronick, 1989) typically demonstrate a blunting of affective display or limited responsivity to affective expressions of others. Thus, their communicative signals may be more subtle or difficult to read. In the case of maltreated children, significant delays in language development may not become apparent immediately, but may be observable beyond emerging language stages (at approximately 31 months) (Cicchetti, 1989). The infant's degree of success in sharing attention and sharing intentions and, for that matter, in sharing affect will

depend largely on the readability of his or her signals, as well as the availability of the primary caregiver in interpreting and responding to these signals (Dunst et al., 1990; Greenspan, 1988).

### Toddlerhood

As young children move into their second year, they develop the representational capacities to reflect and to make decisions based on prior experiences with the social and object world (Stern, 1985). As communicative signaling becomes more persistent, explicit, and sophisticated, toddlers become more successful in regulating social interactions and are more easily read by those interacting with them (Dunst & Lowe, 1986). Thus, the development of mutual (other-directed) and self-regulatory capacities builds on early abilities to regulate emotional states through self- and other-directed behaviors and forms the foundation for the development of more sophisticated communicative capacities and for the ability to participate actively in reciprocal interaction.

Children's first words, which appear during the second year, are mapped onto prelinguistic gestures. At about 13 months, children begin using a small number of words that are symbolic or referential, that is, labels used to refer to an object or class of objects. New word acquisition is very slow during the one-word stage, and it is not unusual for an old word to drop out of the child's vocabulary as a new word comes in, which sometimes causes concern to caregivers. Between 12 and 18 months, children show an increase in the rate of communicating, the use of sounds in coordination with gestures, and the use of consonants in multisyllabic utterances

(Wetherby et al., 1988), thus increasing readability of communicative signals.

At about 18 months, there is a sudden surge in vocabulary growth. Rather than learning about one new word a week, the child learns several new words a day. Language abilities change significantly between 18 and 24 months. During this surge, children begin to produce word combinations and to predicate, or describe states and qualities about agent, objects, and events (Bates et al., 1987). Toward the end of this stage, children begin to request information, to bring up topics about events that are remote in place and time, and to maintain a topic for several turns. Thus, they are truly beginning to engage in conversation.

Major socioemotional developmental achievements during this period include the consolidation of attachment relationships (Cicchetti, 1989), the beginning development of greater autonomy and greater differentiation among persons and between self and others (Lewis, 1987), and, toward the end of this period, further development of the ability to self-regulate emotionally by delaying gratification and tolerating frustration (Cicchetti, 1989). Additionally, toddlers become more aware of their own abilities, of goals to achieve, and of how others can be used to help achieve goals.

The achievement of establishing a secure attachment with a primary caregiver provides the young toddler with a secure base from which to explore the environment (Belsky & Nezworski, 1988), and thus have increased interactions with other people and with the inanimate world. The development of an oral language system during this period serves the toddler well,

as he or she becomes able to communicate more effectively at greater distances, without necessarily requiring the caregiver to be in immediate proximity to interpret nonverbal behaviors or to focus close attention on the child for successful communication (MacDonald, 1989). This is also the period in which the balance of power begins to shift, with toddlers taking greater responsibility in initiating and maintaining communicative interactions (Bronfenbrenner, 1979).

Researchers examining early socioemotional development during the second year have focused on the child's development of a sense of self and increased self-awareness (Greenspan, 1988; Lewis, 1987; Stern, 1985). Stern discussed increased capacities available to toddlers in the second year of life. Due to the emergence of language and symbolic communication, children are increasingly able to refer to themselves as external or objective entities. Additionally, increased representational capacities, such as displayed in deferred imitation, allow children to distinguish between their own subjective experience and more objectively observed experience. Interestingly, first words referring to self appear by the end of this period ("I", "me", "mine"), allowing for more explicit self-reference.

Stern (1985) proposed that with emerging language capacities, a child's developing sense of a verbal self allows for new ways of being with others, in that "meaning, in the sense of the linkage between world knowledge (or thought) and words, . . . is something to be negotiated between the parent and the child" (p. 170). Thus, a child's conceptualization and categorization of personal experiences become influenced by negotiated shared meaning based on interactions with significant others. Language serves to foster autonomy through the toddler's ability to communicate more distally, to refer to self, and to state opinions and preferences. It also "is potent in the service of union and togetherness," as "language is a union experience, permitting a new level of mental relatedness through shared meaning" (Stern, 1985, p. 172).

Toward the end of the second year, the emerging capacity to think and communicate about past and future events may serve both to regulate emotional arousal and to create emotional turmoil. On the one hand, a child's increased capacity to anticipate and communicate about distal events allows for a certain level of cognitive and emotional comfort. The reduction of uncertainty in a child's routines, fostered by greater capacities to relate past experiences to current experiences, aids in maintaining emotional homeostasis. In fact, children begin to request information through language about anticipated events and routines at about 22 to 24 months of age (Halliday, 1975). On the other hand, when changes in anticipated events or routines occur, or when goals of the child conflict with desires of the caregiver, emotional turmoil may result. Unfortunately, language is not sufficiently developed to

---

*Language serves to foster autonomy through the toddler's ability to communicate more distally, to refer to self, and to state opinions and preferences.*

---

serve as a medium for resolving most conflicts during this period.

In summary, during toddlerhood, the development of language as a system for communication and for representing experiences internally is viewed as an essential component of a child's developing sense of self and autonomy. Language also becomes a medium for consolidating relationships with others (Lewis, 1987; Stern, 1985).

### Early childhood

By 24 to 36 months of age, children acquire the basics of sentence grammar—morphology, or word organization, and syntax, or sentence organization. Children's first sentences move from a semantic base to sentence grammar with the increase of grammatical knowledge and words and morphemes that serve a grammatical function (Owens, 1988). Children begin to construct more adult-like sentence forms for declaratives, negatives, imperatives, and interrogatives. With continued rapid vocabulary growth, children acquire semantic relational terms to encode concepts such as position, size, internal state, and time. Children also come to understand and use terms for concepts of conditionality and causality. These advances in grammar and semantics, along with social and cognitive growth, contribute to the child's advancing conversational competence.

Achievements in language development involving the more complete and complex expression of ideas and relationships are paralleled by increased capacities for creativity in play, greater differentiation in experience and expression of emotions, and a broadening social network involving development of relationships with peers and others in addition to primary caregivers. As symbolic play capacities become more complex, emotional themes of conflict, autonomy, and relationships may be introduced (Greenspan, 1988). Furthermore, a child's sense of self-esteem, self-image, and self-efficacy develop during this period as young children develop more complex internalizations of relationships with others, begin to view themselves as part of a broader social network, and become more aware of social standards (Cicchetti, 1989; Rutter, 1987b).

During early childhood, children begin to communicate more clearly about feelings, thoughts, and goals (Greenspan, 1988). More specifically, internal state language expands rapidly. This includes expressions of positive and negative emotions from the perspective of self and others (Bretherton & Beeghly, 1982). Emotions become a topic of communication during this period, allowing for a more objectified view of the emotional experience of self and others. Linguistic expression of emotional states allows for both greater differentiation among emotional categories and forces categorization of emotional experience, which creates "a space between interpersonal experience as lived and as represented" (Stern, 1985, p. 182). Lewis (1977) noted that "In providing the child with a means to put his or her feelings into words, language enhances the child's mastery over feelings and allows greater energy for cognitive growth" (p. 659).

During the child's third year, differences have been reported in children raised in emotionally nonsupportive environments. Cicchetti and Beeghly (1987) reported that maltreated children as com-

pared to nonmaltreated controls matched for low socioeconomic status used fewer internal state words and were more context bound in their use of internal state language. Furthermore, based on maternal report, they found that the maltreated youngsters attributed internal states to fewer social agents when compared with reports of nonmaltreating mothers. Again, these findings point to distortions at the interface of communication and socioemotional development for children raised in high-risk situations.

A child's development of self-esteem, self-efficacy, and self-image is greatly affected by his or her expanding social network and competence in play with other children in early childhood (Cicchetti, 1989; Lewis, 1987). As play becomes a primary medium for development of peer relationships, language and internal representational capacities exert a significant influence on the development of relationships with peers. Children who are able to use language effectively in early childhood to engage in and regulate play interactions with others are able to develop a sense of efficacy and pride relative to their role in peer groups and social networks. Effective use of language also allows for the development of emotional bonding and the capacity for empathy with peers. The important role that language and communication development plays in the development of peer relationships is underscored by the fact that children with language impairment tend to initiate interaction less and to have greater problems establishing positive relationships with peers (Howlin & Rutter, 1987).

Other socioemotional capacities that appear to be closely related to language and communication development during the third year involve children's ability to plan for desirable outcomes in activities, to delay gratification, to control impulses, and thus to self-regulate emotionally to a greater extent than in earlier periods (Greenspan & Porges, 1984). Language becomes a tool for communication about more distant events in time and also for discussing circumstances of conditionality and causality. Thus, language becomes a tool for helping children understand why they may not be able to accomplish ends that they desire and why needs and desires may not be able to be fulfilled immediately, but may be fulfilled at later points in time. The growing capacities for children to obtain information about distant events or about why needs or desires may not be fulfilled aids in emotional regulation toward the end of this period (Cicchetti, 1989).

## DEVELOPMENT IN AT-RISK OR DISABLED CHILDREN

The close relationship between socioemotional development and communication and language development has great implications for children who are biologically and environmentally at risk for communication disorders and emotional and behavioral disorders. It has been demonstrated that childhood disabilities, including communication disorders, have a significant impact on the way caregivers or others interact with the affected child (MacDonald, 1989). Howlin and Rutter (1987) noted that "the failure to develop normal language skills may well have a detrimental affect on parent–child interactions" (p. 287). From the perspective of emotional communication, Greenspan (1988) noted that infants and young children with disabilities

may have difficulties returning their caregivers' wooing and may communicate emotionally in ways that are confusing rather than clear. Caregiver feelings of rejection, anger, or confusion are to be expected and must be understood and responded to in order for caregivers to remain engaged with and emotionally available to their children (p. 15).

These difficulties may place the child with a communication impairment at a greater risk for the development of emotional difficulties.

Howlin and Rutter (1987) added that difficulties in social relationships are strongly predictive of later emotional disturbance, and, as noted, communicatively impaired children have been found to experience such difficulties. A communication impairment may evoke disturbed patterns of interaction, which may then exacerbate the communication difficulties and increase psychosocial stress on the child and family. Thus, in more extreme cases, children experiencing early communication impairments must be considered to be at double risk, because the effects of emotionally stressful environments (i.e., abusive or neglectful environments) on young children may include secondary language and communication delays.

•  •  •

Current attempts to integrate perspectives of socioemotional development and language and communication development remain somewhat speculative. It is likely that investigations with normally developing children, at-risk children, and children with communication and socioemotional disturbances will yield greater insight into the relationships between communication development and socioemotional development. For professionals who work with children with communication disorders and emotional and behavioral disorders, this emerging knowledge will provide a preliminary basis for considering the significant mutual impact and interdependence between these aspects of development.

## REFERENCES

Adamson, L., & Bakeman, R. (1985). Affect and attention: Infants observed with mothers and peers. *Child Development, 56,* 582–593.

Baker, L., & Cantwell, D. (1987). Factors associated with the development of psychiatric illness in children with early speech/language problems. *Journal of Autism and Developmental Disorders, 17,* 499–510.

Bates, E. (1979). *The emergence of symbols: Cognition and communication in infancy.* New York, NY: Academic Press.

Bates, E., O'Connell, B., & Shore, C. (1987). Language and communication in infancy. In J. Osofsky (Ed.), *Handbook of infant development (2nd ed.).* New York, NY: Wiley.

Belsky, J., & Nezworski, T. (Eds.). (1988). *Clinical implications of attachment.* Hillsdale, NJ: Erlbaum.

Bloom, L. (1987). Developments in expression: Affect and speech. In N. Stein (Ed.), *The psychological and biological development of the emotions.* Hillsdale, NJ: Erlbaum.

Blount, B. (1982). The ontogeny of emotions and their vocal expression in infants. In S. Kuczaj (Ed.), *Language development: Vol. 2. Language, thought, and culture.* Hillsdale, NJ: Erlbaum.

Brazelton, T.B. (1982). Joint regulation of neonate–parent behavior. In E. Tronick (Ed.), *Social interchange in infancy.* Baltimore, MD: University Park Press.

Bretherton, I., & Beeghly, M. (1982). Talking about internal states: The acquisition of an explicit theory of mind. *Developmental Psychology, 18,* 906–921.

Bronfenbrenner, U. (1979). *The ecology of human development.* Cambridge, MA: Harvard University Press.

Bruner, J. (1981). The social context of language acquisition. *Language and Communication, 1,* 155–178.

Campos, J., Barrett, K., Lamb, M., Goldsmith, H., & Sternberg, C. (1983). Socioemotional development. In P.H. Mussen (Ed.), *Handbook of child psychology: Vol. 2. Infancy and developmental psychology.* New York, NY: Wiley.

Cicchetti, D. (1984). The emergence of developmental psychopathology. *Child Development, 55,* 1–7.

Cicchetti, D. (1989). How research on child maltreatment has informed the study of child development: Perspectives from developmental psychopathology. In D. Cicchetti & V. Carlson (Eds.), *Child maltreatment: Theory and research on causes and consequences of child abuse and neglect.* New York, NY: Cambridge University Press.

Cicchetti, D., & Beeghly, M. (1987). Symbolic development in maltreated youngsters: An organizational perspective. In D. Cicchetti & M. Beeghly (Eds.), *Atypical symbolic development.* San Francisco, CA: Jossey-Bass.

Dore, J. (1986). The development of conversational competence. In R. Scheifelbusch (Ed.), *Language competence: Assessment and intervention.* San Diego, CA: College Hill Press.

Dunst, C., & Lowe, L. (1986). From reflex to symbol: Describing, explaining, and fostering communicative competence. *Augmentative and Alternative Communication, 2,* 11–18.

Dunst, C., Lowe, L., & Bartholomew, P. (1990). Contingent social responsiveness, family ecology and infant communicative competence. *National Student Speech, Language and Hearing Association Journal, 17,* 39–49.

Early intervention program for infants and toddlers with handicaps: Final regulations. (1989). *Federal Register, 54,* 26306–26348.

Goldberg, S. (1977). Social competence in infancy: A model of parent–infant interaction. *Merrill-Palmer Quarterly, 23,* 163–177.

Greenspan, S. (1988). Fostering emotional and social development in infants with disabilities. *Zero to Three, 8,* 8–18.

Greenspan, S., & Porges, S. (1984). Psychopathology in infancy and early childhood: Clinical perspectives on the organization of sensory and affective-thematic experience. *Child development, 55,* 49–70.

Halliday, M.A.K. (1975). *Learning how to mean.* New York, NY: Elsevier.

Howlin, P., & Rutter, M. (1987). The consequences of language delay for other aspects of development. In W.

Yule & M. Rutter (Eds.), *Language development and language disorders*. Philadelphia, PA: Lippincott.

Kuczaj, S., & Bean, A. (1982). The development of noncommunicative speech systems. In S. Kuczaj (Ed.), *Language development: Vol. 2. Language, thought, and culture*. Hillsdale, NJ: Erlbaum.

Lewis, M. (1977). Language, cognitive development, and personality. *Journal of the American Academy of Child Psychiatry, 16,* 646–661.

Lewis, M. (1987). Social development in infancy and early childhood. In J. Osofsky (Ed.), *Handbook of infant development* (2nd ed.). New York, NY: Wiley.

Luria, A.R. (1961). *The role of speech in the regulation of normal and abnormal behavior*. London, England: Pergamon Press.

Maccoby, E., & Martin, J. (1983). Socialization in the context of the family: Parent–child interaction. In P.H. Mussen (Ed.), *Handbook of child psychology: Vol. 4. Socialization, personality and social development*. New York, NY: Wiley.

MacDonald, J. (1989). *Becoming partners with children: From play to conversation*. San Antonio, TX: Special Press.

Owens, R. (1988). *Language development: An introduction* (2nd ed.). Columbus, OH: Merrill Publishing Company.

Prizant, B.M., Audet, L., Burke, G., Hummel, L., Maher, S., & Theadore, G. (1990). Communication disorders and emotional/behavioral disorders in children. *Journal of Speech and Hearing Disorders, 55,* 179–192.

Rutter, M. (1987a). Continuities and discontinuities from infancy. In J. Osofsky (Ed.), *The handbook of infant development* (2nd ed.). New York, NY: Wiley.

Rutter, M. (1987b). The role of cognition in child development and disorder. *British Journal of Medical Psychology, 60,* 1–16.

Sameroff, A. (1987). The social context of development. In N. Eisenburg (Ed.), *Contemporary topics in development*. New York, NY: Wiley.

Sameroff, A., & Chandler, M. (1975). Reproductive risk and the continuum of caretaking causality. In F. Horowitz (Ed.), *Review of child development research* (Vol. 4). Chicago, IL: University of Chicago Press.

Sameroff, A., & Fiese, B. (1990). Transactional regulation and early intervention. In S. Meisels & J. Shonkoff (Eds.), *Early Intervention: A handbook of theory, practice, and analysis*. New York, NY: Cambridge University Press.

Sroufe, L., & Rutter, M. (1984). The domain of developmental psychopathology. *Child Development, 55,* 1184–1199.

Stern, D. (1985). *The interpersonal world of the infant*. New York, NY: Basic Books.

Tronick, E. (1980). Infant communicative intent. In A. Reilly (Ed.), *The communication game: Perspectives on the development of speech, language, and nonverbal communication skills*. Baltimore, MD: Johnson & Johnson Pediatric Roundtable Series.

Tronick, E. (1989). Emotions and emotional communication in infants. *American Psychologist, 44,* 112–119.

Vohr, B., & Garcia-Coll, C. (1988). Follow-up studies of high-risk low-birthweight infant. In H. Fitzgerald, B. Lester, & M. Yogman (Eds.), *Theory and research in behavioral pediatrics* (Vol. 4). New York, NY: Plenum Press.

Vygotsky, L.S. (1976). Play and its role in the mental development of the child. In J.S. Bruner, A. Jolly, & K. Sylva (Eds.), *Play: Its role in development and evaluation*. New York, NY: Basic Books. (Original work published 1933)

Wetherby, A., Cain, D., Yonclas, D., & Walker, V. (1988). Analysis of intentional communication of normal children from the prelinguistic to the multi-word stage. *Journal of Speech and Hearing Research, 31,* 240–252.

# Delivering communication-based services to infants, toddlers, and their families: Approaches and models

**M. Jeanne Wilcox, PhD**
*Associate Professor*
*School of Speech Pathology and*
  *Audiology*
*Kent State University*
*Kent, Ohio*

ALTHOUGH the vast majority of young children will successfully acquire effective communication skills, some children are at risk for less successful development and others will demonstrate delays or disorders in the acquisition of communication abilities. The critical importance of early communication intervention for these latter children is well established by research concluding that children who demonstrate early communication delays or disorders do not simply outgrow these difficulties. Often their communication problems persist and are related to subsequent academic and social difficulties or deficits (Aram, Ekelman, & Nation, 1984; Aram & Nation, 1980; Hall & Tomblin, 1978; Wallach & Butler, 1984). In addition to this relationship between early and later disabilities, a child's failure to acquire a functional and appropriate communication system is acknowledged as a significant barrier to educational programming within the least restrictive environment, and as a factor that can exert a

*Top Lang Disord*, 1989,10(1),68–79
© 1989 Aspen Publishers, Inc.

strong influence over the course of an individual's entire life (Warren & Kaiser, 1988). In recognition of these facts as well as of recent federal legislative changes (e.g., Public Law 99-457) speech–language pathologists (SLPs) have become increasingly involved in the delivery of communication-based services to infants and toddlers with disabilities and to those who are regarded as being at risk for developing disabilities.

As professionals become more involved in providing services to infants and toddlers, they assume expanded, and in many cases new, professional roles (Campbell & Dunn, 1988; Wilcox, Bashir, Iglesias, Liebergott, & Snyder-McClean, 1989) while also learning to implement new service delivery approaches (Campbell, in press). The primary purpose of this article is to provide an organizational framework for communication-based interventions within the broader context of early intervention by considering various approaches and service delivery models.

# EARLY INTERVENTION APPROACHES

Various approaches have been used to provide services to young children and their families, and they can be classified according to three basic orientations: remediation, prevention, and compensation. These approaches are not new to early intervention, nor are they mutually exclusive. In fact, although the approaches are sometimes used singly, they are most often used in combination. Typically a particular approach is selected in accordance with the point at which a child may be identified as requiring services, with the

degree of disability or developmental delay that is present, and with the intervention goals for a given child.

## Remediation

Most early intervention personnel, including speech–language pathologists, frequently rely on a remedial approach in the design and provision of their services. The goals of remedial approaches usually include improvement of functioning in the delayed or disordered areas that are identified. A child's development is first evaluated with respect to age-appropriate skills; areas of delay or disorder are then determined, and a plan for intervention is formulated and implemented by the professional(s) possessing expertise in the identified deficit areas. For example, a child who demonstrates delays in the acquisition of speech, language, and motor abilities would probably receive the services of a motor therapist (e.g., physical therapist, occupational therapist) and a SLP.

Outcomes of remedial approaches are typically conceptualized in terms of eradication or mitigation. For example, in the case of some early communication disorders (e.g., phonological) remedial efforts often eradicate the diagnosed condition. In other instances, eradication of the deficit may not be possible; however, early intervention efforts may serve to mitigate or prevent longer term effects of a diagnosed problem, and in this sense remedial interventions may have a preventive component.

In remedial approaches, children are eligible for enrollment in early intervention programs from the point of diagnosis of a problem. Optimally, children manifesting developmental delays or disorders are identified during infancy on the basis of medical and biological risk factors. However, early identification of infants with conclusive developmental disorders is a difficult process (Freeman, 1985; Thoman & Becker, 1979; Vietze & Vaughan, 1988). Infants with similar medical difficulties at birth or in the neonatal period, when evaluated as individuals, may demonstrate significantly different behavioral and functional outcomes, although trends toward disability may be projected for the group of infants as a whole.

Because conclusive early identification is difficult, some limitations are imposed on the impact of early intervention instituted from a remedial perspective, particularly for infants and toddlers who are regarded as being at risk. Remedial interventions are provided for the purpose of improving a deficit condition; therefore, children with *diagnosed* delays or disorders are those who receive such intervention services. Children who are considered to be at-risk (i.e., they may develop a problem but have not yet been diagnosed as having one) are not eligible for services provided from a remedial perspective because there is as yet no deficit to eradicate or mitigate. Hence, within remedial approaches, services eligibility is tied to diagnosed conditions. Unfortunately, reliance on formal diagnostic criteria means that by the time a delay or disorder in a single developmental domain is identified it may already have affected other domains, thereby extending the original dysfunction and creating secondary areas of difficulty (Beckman-Bell, 1981). For most developmental skill areas, and particularly for communication, diagnoses of delays or disorders are difficult to make prior to 18

months of age, and even then may not be easy. For example, a 26-month-old child who has not yet begun to use words can readily be diagnosed as in need of the services of a language–communication specialist, but a 17-month-old child who has not yet begun to use words poses a much more difficult case. Although professionals might agree that the latter child is mildly delayed or at risk, they are more likely to recommend reevaluation after six months than intervention. If at the time of reevaluation the child has still not begun to use words, intervention will probably be recommended; however, by this time it is likely that the child has developed additional difficulties in other skill areas that are heavily dependent on or related to communication, such as self-help and social interaction skills.

Another parameter that influences the impact of remedial approaches pertains to programming goals and activities. Remedial programs are typically designed on the basis of age-appropriate skills that a child has not yet mastered. Given this basis, it is important that program goals and procedures focus on the use of skills in functional activities rather than on skills per se. For example, a 24-month-old child who is not producing words requires programming that includes development of a core vocabulary; remedial language intervention efforts would appropriately focus on training an initial lexicon. However, in addition to learning the referential use of specific lexical items, it is essential that a child learn to use the lexicon to convey various meanings (e.g., to request, comment, greet, protest) in typical interpersonal interactions with family members.

The empirical database of remedial approaches to early intervention has received a substantial amount of investigative attention. Extensive reviews have been conducted of the effectiveness of early intervention for children with cognitive and general delays, motor handicaps, language and communication disorders, autism, visual impairments, and hearing impairments (Guralnick & Bennett, 1987). Although data on the efficacy of remedial approaches across all developmental areas conflict and have been confounded by problems with outcome measures as well as other aspects of experimental design (Bennett, 1987; Dunst, 1986; Guralnick & Bricker, 1987; Snyder-McClean & McClean, 1987), early remedial interventions in many areas have been associated with positive developmental gains, at least for children with mild or moderate delays. Less positively, early remedial interventions have been associated with only limited improvements in children with more severe handicaps (Bricker & Dow, 1980; Guralnick & Bricker, 1987; Solomon, Wilson, & Galey, 1982). Moreover, remedial interventions by their nature are focused on improving deficit conditions. This orientation has been found to influence a child's family adversely, in that they tend to dwell on what is "wrong" with the child, an attitude that has been cited as contributing significantly to overall family stress (Turnbull & Turnbull, 1986).

## Prevention

Prevention, as an intervention approach for infants that is independent of remedial interventions, represents a relatively new focus in service delivery, although, as was noted previously, remedial approaches do often serve a preventive function. This orientation is based on the premise that in the course of development there are alterable and unalterable factors. *Unalterable* factors may include biological conditions that cannot be modified, such as brain damage (including that resulting in primary motor and sensory deficits), chromosomal abnormalities, and certain genetic disorders. These unalterable factors may or may not cause various developmental problems, which are regarded as *alterable* factors and include functional communication, sensorimotor, psychosocial, cognitive, and self-help abilities.

Early preventive intervention can assist children with primary deficits in hearing, many of whom demonstrate wide variability in their functional speech and hearing abilities. It has long been recognized that the degree of primary auditory impairment is only one factor influencing functional communication outcomes for this population. Equally, if not more important, are such variables as early identification, early programming, and the availability of assistive devices. Similar effects have been noted for children with primary vision and motor deficits; that is, the degree of deficit is only one factor contributing to functional outcomes (Campbell, 1984; Fraiberg, 1974; Wilcox & Campbell, in press; Wolff, 1982).

As is true with remedial approaches, the early identification of children and their families who are in need of preventive services is critical. However, the criteria for services eligibility in a preventive approach is expanded to include the at-risk population, and so children and their families are eligible for services prior to the diagnosis of a specific developmental prob-

---

*As is true with remedial approaches, the early identification of children and their families who are in need of preventive services is critical.*

---

lem. Hence, early interventionists have the opportunity to prevent the emergence of various alterable or secondary problems and/or to alleviate the effects of a given biological condition across various developmental areas.

Ideally, children who are likely to manifest developmental problems are identified during infancy and receive appropriate preventive programming. However, conflicting data regarding developmental outcomes of at-risk children serve to limit services. Clearly it is not feasible to provide services to all children who are classified as at risk. Therefore, the key issue in delivering preventive services during infancy becomes one of determining those children who are most likely to encounter developmental difficulties and, from the perspective of the SLP, those who are most likely to have problems in the development of communication and language skills or prerequisite oral–motor behavior. In the process of identification, criteria must be developed based on levels of risk as well as the interaction of risk factors. As a rule, the more risk factors that are associated with a given child and his or her family, the greater the adversity for a normal developmental course.

Typically risk factors are categorized as established, biological, or environmental (Liebergott, Bashir, & Schultz, 1984; Ramey, Trohanis, & Hostler, 1982; Tjossem, 1976). *Established* risk factors include diagnosed medical conditions that are known to have an adverse effect on developmental outcome (e.g., Down syndrome, hearing impairment). *Biological* factors include conditions (e.g., very low birth weight, fetal alcohol syndrome, severe asphyxia, grade III or IV brain hemorrhages) that, either singly or in combination, may result in developmental difficulties. *Environmental* factors include psychosocial, familial, and other ecological conditions that may inhibit or interfere with normal developmental progression (e.g., adolescent mothers, parents who are substance abusers, parents with emotional or other mental disturbances).

Given the nature of preventive approaches, interventionists may initially offer services to infants who appear to be developing normally. For example, infants with Down syndrome may demonstrate relatively normal development during the first few months of life. However, such infants are prime candidates for preventive approaches because previous observations of this population indicate that such children eventually demonstrate disabilities/delays in speech, language, and cognition (Stoel-Gammon, 1981). Similarly, full-term infants who survive severe birth asphyxia are likely to manifest a variety of developmental problems, such as spastic quadriplegia, severe mental retardation, optic nerve atrophy, seizures, and hearing impairment (Brann, 1985). Because diagnosis of these conditions may be difficult during the first few months of life, such infants may also seem relatively normal. As a final example, infants delivered between 24 and 28 weeks of gestational age, with very low birth weight (i.e., less than 800 grams) are highly likely to develop significant neuromotor, speech, language, and cognitive problems, although the earliest clinical diagnosis is not likely to be made until around 6 to 12 months (corrected age) for neuromotor difficulties and even later for speech, language, and cognitive difficulties (Bennett, Chandler, Robinson, & Sells, 1981; Ensher & Clark, 1986; Fitzhardinge & Pape, 1981; Nickel, Bennett, & Lamson, 1982; Parmelee, 1981).

Clearly the focus and goals of preventive intervention are quite different from those of the more familiar remedial approaches, of which the primary goal is improvement of functioning in deficit areas. The goals of preventive approaches, in contrast, are focused on facilitating or ensuring acquisition of functional skills in "suspect" areas, with particular consideration given to the fact that one skill deficit is likely to affect other skill areas. For example, consider an infant who has survived severe birth asphyxia and is thus regarded as being at risk for a cluster of developmental disabilities, including primary (e.g., visual, hearing, motor) and secondary (e.g., communicative, linguistic, cognitive) deficits. The infant may demonstrate abnormalities in muscle tone as well as highly variable patterns of motor behavior. Severe abnormalities in muscle tone may present subsequent barriers to the infant's acquisition of motor skills (e.g., sitting, reaching), while also contributing to variability in motoric abilities (Hanson & Harris, 1987). This response variability may in turn create difficulties for consistent and contingent caregiver responses to the infant's behavioral cues. Consistent and contingent caregiver responses are important to communication

and cognition because the opportunity is established for an infant to associate his or her behavior with specific meanings and predictable environmental effects (Bricker & Schiefelbusch, 1984; MacDonald & Gillette, 1986; Wilcox & Terrell, 1985). As can be seen, it is essential to consider the interactive effects of intervention across developmental domains.

Preventive intervention activities that are provided after the diagnosis of an impairment are designed to mitigate the impact of an impairment by assisting a family and their child in the development of strategies to permit a child's participation in appropriate home, school, and community activities. When designing such strategies it is critical that clinicians and teachers examine potential barriers to participation in a broad spectrum of environmental activities. Thus early intervention personnel must focus not only on present conditions surrounding an impairment but also on future difficulties that may be encountered. In order to achieve this goal, observations and evaluations of child behavior must be supplemented by perceived difficulties from the family's perspective. For example, a 2-year-old child who has not yet begun to use words is clearly a child with a communication impairment. Although this child may be participating in typical activities (e.g., play with other 2-year-olds), it is relatively easy to see how failure to acquire language will eventually create barriers to participation. If a program were designed strictly from a remedial perspective, its primary focus would be the acquisition and use of an initial lexicon. However, from a preventive perspective the goal would be expanded to include not only initial lexical training but an examination of the child's ability to convey meaning in any manner and, if necessary, provision of strategies to facilitate his or her communication of meaning in interpersonal settings while learning the language system.

Preventive intervention provided to children with an existing disability is designed to prevent the condition from becoming a handicap, which is defined as the societal disadvantage experienced by the individual with a disability (Beukelman, 1986). The degree of handicap is largely dependent on the attitudes and beliefs of persons in the environments of the individual with a disability. In its more severe form, a handicap results in exclusion from participation in some or all home, school, or community activities. Preventive programming that is instituted for the purpose of inhibiting the onset of a handicap is similar to that designed to inhibit the onset of a disability. The difference is primarily a matter of degree. Children with disabilities have already encountered barriers to participation in environmental activities. As a result of these barriers, such children are at risk for exclusion from various age-appropriate activities. Programming goals, which must be both child-based and environmentally based, can be identified only after a careful analysis of a child's abilities in the context of the various relevant environments.

The effectiveness of preventive approaches for the established risk population has a strong empirical database, although it should be acknowledged that most studies have been conducted with children with Down syndrome. For this population it is relatively clear that early intervention does have the effect of at least

moderating declines in cognitive and communicative abilities (Berry, Gunn, & Andrews, 1984; Clunies-Ross, 1979; Reed, Pueschel, Schnell, & Cronk, 1980). With the exception of infants who demonstrate identifiable primary deficits (e.g., sensory or motor), the effectiveness of early preventive approaches for children regarded as being at risk due to biological and environmental reasons, in terms of specific developmental skill acquisition, is largely unknown at this time, perhaps because preventive intervention is a relatively new option for this population. The bulk of research that can be classified as examining or supporting preventive intervention comes from studies of interventions provided to families and infants regarded as being either environmentally or biologically at risk. Extensive reviews of such research can be found in Bryant and Ramey (1987) and Bennett (1987). As might be expected, efficacy data conflict and are confounded by numerous experimental variables (e.g., subject variation, intensity of interventions, lack of appropriate control groups). However, the following positive conclusions can be drawn: (1) early intervention for at-risk children does prevent or slow a decline from normal development; (2) child-based and family-based services are critical to the effectiveness of early preventive intervention.

What is obviously lacking in research focusing on intervention for the at-risk population is information regarding effects on specific developmental abilities. For example, consider two infants who are at risk for normal acquisition of communication skills for identical biological reasons (e.g., severe asphyxia). If preventive intervention is implemented for one of these infants and focuses on enhancing the acquisition of prelinguistic skills, will the infant who receives preventive programming demonstrate a more positive course of development than the infant who does not? There is no doubt that a strong philosophical rationale can be adduced in support of preventive efforts with at-risk children and their families. Furthermore, efficacy has been established in terms of general enhancement of development. The next step toward the delivery of the best possible preventive services must be a systematic examination of the effects of preventive intervention on specific developmental outcomes.

### Compensatory approaches

Some developmental delays or dysfunctions cannot be substantially improved, regardless of how early intervention begins or which approach is used. In such instances, services are implemented in order to compensate for the degree of disability that is present. For example, some children may never acquire sufficient control of the oral–motor system to communicate functionally using speech. However, these children can learn to communicate effectively through compensatory strategies or devices. Compensatory efforts include the provision of devices and strategies (e.g., hearing aids, augmentative communication systems, prostheses, switches) that are designed to improve such functional abilities as movement, hearing, and communication. Appropriate use of compensatory programming can prevent an impairment from becoming a disability, or prevent a disability from becoming a significant handicap. Compensatory programming approaches may have

a dual focus. Some approaches are child-based, in that devices and strategies are provided directly for a child. Other approaches are environmental and include modifications in both the physical domain (e.g., provision of tables at a height appropriate for a wheelchair) and the interpersonal domain (e.g., talking face to face and close to a child with a hearing impairment).

### SELECTING THE PROGRAMMATIC APPROACH

It should be apparent that remedial, preventive, and compensatory approaches overlap and that they share the overriding goal of improving developmental outcomes. However, each approach offers a unique perspective regarding the processes that will facilitate a positive developmental outcome. Because the programming approaches are not mutually exclusive, they are used most often in combination. The selection of a particular approach is typically dependent on (1) the point at which a child is enrolled in an early intervention program; (2) the type and degree of developmental difficulty that a child is experiencing; and (3) the intervention goals for a particular child. Prevention is the primary service option prior to the actual identification of an impairment. However, after an impairment or a disability has been identified, any one or all of the service approaches may be appropriate. Once a child demonstrates a clear deficit, intervention efforts are most likely to be implemented with the goal of reversing the condition, if possible, through either remedial or compensatory activities.

## SERVICE DELIVERY MODELS

Determining the model that will be used to deliver services to families and their children is as important as selection of the programmatic approach. The term "model" refers to the general structure that will govern the delivery of services. At the most global level, service delivery models can be conceptualized as those in which professionals independently provide services or as those in which the provision of services involves some formal mechanism for interprofessional collaboration (Campbell, 1987; Campbell & Dunn, 1988; Campbell, Stremel-Campbell, & Rogers-Warren, 1985). In the independent model, although interprofessional communication is certainly not precluded, there is no formal mechanism for interaction; professionals provide services relative to their respective areas of expertise. Although this model is commonly used in many areas of service provision to children with disabilities, it can present particular difficulties for the families of infants and toddlers. First, the lack of a formal mechanism for interprofessional cooperation tends to contribute to fragmented services and poor coordination among professionals, thereby creating significant problems for families (Bray, Coleman, & Brackman, 1981). Next, because the interrelatedness of early developmental skills makes it difficult for a single professional to provide intervention without affecting other developmental areas, professionals may inadvertently negate one another's efforts. Finally, the interrelatedness of early developmental skills means that no single discipline can "lay claim" to infant/toddler intervention. In order to provide the best

services, therefore, some sort of interprofessional team effort is required.

The major types of team or collaborative service models include multidisciplinary, transdisciplinary, and interdisciplinary models. In a multidisciplinary model, professionals from various disciplines independently assess and provide services but have a formal mechanism for communication. For example, a SLP, an early childhood special educator, and a physical therapist may each conduct an assessment of a given child and his or her family. These professionals would then convene and share their findings and programming plans. In this way an overall plan is defined, and individual professionals may modify their plans accordingly.

A transdisciplinary model includes cooperative assessment and intervention that may include the concept of role release (Lyon & Lyon, 1980), which involves a commitment to cross disciplinary boundaries and to share roles and responsibilities that may be traditionally associated with a single discipline. Within this model the function of an early intervention professional may be altered from that of direct service provider to that of a consultant, or indirect provider. Indirect service providers identify children's programming needs, design intervention programs, and train others (e.g., other early intervention personnel, parents, day care personnel, preschool teachers) to carry out those programs.

The interdisciplinary model falls somewhere between the other team models. The collaborative commitment is stronger than that associated with the multidisciplinary model but does not typically include the role release associated with the transdisciplinary model. As members of an interdisciplinary team, professionals typically conduct individual assessments and then convene to identify joint intervention goals and create intervention strategies.

No single team model is ideally suited to delivering services to families and their infants and toddlers. Different models are appropriate in accordance with different conditions. For example, although the interdisciplinary model appears to be the most compatible with the focus of Public Law 99-457, it may not be the most compatible with identified family needs, or its implementation may not be possible in certain geographically isolated areas. Ultimately team structures must be designed to ensure maximum flexibility in professional representation. Professionals from many disciplines, including speech–language pathology, audiology, early childhood special education, physical and occupational therapy, developmental psychology, developmental nursing, nutrition, and others may have a role to play on the team. Team membership must be defined in response to individual child and family needs, because no set composition formula can be regarded as suitable for all

children and families who might benefit from early intervention services.

•  •  •

The acquisition of communication skills represents one of the most important developmental tasks that children must accomplish. Failure to acquire appropriate and effective communication skills has lifelong effects. Early identification and programming are essential for children who may or do encounter difficulties in the acquisition of communication abilities. Given the central role of communication and the interrelatedness of developmental abilities during the first years of life, discussions of early communication-based programming cannot be conducted independent of early intervention in general. The most appropriate model for delivery of early intervention services is that which includes a programming team. Each of the identified programming approaches (i.e., prevention, remediation, compensation) have advantages and limitations. Early intervention personnel should be well versed in each of the approaches and make decisions in accordance with the needs of individual infants, toddlers, and families.

## REFERENCES

Aram, D., Ekelman, B., & Nation, J. (1984). Preschoolers with language disorders: 10 years later. *Journal of Speech and Hearing Research, 27*, 232–244.

Aram, D., & Nation, J. (1980). Preschool language disorders and subsequent language and academic difficulties. *Journal of Communication Disorders, 13*, 159–170.

Beckman-Bell, P. (1981). Child-related stress in families of handicapped children. *Topics in Early Childhood Special Education, 1*, 45–54.

Bennett, F. (1987). The effectiveness of early intervention for infants at increased biologic risk. In M. Guralnick &

F. Bennett (Eds.), *The effectiveness of early intervention for at-risk and handicapped children* (pp. 79–114). New York: Academic Press.

Bennett, F., Chandler, L., Robinson, N., & Sells, C. (1981). Spastic diplegia in premature infants. *American Journal of Diseases of Children, 135*, 732–737.

Berry, P., Gunn, V., & Andrews, R. (1984). Development of Down's syndrome children from birth to five years. In J. Berg (Ed.), *Perspectives and progress in mental retardation: Vol. 1. Social, psychological, and educational aspects* (pp. 167–177). Baltimore: University Park Press.

Beukelman, D. (1986). Evaluating the effectiveness of intervention programs. In S. Blackstone (Ed.), *Augmentative communication: An introduction* (pp. 423–446). Rockville, MD: American Speech–Language–Hearing Association.

Brann, A.W. (1985). Factors during neonatal life that influence brain disorders. In J.M. Freeman (Ed.), *Prenatal and perinatal factors associated with brain disorders* (pp. 263–358). Washington, DC: U.S. Department of Health and Human Services. (NIH Publication No. 85-1149).

Bray, N., Coleman, J., & Brackman, M. (1981). Critical events in parenting handicapped children. *Journal of the Division for Early Childhood, 3,* 26–33.

Bricker, D.D., & Dow, M.G. (1980). Early intervention with the young severely handicapped child. *Journal of the Association for Persons with Severe Handicaps,* 5(2), 130–142.

Bricker, D., & Schiefelbusch, D. (1984). Infants at risk. In L. McCormick & R. Schiefelbusch (Eds.), *Early language intervention* (pp. 243–266). Columbus, OH: Charles E. Merrill.

Bryant, D., & Ramey, C. (1987). An analysis of the effectiveness of early intervention programs for environmentally at-risk children. In M. Guralnick & F. Bennett (Eds.), *The effectiveness of early intervention for at-risk and handicapped children* (pp. 33–78). New York: Academic Press.

Campbell, P. (In press). Service delivery approaches for infants and toddlers. In M. Wilcox & P. Campbell (Eds.), *Communication programming from birth to three.* Boston: Little, Brown.

Campbell, P. (1987). The integrated programming team: An approach for coordinating professionals of various disciplines in programs for students with severe and multiple handicaps. *Journal of the Association for Persons with Severe Handicaps, 12,* 85–92.

Campbell, P., & Dunn, W. (1988, December). The role of integrated therapy in programs for young children. Paper presented at the annual meeting of the Association for Persons with Severe Handicaps, Washington, DC.

Campbell, S. (1984). *Pediatric neurologic physical therapy: Vol. 5.* New York: Churchill Livingston.

Campbell, R., Stremel-Campbell, K., & Rogers-Warren, A. (1985). Programming teacher support for functional language. In S. Warren & A. Rogers-Warren (Eds.), *Teaching functional language* (pp. 309–340). Baltimore: University Park Press.

Clunies-Ross, G. (1979). Accelerating the development of Down's syndrome infants and young children. *The Journal of Special Education, 13,* 169–177.

Dunst, C. (1986). Overview of the efficacy of early intervention programs. In L. Bickman & D. Weatherford (Eds.), *Evaluating early intervention programs for severely handicapped children and their families* (pp. 79–148). Austin, TX: Pro-Ed.

Ensher, G., & Clark, D. (1986). *Newborns at risk: Medical care and psychoeducational intervention.* Rockville, MD: Aspen Publishers.

Fitzhardinge, P., & Pape, K. (1981). Follow-up studies of the high risk newborn. In G. Avery (Ed.), *Neonatology: Pathophysiology and management of the newborn* (2nd ed., pp. 350–367). Philadelphia: J.B. Lippincott.

Fraiberg, S. (1974). *Insights from the blind: Comparative studies of blind and sighted infants.* New York: Basic Books.

Freeman, J.M. (Ed.). (1985). *Prenatal and perinatal factors associated with brain disorders.* Washington, DC: U.S. Department of Health and Human Services: NIH Publication No. 85-1149.

Guralnick, M., & Bennett, F. (Eds.). (1987). *The effectiveness of early intervention for at-risk and handicapped children.* New York: Academic Press.

Guralnick, M., & Bricker, D. (1987). The effectiveness of early intervention for children with cognitive and general developmental delays. In M. Guralnick & F. Bennett (Eds.), *The effectiveness of early intervention for at-risk and handicapped children* (pp. 115–174). New York: Academic Press.

Hall, P., & Tomblin, B. (1978). A follow-up study of children with articulation and language disorders. *Journal of Speech and Hearing Research, 43,* 227–242.

Hanson, M. (1982). Issues in designing intervention approaches from developmental theory and research. In D. Bricker (Ed.), *Intervention with at-risk handicapped infants: From research to application* (pp. 249–268). Baltimore: University Park Press.

Hanson, M., & Harris, S. (1987). *Teaching the young child with motor delays.* Austin, TX: Pro-Ed.

Liebergott, J., Bashir, A., & Schultz, M. (1984). Dancing around and making strange noises: Children at-risk. In A. Holland (Ed.), *Language disorders in children* (pp. 37–58). San Diego: College-Hill Press.

Lyon, S., & Lyon, G. (1980). Team functioning and staff development: A role release approach to providing integrated educational services for severely handicapped students. *Journal of the Association for Persons with Severe Handicaps, 5,* 250–263.

MacDonald, J., & Gillette, Y. (1986). Communicating with persons with severe handicaps: Roles of parents and professionals. *Journal of the Association for Persons with Severe Handicaps, 11,* 255–265.

Nickel, R., Bennett, F., & Lamson, F. (1982). School performance of children with birth weights of 1,000 grams or less. *American Journal of Diseases of Children, 136,* 105–110.

Parmelee, A., Jr. (1981). Auditory function and neurological maturation in preterm infants. In S. Friedman & M. Sigman (Eds.), *Preterm birth and psychological development* (pp. 127–155). New York: Academic Press.

Ramey, C., Trohanis, P., & Hostler, S. (1982). An introduction. In C. Ramey & P. Trohanis (Eds.), *Finding and educating high-risk and handicapped infants* (pp. 1–13). Baltimore: University Park Press.

Reed, R., Pueschel, S., Schnell, R., & Cronk, C. (1980). Interrelationships of biological, environmental and competency variables in young children with Down's syndrome. *Applied Research in Mental Retardation, 1,* 161–174.

Snyder-McClean, L., & McClean, J. (1987). Effectiveness of early intervention for children with language and communication disorders. In M. Guralnick & F. Bennett (Eds.), *The effectiveness of early intervention for at-risk and handicapped children* (pp. 213–274). New York: Academic Press.

Solomon, G.S., Wilson, D.O., & Galey, G.S. (1982). Project DEBT: Attempting to improve the quality of interaction among handicapped children and their parents. *Journal of the Association for Persons with Severe Handicaps, 7,* 28–35.

Stoel-Gammon, C. (1981). Speech development of infants and children with Down's syndrome. In J. Darby, Jr. (Ed.), *Speech evaluation in medicine* (pp. 341–360). New York: Grune & Stratton.

Thoman, E.B., & Becker, P.T. (1979). Issues in assessment and prediction for the infant born at risk. In T.M. Field (Ed.), *Infants born at risk: Behavior and development* (pp. 461–484). New York: Spectrum Publications.

Tjossem, T (1976). Early intervention: Issues and approaches. In T. Tjossem (Ed.), *Intervention strategies for high-risk and handicapped children.* Baltimore: University Park Press.

Turnbull, A., & Turnbull, H. (1986). Stepping back from early intervention: An ethical perspective. *Journal of the Division for Early Childhood, 10,* 106–117.

Vietze, P., & Vaughan, H. (Eds.). (1988). *Early identification of infants with developmental disabilities.* New York: Grune & Stratton.

Wallach, G., & Butler, K. (Eds.). (1984). *Language learning disabilities in school-age children.* Baltimore: Williams & Wilkins.

Warren, S., & Kaiser, A. (1988). Research in early language intervention. In S. Odom & M. Karnes (Eds.), *Early intervention for infants and children with handicaps* (pp. 89–108). Baltimore: Paul H. Brookes.

Wilcox, M., & Terrell, B. (1985). Child language behavior: The acquisition of social communicative competence. In C. McLaughlin & D. Gullo (Eds.), *The young child in context* (pp. 40–65). Springfield, IL: Charles C. Thomas.

Wilcox, M, Bashir, A, Iglesias, A, Liebergott, L, & Snyder-McClean, L. (1989). Communication-based services for at-risk and handicapped infants, toddlers, and their families. *Asha, 31,* 32–34.

Wilcox, M., & Campbell, P. (In press). Sociocommunicative intervention for infants and toddlers with disabilities In M Wilcox & P. Campbell (Eds.), *Communication programming from birth to three.* Boston: Little, Brown.

Wolff, P.H. (1982). Theoretical issues in the development of motor skills. In M. Lewis & L. Taft (Eds.), *Developmental disabilities: Theory, assessment, and intervention* (pp. 117–134). New York: Spectrum Publications.

# Part II
# Assessment Strategies: Implications from Practice and Research with Normal and Disordered Populations

# Ins and outs of the acquisition of spatial terms

Cheryl K. Messick, PhD
*Early Childhood Program Director*
*Family Child Learning Center*
*Children's Hospital and Medical*
*Center of Akron*
*Akron, Ohio*

THE ACQUISITION of spatial terms occurs as a gradual process involving the integration of complex conceptual and linguistic knowledge. Spatial terms include prepositions that express locative relations (e.g., *in, on, under, between*); nouns labeling position (e.g., *top, bottom, side*); as well as adjectives that convey attribution characteristics (e.g., *tall, long, narrow*). The conceptual knowledge of spatial terms is abstract and refers to a relationship within an item or between items (Cox & Richardson, 1985). For example, *in* includes the notion of containment, while *on* refers to a relation of support between two objects (Johnston & Slobin, 1979). These concepts are more ambiguous, if not more complex, than those required in the acquisition of a label for a concrete referent (Cox & Richardson, 1985).

To complicate matters further, the relationships involved in spatial terms are not absolute (Cox & Richardson, 1985). Selec-

*Top Lang Disord*, 1988, 8(2), 14–25
© 1988 Aspen Publishers, Inc.

tion of the appropriate term is influenced by contextual characteristics such as the viewpoint of the speaker–listener, as well as object characteristics such as size, shape, and positioning (e.g., Bernstein, 1984; E.V. Clark, 1973b; Harris & Folch, 1985). The spatial term used in one situation may not be appropriate in a slightly different context. For example, a particular object may be labeled with the spatial adjective *big* in one context and *small* in another (e.g., *mommy's shoe* versus *baby's shoe*; *mommy's shoe* versus *daddy's shoe*).

The ambiguity of contextual influences can be further illustrated by examining the use of the prepositions *in front of/in back of* in the context of a box with sides equal in length, width, and height. Designation of the *front/back* of the box is determined by the orientation of the box in relation to the speaker. Typically the *front* will be considered the side closest to the speaker or between the speaker and the object. *Back* will be considered the far side or the hidden side. If the orientation of the box is shifted 45 degrees, a different side will be designated as *front*.

The appropriate use of spatial terms involves the gradual acquisition of abstract relational concepts as well as knowledge of the influence of contextual factors. As noted by Johnston & Slobin (1979), there is a gap between the emergence of the conceptual notion of a specific spatial term and correctly encoding the notion linguistically. The process of spatial term acquisition is explored here. A review of two primary theories of word meaning and concept acquisition is presented, followed by a summary of current developmental research on spatial terms and a discussion of the factors influencing

acquisition. Finally, guidelines for the assessment and teaching of spatial terms are presented.

## THEORETICAL BACKGROUND

Two basic approaches to word meaning are the most relevant to spatial-term concepts: an intensional approach and an extensional approach. Intensional approaches, such as E.V. Clark's (1973b) feature or componential approach, focus on defining the appropriate set of components to define a concept. Extension approaches, such as the prototype theory, focus on defining the set of all exemplars referred to by a concept.

The feature approach, originally described by E.V. Clark (1973b), provided the initial testing ground for determining the order of acquisition of spatial terms. E.V. Clark (1973b) proposed that the semantic "sense" of a lexical item is composed of a bundle of semantic features. Together these features define the meaning of a word and differentiate it from words that are related but not equal in meaning. For example, *above* and *on top of* include the following set of common features: locative term, vertical dimension, and height. Two terms that are not equal in meaning must possess at least one feature that serves to differentiate the two meanings. In the case of *above* and *on top of*, "contact with surface" is a differentiating feature for *on top of*.

Differences between a child's use of a word and the appropriate adult use occur when there is a mismatch in the set of semantic components. Mismatching may be caused by the absence of critical semantic features or the inclusion of incorrect components (E.V. Clark, 1973a; Carey, 1982). Children use hypothesis testing to determine the appropriate subset of semantic components of a word. Before determining the critical features of a term, they may use a term correctly in some situations and incorrectly in others (Anglin, 1977; E.V. Clark, 1973a; H.H. Clark & E.V. Clark, 1977). The feature approach to word concepts examines intension, focusing on defining the appropriate set of components to express the concept. Intension then determines word extension (Bridges, Sinha, & Walkerdine, 1981; Greenberg & Kuczaj, 1982).

As indicated earlier, prototype theory is based primarily on extension or inclusion (Greenberg & Kuczaj, 1982; Rosch, 1973; 1978). Concept extension defines the set of all exemplars referred to by a concept (Bridges et al., 1981). The set is determined by a member's central tendency toward a prototype or nuclear exemplar. Initially, the first object the child experiences with the label is considered the prototypical member (Anglin, 1977). As the child experiences additional instances of the concept, the prototype becomes a mental representation of the properties that have been found to cooccur across a large number of exemplars (Rosch, 1978).

Membership in a set in the prototype approach is determined by a "best fit" criterion (Palmer, 1978). Some members of the set are "good" exemplars, while others are "poorer" exemplars, as determined by similarity to the prototype. For example, a container such as a box may be a better exemplar for the concept *in* than a pocket on a shirt. Similarly, a container may be more prototypical for the concept *in*, while a support surface (e.g., table top)

may be more prototypical for the concept *on*.

## DEVELOPMENTAL PROGRESSION OF SPATIAL-TERM ACQUISITION

A review of the literature in the area of spatial-term acquisition reveals numerous gaps in the knowledge base. As a whole, the studies have included a variety of different methods and tasks for measuring acquisition. Some have assessed comprehension only (e.g., Bernstein, 1984; Cox, 1979; Harris & Folch, 1985), while others have focused entirely on production (e.g., Cox & Richardson, 1985; Johnston, 1984; Johnston & Slobin, 1979). Several spatial terms that have been examined superficially, or not at all include *deep/shallow*, *thick/thin*, *out*, and *around*. In contrast, a number of terms have been examined cross-linguistically to determine universal influences on acquisition as opposed to language-specific influences (Harris & Folch, 1985; Harris, Morris, & Terwogt, 1986; Johnston & Slobin, 1979).

### Contextual influences on acquisition

Children as young as 18 months use contextual information to decipher the meanings of *in*, *on*, and *under* (E.V. Clark, 1973b; Hoogenraad, Grieve, Baldwin, & Campbell, 1978; Wilcox & Palermo, 1974). That is, before children actually understand the conceptual distinctions among these terms, they give the appearance of word comprehension (Chapman, 1978; Chapman & Kohn, 1978). Children use different kinds of contextual information to differentiate among spatial terms, including the physical characteristics of an object and the typical use or function of the object. For example, if the referent object is a container, the typical response would be to *put X inside*. In contrast, if the referent has a supporting surface, the typical response would be to *put X on*. When responses are determined by the physical characteristics of the object, rather than comprehension of the actual spatial term, a child is likely to show comprehension of the terms *in* and *inside* but not understand *under*, *behind*, and *above*.

Task factors (e.g., pointing to a picture or placing objects in position) have a considerable influence on children's comprehension of spatial terms. For example, Washington and Naremore (1978) evaluated children's comprehension of nine prepositions using both picture and object stimuli. The children (ages 3;0–4;11 years) performed better with object stimuli than picture stimuli. Bernstein (1984) supplemented these data further in a study that used objects to measure comprehension of *in*, *on*, and *under*. Bernstein used box-like stimuli that varied in the shape and in the location of the opening. Some boxes opened on the top, while others opened on the front, bottom, or sides. His subjects (ages 1;5–3;3 years) performed better when they did not have to manipulate the objects but could instead give a simple pointing response. When object manipulation was required, responses seemed to be influenced by object characteristics.

Children's performance in pointing tasks can be influenced by a number of additional factors. The influence of direction of movement was measured in several studies focusing specifically on comprehension of *big/tall* (Harris & Folch, 1985; Maratsos, 1974). Children's performance on comprehension tasks decreased when they observed a vertical change in object location, but not when they observed a horizontal movement. Children's understanding of terms such as *front/back* and *big/tall* can also be influenced by the size of the objects used. For example, *behind* is initially comprehended as if it means "not visible" (Johnston, 1984) or hidden. Thus, a child may demonstrate comprehension of *behind* when a small car is placed behind a big car, but will not comprehend the term if the big car is behind the small car. Children's comprehension of spatial terms is influenced by their conceptual understanding of the terms. Initially their concept may include variables (i.e., size of stimuli) that are not relevant in the adult concept of the term.

The inherent characteristics of stimuli have also been examined as an influencing factor when measuring knowledge of *front/back*. Objects with inherent *fronts* or *backs*, such as a face, television set, or dresser, are passed-on comprehension tasks before objects without inherent *fronts/backs* (e.g., drinking glass, orange, ball).

## Developmental order of acquisition

As noted earlier, there are many gaps in the literature on spatial-term acquisition. However, a review of the research does reveal some general developmental consistencies among these terms. Children acquire spatial terms gradually and show an increase in spatial-term knowledge with age (E. Clark, 1980; Cox & Richardson, 1985; Johnston, 1984; Johnston & Slobin, 1979; Washington & Naremore, 1978). By 4 years of age, children have acquired most spatial terms, although some word concepts held by children continue to change in meaning until the children are around 7 years of age (Cox & Richardson, 1985). Most of the studies define order of acquisition across a small set of spatial terms, although a few studies define chronological age expectations.

### Spatial adjectives

Information on spatial adjectives is relatively sparse. Carey (1982) defined the following general order of acquisition across spatial adjectives, based on a review of several studies (e.g., Bierwisch, 1967; Clark, 1973): stage one, big/little; stage two, long/short, tall/short, high/low; stage three, wide/narrow, deep/shallow, thick/thin. There appear to be a number of factors relating to this order of acquisition. For example, *big* is acquired early because it is semantically simple. It refers to size in any dimension. In contrast, *wide* is acquired later because it refers specifically to one dimension of size (E.V. Clark, 1973b). This general order of emergence of terms also supports H.H. Clark's (1973) predictions concerning the complexity of spatial dimensions: height and length precede width, which precedes thickness. It is also possible that the levels reflect frequency of occurrence in parental speech to children. Ravn and Gelman (1984) have noted that *big/little* is frequently used in speech to young children. Also, the spatial adjectives of the third stage (*wide/narrow*, *deep/shallow*, and *thick/thin*) are probably used less frequently with young children.

H.H. Clark (1973) has suggested that positive terms in polar pairs of adjectives are usually acquired before negative

*More detailed examination of the acquisition of* big *has revealed that many positive adjective terms are considered as equivalent to* big *when they are initially learned by children.*

terms. More detailed examination of the acquisition of *big* has revealed that many positive adjective terms are considered as equivalent to *big* when they are initially learned by children. Thus, in acquiring the polar terms, children initially view the adjectives as referring to a general dimension of size, and later learn the specific dimension characteristics. Thus, at various points in children's development, *long, thick, wide,* and *high* are all considered to be equivalent to *big*. Children initially seem to view the adjective pairs as generally contrastive in meaning and later learn that the terms refer to specific aspects of dimensional contrast (Carey, 1982; Gathercole, 1982).

### Spatial prepositions

The literature on acquisition of spatial prepositions is more extensive than that for spatial adjectives. Most of the studies have examined production of spatial prepositions. A study by Washington and Naremore (1978) is one of the few that included both comprehension and production tasks. The following prepositions were evaluated: *inside, on, under, around, behind, front, between, beside,* and *over*. Subjects were 80 children ranging in age between 3;0 and 4;11 years. Not surprisingly, comprehension and production of the prepositional terms increased with age. In general, more terms were comprehended than were produced. Table 1 provides a listing of the age levels at which each preposition was comprehended and produced with 70% accuracy.

Examination of the Washington and Naremore (1978) data reveals some variability across words in comprehension versus production. Some words were produced several months after they were comprehended (e.g., *around, between, beside*), whereas others were comprehended and produced around the same time (e.g., *in, on, behind*).

The production findings of Washington and Naremore (1978) are interesting to compare with those of Johnston (1984) and Johnston and Slobin (1979). Johnston and Slobin collected data from English-, Italian-, Serbo-Croatian-, and Turkish-speaking children ranging in age from 2;0 to 4;8 years. Children were asked to describe where an object was. Johnston (1984) used a slightly different procedure. Children varying in age from 2;7 to 4;7 years were asked to tell a puppet where to

---

**Summary of Order of Production Acquisition of Spatial Prepositions Across Two Studies**

| Johnston & Slobin (1979) | Johnston (1984) |
|---|---|
| I. in, on, under, beside | I. on, in |
| II. between, back and front (featured objects) | II. under, next to |
| III. back, front (nonfeatured objects) | III. back (tall)<br>back (featured) |
| | IV. front (featured)<br>back (nonfeatured) |
| | V. front (tall)<br>front (nonfeatured objects) |

*Note:* Johnston & Slobin, 1979; Johnston, 1984.

---

find hidden objects. Despite the different methodologies, children in the three studies (Washington & Naremore, 1978; Johnston & Slobin, 1979; and Johnston, 1984) demonstrated a similar order of acquisition pattern (see box). In all three studies, *in/inside, on,* and *under* were the first prepositions acquired. Two of the studies

---

**Table 1.** Listing by age levels of acquisition of prepositions in comprehension and production as tested with three-dimensional stimuli

| Age level° | Comprehension | Production |
|---|---|---|
| 3;0–3;5 | inside, in, on, under, between, around | in, inside, on, under |
| 3;6–3;11 | behind, in front of, between, beside | behind |
| 4;0–4;5 | | beside, around |
| 4;6–4;11 | | between |

*Note:* Washington & Naremore (1978).
°70% accuracy.

(Johnston, 1984; Johnston & Slobin, 1979) found that *beside/next to* emerged next. *Between* emerged before *back/front* (nonfeatured where nonfeatured refers to objects without inherent backs or fronts, e.g., a drinking glass, a key, or a ball).

There are several stages of acquiring *back/front* (Johnston, 1984; Johnston & Slobin, 1979). Children initially used the terms to refer to their own anatomical *front* and *back* (Kuczaj & Maratsos, 1975). At this time, children successfully convey the notion of *back/front* through the use of deictic terms *(here/there)* or environmental cues to describe object location (e.g., by the door; close to the floor/ceiling) (Cox & Richardson, 1985). The appropriate linguistic use of *back* emerges first to describe objects that have intrinsic fronts and backs (e.g., a television set, car, or doll) (Johnston, 1984; Johnston & Slobin, 1979). *Front/back* are also used at this time to describe a relation with a large object of reference, for which the concept of *back/front* may be more salient. At this level, *back* seems to convey the meaning of hidden object. Later uses of *front/back* occur in contexts without intrinsic front and back features and with variation in the speaker's or listener's point of view (Johnston & Slobin, 1979). Cox (1979) found the same order of acquisition using a comprehension task.

## ASSESSMENT

A review of common language assessment instruments confirms that spatial terms are an important aspect of language ability. Spatial terms provide a context for examining abstract conceptual knowledge. Many spatial terms are semantically complex because they refer to ever-changing relations between objects. Syntactically, they occur as nouns (e.g., *top, side, corner*), adjectives (e.g., *tall, short*), and prepositions.

Many language tests and a number of developmental tests assess children's knowledge of spatial terms. The specific terms assessed, however, vary from test to test. Tests also vary in their assignment of ages of mastery. For example, the Denver Developmental Screening Test (Frankenburg & Dobbs, 1967) places comprehension of *on, under, in front of,* and *behind* at the 4-to-4½-year level, while the Receptive Expressive Emergent Language Scale (Bzoch & League, 1971) places the same terms at the 33-to-36-month level. Not one of the assessment instruments appears to gauge spatial-term acquisition in relation to levels of acquisition, as suggested by recent research in this area.

There are numerous weaknesses in the specific procedures used to obtain measures of spatial-term knowledge. Most language assessment tests use picture stimuli to elicit both comprehension and production responses. As noted earlier, research has suggested that children perform better with object stimuli than picture stimuli (Washington & Naremore, 1978). On most tests, each spatial term is assessed on the basis of only one item. But observations of children's actual word categories in relation to contextual variation are possible only if a term is assessed several times in different contexts. At best, traditional language tests screen spatial-term knowledge and should therefore be supplemented by more in-depth probing.

Children's knowledge of spatial concepts should be examined independently from their knowledge of the linguistic use of spatial terms. Levine and Carey (1982) provide a simple methodology for observing children's concept of *front/back* orientation. The examiners lined up three dolls, animals, or vehicles and then asked children to complete the parade line using the remaining objects. A second task involved placing nine objects, one at a time, in position to talk with a "conversational doll." These two tasks allowed Levine and Carey (1982) to distinguish between children's understanding of *front/back* orientation and their ability to comprehend and produce the terms linguistically.

Assessment of linguistic knowledge should include measures of both comprehension and production. To optimize linguistic performance, controls must be placed on variables that influence spatial-term performance. Object stimuli should be used rather than picture stimuli. The child should not be required to manipulate the objects, because object manipulation can influence linguistic performance (Cox & Richardson, 1985). Rather, the child's task should strictly be one of linguistic judgment (comprehension) or description (production). On comprehension measures, for example, the child should be required merely to point to the objects depicting the targeted spatial relation from several presented choices. Between trials, a screen should be used to block the child's vision of stimulus items, because object movement has also been found to influence performance (Harris, Morris, & Terwogt, 1986).

Each spatial term tested should be assessed in a number of different contexts in which the variables are controlled appropriately. For example, when testing a child's comprehension of *in*, the examiner should vary the contextual cues (physical characteristics of the objects). Objects that invite putting things in should be used (e.g., containers), as well as objects that require strictly linguistic comprehension for correct placement. Likewise, when testing knowledge of *front/back*, the examiner should use objects with and without inherent *front/back* characteristics (e.g., *radio* versus *shoe box*).

Table 2 is an example of a probe for assessing a child's comprehension of *on*. The stimulus items chosen include words that are familiar to young children. Each spatial term should be tested at least five times using different stimulus items to determine the child's consistency of response. Note that the stimulus items used in the task could also be used to assess a number of different spatial terms (e.g., *in, under, beside, behind, in front of*). Also, there should be three identical objects for each stimulus so that foils vary only in terms of the spatial relation being depicted.

When limitations in production are noted for specific spatial terms, it is important to determine whether the child is able to convey the semantic aspects of the term in an alternative form. For example, is the child able to use word order, deictic terms, or environmental cues to convey a notion of locative relations?

When choosing which spatial terms to assess, the examiner should consider the developmental order of acquisition. For very young children, the examiner's focus may be restricted to earlier developing spatial terms such as *big/little, in, on,* and

**Table 2.** Example of items for assessing comprehension of *on*

| Stimulus items | | |
|---|---|---|
| car | | block |
| cereal/cracker box | | Fischer-Price man |
| miniature chair | | doll shoe |
| cup with a lid | | doll spoon |
| jewelry box on short legs with a hinged lid | | folded piece of paper |

| Instructions to child | | Placement of stimulus items (foils and target) | |
|---|---|---|---|
| Show me block on car | block *in* car | block *in front of* car | block *on* car |
| Show me man on box (use a cereal/cracker carton) | man *on* box | man *beside* box | man *under* box |
| Show me shoe on chair | shoe *under* chair | shoe *on* chair | shoe *behind* chair |
| Show me spoon on cup | spoon *on* cup | spoon *in* cup | spoon *behind* cup |
| Show me paper on box | paper *beside* | paper *in front of* box | paper *on* box |

*under.* For an older child, more time may be spent on determining the level of *front/back* knowledge. In some cases, it may not be necessary to evaluate a child's knowledge of all spatial terms. The focus instead will be on obtaining in-depth knowledge of a subset of spatial terms (e.g., *over* and *above*), when, for example, a child has demonstrated adequate knowledge of some spatial terms. For a child functioning at beginning levels of language the focus would be on early developing spatial terms.

## INTERVENTION

Before teaching spatial terms it is important to ensure that the child has the underlying conceptual knowledge required for the spatial term. If there are no indications that the underlying concepts exist, the child should be given experiential activities to build such concepts prior to linguistic training. If the child does not have an underlying concept of the term, it is unlikely that he or she can successfully be taught to produce the form.

An additional factor to consider when selecting spatial terms for training is to examine the child's current method of

*Before teaching spatial terms it is important to ensure that the child has the underlying conceptual knowledge required for the spatial term.*

conveying spatial relations. If the child successfully conveys the concept of *in* nonverbally (e.g., through a gesture or sign), it is advisable to initially choose a target item for teaching that is not being successfully conveyed in any manner, thus expanding the child's options for conveying spatial meanings rather than providing an alternative form for noting concepts already communicated nonlinguistically. Alternatively, other linguistic deficits (e.g., phonological or syntactical) may sometimes outweigh spatial-term difficulties. In such a situation strategies for bypassing the need for specific spatial terms may be taught. The child may learn to use deictic markers or environmental cues to convey spatial concepts nonlinguistically. Later, the clinician may teach the appropriate spatial terms.

In general, the developmental order of acquiring spatial terms will provide the guidelines for teaching these words. In most cases, earlier developing terms should be trained before later developing items. Thus, if a child is not using any spatial prepositions, stage one (*in, on, under,* or *beside*) prepositions should be trained before later developing terms (i.e., *front/back, deep/shallow*).

In some cases, however, a spatial term that is functionally communicative for the child should be chosen over an earlier developing spatial term. For example, if the child spends considerable time during play lining up objects, *front/back* may be an appropriate target for teaching, depending on the child's conceptual level. Communicative relevance to the child can potentially facilitate the acquisition of these terms.

An additional example of deviating from a developmental model occurs when teaching a spatial term that is acquired by normally developing children through several stages. For example, normal children go through a stage when they use positive polar adjective terms as if they were equivalent to *big*. Rather than taking

a language-delayed child through the incorrect use of an adjective (e.g., *big* for the concept of *tall*), the child may learn to contrast the two forms. Similarly, if a child is not using contextual information to interpret *in* or *on*, training could focus on contrasting these two terms by using objects that promote use of both concepts (e.g., table with a drawer, box with a lid, or bucket with a lid). Stimuli that reflect the contrast between the terms should be used in training. By selecting contrastive stimuli, the child may learn to use *in* and *on* correctly without going through the stage of using the two terms interchangeably.

In general during intervention, object stimuli should be used initially rather than picture stimuli. Training should begin in contexts that do not require the child to manipulate objects. However, the child should not be a passive participant in the intervention process. The child may manipulate the objects, but should experience occasions when manipulation is not required. The literature on the effects of object manipulation (Harris & Folch, 1985; Maratsos, 1974; Washington & Naremore, 1978) suggests that learning of spatial terms may be facilitated in contexts that do not require object manipulation. The child's body may also be used as a referent in teaching. For example, the child may initially be asked to place objects *in front/in back* of his or her own body.

Training stimuli should vary in terms of the actual items and in features such as size, inherent marking, and shape. Because of the abstract nature of the terms, concept learning requires a variety of stimuli. Variety decreases the chances that the child will focus on the referents rather than the relationships among referents. For example, when training *front/back*, it is important to initially use large objects that have inherent fronts.

A number of recent research studies on spatial terms provide interesting tasks that could be used during the intervention process (Bernstein, 1984; Cox & Richardson, 1985; Johnston, 1984). Bernstein used a set of geometrical constructions that allowed placement of objects in a variety of spatial positions. His constructions consisted of containers varying in shape, including cubes and trapezoid-type containers. Many of them were raised on a platform. Such containers are ideal for training concepts such as *in, on,* and *under,* because each of the concepts can be contrasted using the same stimulus item. Cox and Richardson (1985) built a hollow plexiglass construction that allowed for the placement of small balls in a variety of positions including *top, bottom, front/back, next to, above,* and *below.*

The puppet task by Johnston (1984) provides a more naturalistic context for teaching spatial terms and could be used for training both spatial adjectives and prepositions. The task involves using props in a defined scenario (e.g., going to the park) that incorporates spatial terms in a naturalistic context. For example, the puppet may drive "in front of a store," and then go "behind the bus." This format can be used during structured play with a child to allow training of both comprehension and production, using a variety of controlled stimuli.

•　　•　　•

As information regarding spatial-term acquisition grows, it should be incorporated into clinical techniques of assessment and intervention. When focusing on spatial terms, it is important to remember that such terms require abstract conceptual knowledge for appropriate use in comprehension and production. The job of the speech-language pathologist is to examine the child's conceptualization as well as linguistic comprehension and production of spatial terms. Such an examination will yield areas and methods for training spatial knowledge. The abstract nature of the terms suggests that intervention may include direct training of spatial terms or indirect training through experiential activities where therapy is aimed at other areas of deficit. The training of spatial terms requires carefully planned strategies and activities to maximize intervention effectiveness.

## REFERENCES

Anglin, J.M. (1977). *Word, object and conceptual development.* New York: Norton.

Bernstein, M.E. (1984). Non-linguistic responses to verbal instructions. *Journal of Child Language, 11,* 293–311.

Bierwisch, M. (1967). Some semantic universals of German adjectivals. *Foundations of Language, 3,* 1–36.

Bridges, A., Sinha, C., & Walkerdine, V. (1981). The development of comprehension. In G. Wells (Ed.), *Learning through interaction* (pp. 116–156). Cambridge, MA: Cambridge University Press.

Bzoch, K., & League, R. (1971). The Receptive Expressive Emergent Language Scale. Gainesville, FL: Tree of Life Press.

Carey, S. (1982). Semantic development: The state of the

art. In E. Wanner & L.R. Gleitman (Eds.), *Language acquisition: The state of the art* (pp. 347–389). Cambridge, MA: Cambridge University Press.

Chapman, R.S. (1978). Comprehension strategies in children. In J.F. Kavanagh & W. Strange (Eds.), *Speech and language in the laboratory, school, and clinic* (pp. 308–326). Cambridge, MA: MIT Press.

Chapman, R.S., & Kohn, L.L. (1978). Comprehension strategies in two and three year olds: Animate agents or probable events? *Journal of Speech & Hearing Research, 21,* 746–761.

Clark, E.V. (1972). On the child's acquisition of antonyms in two semantic fields. *Journal of Verbal Learning & Verbal Behavior, 11,* 750–758.

Clark, E.V. (1973a). Non-linguistic strategies and the acquisition of word meaning. *Cognition, 2,* 161–182.

Clark, E.V. (1973b). What's in a word? On the child's acquisition of semantics in his first language. In T. E. Moore (Ed.), *Cognitive development and the acquisition of language* (pp. 65–110). New York: Academic Press.

Clark, E. (1980). Here's the top: Non-linguistic strategies in the acquisition of orientational terms. *Child Development, 51,* 329–338.

Clark, H.H. (1973). Space, time, semantics, and the child. In T.E. Moore (Ed.), *Cognitive development and the acquisition of language.* New York: Academic Press.

Clark, H.H., & Clark, E.V. (1977). *Psychology and language.* New York: Harcourt Brace Jovanovich.

Cox, M.V. (1979). Young children's understanding of "in front of" and "behind" in the placement of objects. *Journal of Child Language, 6,* 371–374.

Cox, M.V., & Richardson, J.R. (1985). How do children describe spatial relationships? *Journal of Child Language, 12,* 611–620.

Frankenburg, W., & Dobbs, J. (1967). *Denver Developmental Screening Test.* Denver: University of Colorado Medical Center.

Gathercole, V.C. (1982). Decrements in children's responses to big and tall: A reconsideration of the potential cognitive and semantic causes. *Journal of Experimental Child Psychology, 34,* 156–73.

Greenberg, J., & Kuczaj, S.A. (1982). Towards a theory of substantive word-meaning acquisition. In S. Kuczaj (Ed.), *Language development: Vol. 1. Syntax and semantics* (pp. 275–311). Hillside, NY: Erlbaum.

Harris, P.L., & Folch, L. (1985). Decrement in the understanding of big among English- and Spanish-speaking children. *Journal of Child Language, 12,* 685–690.

Harris, P.L., Morris, J.E., & Terwogt, M.M. (1986). The early acquisition of spatial adjectives: A cross-linguistic study. *Journal of Child Language, 13,* 335–352.

Hoogenraad, R., Grieve, R., Baldwin, P., & Campbell, R. (1978). Comprehension as an interactive process. In R.N. Campbell & P.J. Smith (Eds.), *Recent advances in the psychology of language—Language development and mother-child interaction* (163–186). New York: Plenum.

Johnston, J.R. (1984). Acquisition of locative meanings: Behind and in front of. *Journal of Child Language, 11,* 407–422.

Johnston, J.R., & Slobin, D.I. (1979). The development of locative expressions in Englih, Italian, Serbo-Croatian, and Turkish. *Journal of Child Language, 6,* 529–545.

Kuczaj, S.A., & Maratsos, M.P. (1975). On the acquisition of front, back, and side. *Child Development, 46,* 202–210.

Levine, S.C., & Carey, S. (1982). Up front: The acquisition of a concept and a word. *Journal of Child Language, 9,* 645–657.

Maratsos, M.P. (1974). When is the high thing the big one? *Developmental Psychology, 10,* 367–375.

Palmer, S. (1978). Fundamental aspects of cognitive representation. In E. Rosch & B. Lloyd (Eds.), *Cognitive and categorization.* Hillsdale, NJ: Erlbaum.

Ravn, K.E., & Gelman, S.A. (1984). Rule usage in children's understanding of "big" and "little." *Child Development, 55,* 2141–2150.

Rosch, E. (1973). On the internal structure of perceptual and semantic categories. In T. Moore (Ed.), *Cognitive and the acquisition of language.* New York: Academic Press.

Rosch, E. (1978). Principles of categorization. In E. Rosch & B. Lloyd (Eds.), *Cognitive and categorization.* Hillsdale, NJ: Erlbaum.

Washington, D.S., & Naremore, R.C. (1978). Children's use of spatial prepositions in two- and three-dimensional tasks. *Journal of Speech and Hearing Research, 21,* 151–165.

Wilcox, S., & Palermo, D.S. (1974). 'In', 'on', and 'under' revisited. *Cognition, 3,* 245–254.

# Freeing talk from the here-and-now: The role of event knowledge and maternal scaffolds

*Joan Lucariello, PhD*
*Assistant Professor of Psychology*
*Graduate Faculty—Psychology*
*New School for Social Research*
*New York, New York*

AT LEAST TWO sources of language acquisition, the cognitive and the social-interactive, relate to the acquisition of temporally displaced (TD) speech, defined as talk about objects and events displaced in time from the present situation. The ability to talk about the nonpresent, that is, past and future happenings and persons and things not in the perceptual field, is one of the most important characteristics of linguistic communication, indeed setting it apart from other forms of communication. Displaced reference emerges in children in the second half of the second year, at approximately 20 to 24 months of age (Eisenberg, 1985; Sachs, 1983). How might cognition and social interaction serve as a basis for its acquisition?

The contribution of cognition may be tied to a predominant form of knowledge organization for very young children: event representations or schemata (Nelson, Fivush, Hudson, & Lucariello, 1983; Nelson & Gruendel, 1981). Event representations

*Top Lang Disord*, 1990,10(3),14–29

specify the sequence of actions, the goal organizing those actions, and the actors/roles and props appropriate to a particular spatial/temporal context. For example, the schema for the restaurant event incorporates the goal of eating; actions such as being seated, reviewing the menu, ordering, eating, and paying; roles such as hostess and waiter; and props such as menus. Event representations may account for the emergence of TD talk in terms of its context of occurrence, that is, where it takes place, and in terms of its content, that is, what it is about.

As to where TD talk occurs, its emergence may be context dependent. Such talk may be more likely to occur in contexts for which children have event representations. These contexts may be termed routine or scripted. This proposal is based on an information processing perspective on the deployment of linguistic skills (Shatz, 1978, 1983). In situations where an event representation can be instantiated to guide here-and-now physical activity, processing capacity can be allocated to linguistic behavior, and, in particular, to complex linguistic skills such as displaced reference.

Event knowledge may also serve to explain what early TD talk is about. Mothers and children share knowledge not only of the routine/scripted activity in which they are currently involved, but also of a host of noncurrent routine activities that may serve as topics for displaced speech. Such a situation occurs when we ask one another, "What happened at work or school?" Eisenberg (1985) found that mother–child talk about the past was often based on shared knowledge about scripted events. It may be expected that the event

knowledge of young children would support talk about the future as well.

Interest in the contribution of social-interactive factors to child language acquisition may be traced to the work of Vygotsky (1978) and, more specifically, to his conception that higher mental functions develop within the context of the child's interactions with others. The "zone of proximal development" (ZPD) characterizes the child's potential level of development as psychological functions that can be elicited by others through means such as leading questions. Bruner applied the ZPD notion to child language acquisition, with his concepts of "scaffolding" (Bruner, 1978) and language acquisition support system (LASS) (Bruner, 1983). Scaffolding or LASS entails the mother's reducing the degrees of freedom with which the child has to cope, concentrating the child's attention into a manageable domain, providing models of expected language from which the child can extract selectively what is needed to fulfill a role in discourse, and creating linguistic formats or routines. LASS or scaffolding has been found to play a role in the child's acquisition of the linguistic skills of reference and requesting (Bruner, 1983).

Social-interactive factors may be highly related to the question of how TD talk occurs. It is expected that the child's early forays into displaced reference will be highly scaffolded by the mother. There is some evidence suggesting that maternal language plays such a role. Sachs (1983) has shown that when adults structure talk about the past into conversational routines, children benefit. Indeed, she found that the child's ability to talk about displaced events emerged in such linguistic routines. Such structuring may, in fact, be critical. Eisenberg (1985) notes that the minimal participation of the adults she observed in conversations on displaced topics may have been responsible for the disorganization observed in children's descriptions of past events.

These hypotheses on the role of cognition and social interaction in child language acquisition have important implications for the language clinician in the areas of intervention/training and assessment. For example, with regard to intervention, if the acquisition of TD speech were found to have a social-interactive basis, then how that social-interactive base might best be arranged or organized to serve an instructional function becomes key. Moreover, if child cognition has the proposed effect on TD speech, that is, if there is situational variation in the acquisition and manifestation of such speech, this has serious ramifications for assessment.

The proposals on the contributions made by event knowledge and maternal scaffolding to the acquisition of TD talk were investigated in the present research. The general framework of the study involved the observation of children and mothers in three different contexts. The first was defined as a scripted context, consisting of a commonly occurring routine activity that was highly familiar and predictable to both mothers and children. The other two contexts were not predictable, that is, they had no predetermined structure, but they varied on the dimension of familiarity to the child, one being a free-play situation with age-appropriate toys, and the other a situation involving novel materials and scenario.

There were several foci of the analyses. One focus was to determine in what contexts talk about the past and future occurred. Moreover, because event knowledge might be expected to have an effect on displaced talk not only in terms of situation of occurrence, but also in terms of content, TD talk was subjected to a content analysis as well. Additional thrusts of the analyses entailed the characterization of maternal contributions to TD talk to determine if mothers are attempting to scaffold such talk, and the characterization of child contributions to determine the role of the child in the production of this talk, and possible effects of scaffolding.

## METHOD

### Subjects

Ten children, 6 boys and 4 girls, aged 2 years, 0 months to 2 years, 5 months and from middle-class families in a suburb of New York, and their mothers, participated in this study. All were within normal ranges of language development for their age, with mean length of utterances (MLUs) (words) between 1.23 and 2.76. All children were first-born and, at the time of the study, only children.

### Procedure

Children were visited in their homes on four occasions. On the first visit, the dyad

*One focus was to determine in what contexts talk about the past and future occurred.*

became acquainted with the experimenter/visitor and was informed that the study concerned children's language and would involve videotaping the child in the home during three different activities. Mothers were asked to identify one highly familiar, routine activity that the child participated in and that occurred at least three times a week. This was designated the scripted context and was the focus of observation on one of the three subsequent visits. Five dyads were observed in a lunch routine, three in a getting-dressed-in-the-morning routine (which twice included bathing), and two in a bathing/getting-ready-for-bed routine. On each of these three visits, the dyads were audio- and videotaped for approximately 15 minutes in a different context each time, the order of contexts counterbalanced across subjects.

In addition to the scripted context, a free-play context was established on one visit by presenting the pair with five toys appropriate to children of this age, but that the children did not already possess. This was to ensure that no particular sequence of actions or distribution of roles would be readily anticipated by the child based on scripts formed in prior play experiences with the mother. These toys were a hand puppet, tea set, pull-along-train, stack-toy dog, and shape register. The third situation was a novel context established by presenting the dyad with a model castle with associated toy figures such as knights and a princess. It was ascertained on the first home visit that the children were unfamiliar with both the castle objects and an appropriate scenario for engaging with them. The free-play situation differed from the novel situation

in that no particular scenario was involved in the free-play context, and although the toys used in that context were unfamiliar, they were of the type usually offered to children of this age.

## RESULTS AND DISCUSSION

Video- and audiotapes were transcribed and subjected to analysis. For the purposes of this article, episodes involving reference to temporally displaced events were identified. Temporal displacement was defined as reference to past events, that is, events that had occurred prior to the recording session, and reference to future events, defined as events that would or might occur after the completion of the recording session. A TD episode was defined as an utterance or set of utterances by mother or child or both that referred to a single past or future event. There were a total of 38 episodes of past talk and 44 episodes of future talk. These episodes were subjected to further analyses.

### Cognitive contribution: The role of event knowledge

#### Where TD talk occurs

One way to examine the role of the knowledge base, or shared knowledge, in TD talk is to determine whether there is situational variation in the occurrence of TD talk, given that situations varied in the extent to which the child and the dyad had knowledge about them. The number of TD episodes in each context and the number of dyads contributing these episodes are presented in Table 1. These data indicate that the vast majority of TD talk occurred in the scripted context—89% of

**Table 1.** Total number of episodes and dyads contributing by context

| Context | Past (%) | Future (%) | Total (%) |
|---|---|---|---|
| Routine/scripted | | | |
| No. dyads | 9 | 9 | 10 |
| No. episodes | 32 (84) | 39 (89) | 71 (87) |
| Free play | | | |
| No. dyads | 2 | 2 | 4 |
| No. episodes | 2 | 5 (11) | 7 (9) |
| Novel play | | | |
| No. dyads | 2 | 0 | 2 |
| No. episodes | 4 (11) | 0 | 4 (5) |

Note: Percentage of episodes by context in parentheses
Reprinted with permission from Lucariello, J. & Nelson, K. (1987). Remembering and planning talk between mothers and children. *Discourse Processes, 10*(3), 223. © 1987, Ablex Publishing Corporation.

future talk and 84% of past talk, with nine dyads contributing to each type. Thus, the hypothesis that displaced reference would occur most frequently in the scripted context was strongly supported.

It should be noted that displaced talk was found across all 10 dyads in the contexts serving as scripted in the present research. Specifically, the lunch context elicited 22 episodes of past talk and 18 episodes of future talk across five dyads. The getting-ready-in-the-morning context elicited six past-talk episodes across two dyads, and 18 future-talk episodes across three dyads. The bathing/getting-ready-for-bed context yielded four past-talk episodes across two dyads, and three future-talk episodes for one dyad. Thus, displaced speech occurred across a range of scripted contexts, and not simply in one form of routinized activity.

Moreover, the scripted context served as the arena for the emergence of these

linguistic skills. Sachs (1983) has pointed out that displaced reference is just coming to the fore in children of the age studied, and the present data support that observation. A calculation of the mean percentage of maternal and child utterances in the routine context involving displacement revealed that such talk accounted for less than 10% of the speech ($M$ mother $= 8.9\%$, $M$ child $= 6.2\%$). Thus, "here-and-now" talk was still predominant in dyadic speech, with "there-and-then" talk making its breakthrough in routine/scripted contexts.

### What TD talk is about

The analysis of situational variation in the occurrence of TD talk speaks to the importance of the knowledge base in supporting such talk. Additionally, the knowledge base may play a role in TD talk by providing topics, thereby contributing to the content of such talk. Mothers and children may be presumed to have knowledge of a range of routine activities in which they are not currently participating. These events may serve as TD conversational topics. To explore this possibility, four topic categories were defined as follows:

1. Verbal activity—Episode topic is language behavior. Examples: "Remember when we talked about whining?" "And when everybody asks you how old you are tomorrow, what are you gonna say?"
2. Specific activity—Episode topic is a unique or an infrequently occurring event idiosyncratic to the mother, child, or dyad. Examples: "What did the baby squirrel eat for lunch

today?" "Will you miss her when you go to California?"

3. Routine activity—Episode topic is a routine, frequently occurring event. Examples: "So what did you do at the Hudson School today?" "You gonna take a nap after lunch?"

4. Pretense activity—Episode topic is a pretense event, defined according to criteria outlined by Fein (1981). Example: "Should we save the tea (imaginary object) for daddy when he comes home?"

Intercoder reliability in terms of percentage agreement between two coders was 98% for future and 92% for past episodes. The distribution of past and future talk episodes across these topics can be found in Table 2. The most striking result in this table is the difference between past and future talk with respect to focus on routine or specific activities. As can be seen, past talk was concerned with specific activities more than half (55%) of the time, whereas future talk rarely (14%) concerned such topics. In contrast, future talk concerned routine activities 77% of the time, whereas past talk concerned these much less frequently (24%). The

**Table 2.** Episodes of talk by topic category

| Topic | Past | Future | Total |
|---|---|---|---|
| Routine activity | 9 | 29 | 38 |
| Pretense routine activity | 0 | 5 | 5 |
| Specific activity | 21 | 6 | 27 |
| Verbal activity | 7 | 3 | 10 |
| Uncodable | 1 | 1 | 2 |

Reprinted with permission from Lucariello, J. & Nelson, K. (1987). Remembering and planning talk between mothers and children. *Discourse Processes, 10* (3), 225. © 1987, Ablex Publishing Corporation.

difference in the distribution of past and future talk across these two activity types was highly significant, $\chi^2$ (1) = 19.49, $p < .001$. If episodes of pretense talk were included in this analysis, the outcome would be even more striking, because all the pretense episodes involved routine activities, such as mealtime or daddy's homecoming, and all of them were also future-talk episodes.

Hence, across a total of 82 (38 past and 44 future) TD episodes, 43 (including pretense episodes as routine activities) or 52% relied on event knowledge for a topic. These findings speak to the strong influence of the knowledge base on TD talk, with event knowledge accounting for just more than half of all TD topics, and for more than three-quarters of future-talk topics. Thus, event knowledge served as a major topic source, with knowledge of routine activities in which dyads are not presently engaged supporting many of their early forays into displaced talk. Given that most TD talk occurred in the routine context, it may be that the routine itself suggests topics about routines to come next (for example, napping or going to the park after lunch) or that went before (for example, preschool morning activities). These findings are in accord with the findings of Eisenberg (1985), who found an entire phase in the development of displaced talk, specifically past talk, to be characterized by a dependency on event knowledge.

### Time-frame of TD episodes

TD episodes were coded for whether they were same-day, that is, referred to an event that had occurred or might occur on the day of observation, or distant, that is, referred to an event that had occurred prior to the day of observation or might occur after the day of observation. The results of this analysis are presented in Table 3. Considering only those episodes for which temporal reference could be determined, it can be seen that future talk was used almost exclusively (95%) for same-day activities, whereas more than half (63%) of past talk involved reference to the distant past. This difference is highly significant ($\chi^2 (1) = 27.28$, $p<.001$).

## Social-interactive contribution: Maternal scaffolding

### Child contributions to TD episodes

Child contributions to TD episodes were coded as substantive or nonsubstantive. Substantive contributions provided information about the event through spontaneous comments or responses to wh-questions. Nonsubstantive contributions consisted of imitations, fillers (e.g., yeah, mm-huh), responses to yes/no questions, and questions that sought, but did not contain, information. An example containing nonsubstantive contributions is the following:

*M:* And where did we get the zucchini?
*C:* Huh?
*M:* Who gave us the zucchini?
*C:* Huh? Huh? Huh?
*M:* **Who gave us the zucchini?**
*C:* Who?
*M:* Gail.
*C:* Gail.

As this example illustrates, in nonsubstantive episodes, children, although they may be attempting to stay in the conversation, are unable to contribute information

**Table 3.** Episodes of talk by time-frame

| Time-frame | Past | Future | Total |
|---|---|---|---|
| Same day | 10 | 39 | 49 |
| Distant | 17 | 2 | 19 |
| Indeterminate | 11 | 3 | 14 |

Reprinted with permission from Lucariello, J. & Nelson, K. (1987). Remembering and planning talk between mothers and children. *Discourse Processes, 10* (3), 226. © 1987, Ablex Publishing Corporation.

to it. In contrast, an example of a substantive contribution is evidenced in the following TD talk segment:

*M:* You did get a boo boo.
       Look at that foot.
       How'd you do that?
*C:* Door.
*M:* On the door?
*C:* Yeah.

Here, the child is providing information about a previous occurrence, information that the mother does not already have. To be counted as substantive, the child contribution might refer to information that the mother also knows with the stipulation it had not previously been mentioned by the mother in that episode.

As shown in Table 4, children made substantive contributions to 17 (21%) of the total 82 TD episodes, that is, to 24% of the past TD episodes and 18% of the future TD episodes. The limited number of episodes to which children make substantive contributions as well as the small number of children contributing, 6 in all (see Table 4), supports the observation that children of this age are just beginning to acquire the ability to engage in displaced reference (Sachs, 1983). The vast majority of substantive contributions made by the

**Table 4.** Child substantive contributions by episodes and subjects

| Contributions | Past | Future |
|---|---|---|
| Total no. contributions | 16 | 13 |
| No. subjects | 5 | 4 |
| Total episodes with child contributions | 9 | 8 |
| M contributions per episode | 1.78 | 1.63 |
| M contributions per child | 3.20 | 3.25 |

Reprinted with permission from Lucariello, J. & Nelson, K. (1987). Remembering and planning talk between mothers and children. *Discourse Processes, 10* (3), 227. © 1987, Ablex Publishing Corporation.

child occurred in TD episodes from the routine or scripted context. For past talk, 3 of the 16 contributions derive from one episode in the novel play context, with the rest deriving from the scripted context. For future talk, 1 of the 13 substantive contributions derived from a single TD episode in the free-play context, with the remaining contributions belonging to the scripted context.

Child contributions to TD episodes did not differ across past and future talk in terms of the number of subjects contributing, the total number of contributions, and the mean number of contributions by child and episode, as Table 4 indicates. However, there was some suggestive evidence that children were more facile with talk about the future than with talk about the past. First, in contrast to none in past

---

*The vast majority of substantive contributions made by the child occurred in TD episodes from the routine or scripted context.*

---

talk, there were three instances of child-initiated talk about the future. Second, an analysis involving the breakdown of substantive contributions into spontaneous comments and responses to wh-questions revealed that for future talk, 69% (9 of 13) of substantive contributions were spontaneous comments, and only 31% were responses to wh-questions. For past talk, however, the story was reversed, with only 37.5% (6 of 16) of substantive contributions being spontaneous, and 62.5% being answers to wh-questions.

Child ability to contribute to TD episodes did not appear to be related to the topic of such episodes, in terms of whether the topic was a routine or specific activity. For past talk, four episodes on specific activities and four episodes on routine activities included child substantive contributions. These data provide additional evidence that children can recall information pertaining to specific, unusual happenings, as well as the details of commonly occurring events. For future talk, two episodes on specific activities and five episodes on routine activities included child substantive contributions. The greater number of routine activity episodes here containing child substantive contributions probably reflects the greater preponderance of routine activity topics in future talk (see Table 2).

Children had difficulty, however, with verbal activity topics. In general, they were unable to contribute to episodes about such topics. Children were apparently unable to remember utterances from the past or the occasion of particular verbal exchanges; whether this was due to the information being unavailable or inaccessible is not known. Moreover, children were not able to formulate utterances for future occasions. Linguistic experiences may be less memorable, less accessible, and less manipulable than knowledge about the nonverbal behaviors that comprise an event, such as physical actions.

Child ability to make substantive contributions to TD episodes did not appear to be affected by episode time-frame. Child substantive contributions were made in four episodes of distant past talk, three episodes of same-day past talk, and two episodes of indeterminate talk. Future-talk episodes were not analyzed because they were concerned almost exclusively with same-day activities.

### How TD talk occurs: Maternal contributions to episodes

Because child contributions to TD episodes were fairly restricted, the production of TD talk rested primarily with the mother. A detailed examination of maternal talk revealed four important uses of language by mothers: (a) temporal language, (b) conditional/hypothetical language, (c) conversational formats/routines, and (d) wh-questions. Wh-questions and conversational routines reflect general properties of scaffolding, that is, properties applicable across a wide range of topics, whereas the use of temporal and conditional/hypothetical language by mothers represents scaffolding specific to TD topics.

#### Temporal Language

As might be inferred from the MLU level of the children in this study, children's contributions to TD episodes were for the most part elliptical. The burden of establishing the time-frame fell on the mother's part of the conversations. Few of the child's utterances contained verbs, and

when they did they were almost always simple present tenses, with only two instances of past-tense forms, and two each of "wanna" and "gonna" observed in these episodes. Nor were the temporal adverbials used by these children to mark future or past. One instance of "now" and one of "later" were the only such forms to appear. Thus, it is clear that the children had not yet acquired the language forms and structures appropriate for reference to past and future events. It might be, however, that TD episodes provide occasions on which children can learn the appropriate language. To that end, maternal use of language in these episodes, in particular, use of adverbial temporal markers, was examined. (Tense use by mothers would be uninformative in that mothers can be expected to use the appropriate tense form in all obligatory contexts.)

In past TD episodes the most commonly occurring lexical term was "remember," which occurred 10 times. This word may come to serve as a flag to the child that a past episode that he or she has taken part in is the topic. Mothers frequently identified specific times or dates by the use of terms such as "today" (eight times), and "last night" (seven times). They less frequently used relative markers of time. Such usage was primarily restricted to "before" (two) and "when" (three). Thus, in keeping with the observation that past talk was concerned with specific episodes, mothers identified specific times of occurrence in their talk about those episodes.

In contrast, future TD talk emphasized relative terms rather than dates. "Later" was the most common form used (10 times). Other common forms included "after" (seven), "when" (six), and "then" (five). Ways of specifying when an event would occur were varied. The most common were "tomorrow" (five), "today" (four), and "this afternoon" (three). "When" and "then" often occurred together, in phrases expressing conditionality as well as future reference.

Maternal use of such linguistic forms, before the child's being able to use them productively, reflects an important feature of scaffolding behavior. Mothers are providing a model of appropriate displaced speech, from which the child may come eventually to select what is needed to fulfill a role in discourse. In this way, such TD episodes may play an important part in the child's learning of the form of TD talk.

### Conditional/Hypothetical Language

Future events commonly have at least two characteristics. One is that they may be contingent on some factor, that is, conditions may be placed on future activity or events. Second, such activities are not always predetermined, thus affording speculation or hypothesizing about them. Just as maternal use of appropriate temporal language may provide an occasion for the child to learn aspects of the form of TD talk, so too may maternal use of language expressing conditionality or hypotheticalness provide a means for the acquisition of the form of TD talk.

Accordingly, TD episodes were examined for hypothetical and conditional expressions. In some cases, specific lexical items signal such meanings, for example, "might" or "maybe" signaling hypotheticalness, and "if-then" clauses signaling conditionality. In other cases, these meanings are formulated in larger discourse segments (e.g., "We can have an orange

after a nap."). A second coder independently rated TD episodes for the presence of such expressions, and an interrater reliability of 90% was achieved. The results of this analysis indicated that 39% (17 of 44) of future TD episodes incorporated language expressing one or both of these meanings, and in all cases the mother was the one responsible for generating the expressions. Two examples of such episodes are as follows:

*Hypothetical*
M: You could go out and play later with your jeans on.
C: And Barbara?
M: Maybe Barbara'll come and Stacey.
C: Okay.

*Conditional*
M: You have to get dressed if you wanna go out.

Maternal use of language in these ways provides a potential source of the child's understanding of and linguistic expression of hypothetical and conditional relations. Here again, maternal use of language to convey such meaning before the child's being able to fully express these meanings indicates scaffolding. Mothers are modeling appropriate form, making it available for extraction by the child for later discourse use, and in this way TD episodes may enable child acquisition of the form of TD talk.

### Conversational Formats/Routines

Conversational routines have been found to play a significant role in language acquisition. They can account, at least in part, for the acquisition of reference and requesting (Bruner, 1983), and lexical items and constructions used to talk about pictures in book-reading sessions (Snow & Goldfield, 1983). More importantly for the present research, such linguistic formats or routines have been found to facilitate the emergence of displaced reference in child speech (Sachs, 1983). To determine if they were operating here, an analysis was conducted on the extent to which mothers engaged in the "routinization" or "formatting" of TD episodes. A conversational routine was defined as the repeated reference to the same event in different episodes, that is, episodes separated by non-TD discourse or TD discourse on other activities. An example of this with reference to the past is as follows:

1. *M:* Oh the balloons.
   I got those balloons for you last night at the meeting.
2. *M:* Those (balloons) are special cause I got them just for you.
   *C:* Oh, at the meeting.
   *M:* At the meeting, that's right.

An example referring to a future event is the following:

1. *M:* Then we'll go to the club and go see Diane.
   *C:* Yeah.
2. *M:* You wanna go to the club, don't you?
3. *M:* Wanna get dressed to go to the club?
4. *M:* We're gonna go see Kevin at the club, Jimmy.
5. *M:* Where we going today, Jimmy?
   *C:* Club.
   *M:* We're going to the club?
   *C:* Yeah.

For future talk, seven mothers each showed 1 episode whose event content was repeated in 1 or more of their subsequent TD episodes, leading to a total of 23 formatted episodes. All these episodes occurred in the routine context. Thus, of 44 total future-talk episodes, more than half (52%) were formatted. For past talk, four mothers showed either one or more episodes whose event content was repeated in one or more of their subsequent TD episodes. There was a total of 16 formatted episodes. Thus, almost half (42%) of the 38 total past-talk episodes were formatted. For both past and future talk, this is a high incidence of use of such formats, especially given that the period of observation per mother was of a relatively limited duration.

Formatting displays the following characteristics of scaffolding behavior. First, such TD episodes represent linguistic routines. Second, they provide a model for the child of how to talk about events and provide information that the child can use to take part in the conversation when the topic is raised another time. Moreover, formats serve to reduce the degrees of freedom with which the child has to cope, focusing child attention into a manageable domain.

Such scaffolding appeared to be somewhat effective in supporting or eliciting child TD talk. Of the 14 original episodes whose event content was repeated in subsequent TD episodes, 3 child substantive contributions to TD talk (2 future, 1 past) occurred in the final rendition of each of the appropriate episodes.

### Wh-Questions

Mothers employed at least one wh-question in almost half (47%) of past-talk episodes, and in 28% of future-talk episodes. Thus, mothers are asking more than is being answered (see Table 4). Many of the child's substantive contributions to TD episodes involved answers to maternal wh-questions, particularly for past-talk episodes—63% for past talk and 31% for future talk. Maternal demands for such information (who, what, when, where, and how) in these accounts may and should serve to indicate to the child what elements of an event are important to talk about. Through the use of this linguistic form, mothers scaffold. Wh-questions enable the mother to reduce the degrees of freedom with which the child has to cope, and key the child into the critical elements. The following example illustrates the mothers' use of wh-questions to ascertain information essential to an activity. This episode occurred during lunch:

M: So what did you do at the Hudson School today?
C: I don't know played.
M: You played?
C: Yes.
M: Who did you play with?
C: I don't know Steven.

Wh-questions scaffold also by imposing a model organization on TD descriptions, an organization adopted by the child through limited responding to these questions, and an organization that the child may come spontaneously to impose on his or her own future accounts by providing statements containing such information (see Eisenberg, 1985, for similar proposals about the relation between adult and child TD talk).

### General scaffolding techniques and child contributions to TD episodes

The data on maternal wh-questions and conversational formats indicate that moth-ers are engaging in the scaffolding of TD talk to a substantial degree. To obtain an overall picture of the effectiveness of scaffolding for the child's learning of TD talk, it was determined how many child substantive contributions could be attributed to scaffolding by virtue of being answers to wh-questions or by virtue of occurring within formatted episodes.

For past talk, 11 of 16 (69%) of child substantive contributions were attributable to scaffolding. For future talk, 5 of 13 (39%) of child substantive contributions were accounted for by scaffolding. These findings indicate that maternal scaffolding plays a significant role in supporting past TD talk by children, and is fairly effective in supporting their future TD talk. Wh-questions appear to be the more effective scaffolding technique; however, the facilitative effects of formatting in general may not be fully seen in nonlongitudinal designs. The work of Sachs (1983) has shown that conversational routines on TD topics are often established and elaborated over the course of several months.

## IMPLICATIONS FOR THE LANGUAGE CLINICIAN

The present study holds some implications for language specialists. These implications lie in two areas: assessment and

---

*The data on maternal wh-questions and conversational formats indicate that mothers are engaging in the scaffolding of TD talk to a substantial degree.*

intervention/training. Each of these will be discussed in turn.

## Assessment

Two factors require consideration in the achievement of accurate assessment: how to assess, and what to assess.

First, with regard to the "how" of assessment, the study reported here highlights the important contribution of the child's cognitive system to the language acquisition process. The manifestation of linguistic skills was context-sensitive. Children showed displaced speech almost exclusively in one context, the routine/ scripted one, although they were observed in two others as well. This context was a familiar one, that is, one for which children had knowledge.

There is considerable research showing that the display of both linguistic and cognitive skills is contextually dependent. In contexts that are meaningful to the child, cognitive and linguistic behaviors, absent in other less familiar situations, often emerge. For example, additional analyses of the present database revealed that conversational behavior was richest, in terms of length and complexity of topic, in the scripted context (Lucariello, Kyratzis, & Engel, 1986). Moreover, one of the most important triggers for the revision of Piagetian theory was the finding that the manifestation of logical ability was highly contingent on context. Children considered too cognitively immature to show such abilities did so when tested in known, hence meaningful, contexts (see for example Donaldson, 1978).

Quite importantly, in the present case, the context in which children showed more advanced language, as indexed by TD speech, was not the one highly typical of language research in general. That is, to a large extent, language research is conducted in the laboratory, using a free-play situation. However, in the present investigation, reliance on the free-play context alone would have led to a misassessment of child linguistic ability with regard to displaced reference as well as other linguistic behaviors. Important and advanced linguistic behaviors emerged almost exclusively in the routine/scripted context. A reliance on the free-play setting alone would have led to missing emerging linguistic skills, such as displaced speech and complex conversational ability.

This state of affairs prompts two suggestions for assessment. One is the use of multiple means for assessing any given ability. This may entail the use of multiple observational contexts, multiple tests or scales, or multiple methods. Second, when selection of the means for assessment is made, the selection process should be guided by a rationale for why specific child behaviors might or might not be manifested in any given context. For this rationale to lead to a successful outcome, it must take into account the knowledge of the child.

In terms of what to assess, the present research targets an important aspect of intellectual functioning, rooted in the ZPD principle. The ZPD is based on the premise that a more informative assessment of child ability may be garnered when there is measurement of what the child can accomplish with the help of others rather than what can be accomplished independently. That is, children may vary in the extent to which they can benefit from aids or avail themselves of help. Hence, there is a need for dynamic, as well as static, measures of child ability. In the present study, child language was observed as it occurred in interaction with the mother. These children were able to take advantage of the instructional nature of maternal speech to some degree. A similar situation is found in the work of Brown and Ferrara (1985). They demonstrated that an "inter/psychological learning score" (consisting of the number of hints needed to solve IQ problems that could not be solved independently) provided considerably more information on grade-schoolers' cognitive ability than did the standard IQ score alone.

Hence, an important facet of child intellectual functioning is the ability to be boosted. In assessing child language ability, it is important to assess this aspect of cognitive functioning. Moreover, such an assessment could be of great significance in the formulation and modification of instructional techniques.

## Intervention/training

The data reported earlier in this article suggest that language acquisition may indeed have a social-interactive base. Mothers were highly involved in the child's learning of TD talk. An examination of maternal speech shows such language to exhibit some important characteristics of instruction or training. There are three very striking features.

One pertains to the relation between instruction and development. Vygotsky (1978) has proposed that instruction should be ahead of development; that is, it should serve an awakening function for cognitive processes that have not yet matured. In Vygotsky's view, training ought to be directed at the buds instead of the fruits of development. For example, Vygotsky (1978) was critical of contemporaneous educational plans for the retarded. On the assumption that retarded children could not engage in abstract thinking, curricula employed concrete, look-and-do methods. Vygotsky argued that such methods not only failed to aid retarded children in overcoming their handicaps, but actually reinforced these handicaps by accustoming children exclusively to concrete thinking, and suppressing rudiments of any abstract thought.

In the present case, child talk was predominantly bound to the here-and-now. Primarily through maternal initiative, displaced topics were introduced. Even then, however, children were often weak contributors. Yet mothers engage in displaced speech. Hence, their use of semantic and syntactic devices is not restricted to the child's current level of expertise, but is aimed at the child's potential level of expertise. This proved facilitative of child TD speech, and such an alignment between teacher and learner has proved beneficial in other situations as well. For example, Palincsar and Brown (1984) have shown the beneficial effects of tutoring aimed toward the upper-bound (i.e., the level of competence that can be achieved under the most favorable circumstances), with children characterized by severe reading comprehension problems.

An additional characteristic of maternal speech, and one that would appear important for instruction in general, is its scaffolded quality. Mothers observed here were speaking about the nonpresent in a highly fashioned way, with their talk exhibiting certain properties. They focused the child's attention, that is, reduced the degrees of freedom with which the child had to cope. This was accomplished primarily through the use of formatting and wh-questions. They modeled appropriate speech forms through the use of temporal and conditional and hypothetical language. They imposed the appropriate organization on the speech through the use of wh-questions and formatting. Scaffolding was effective here, and, as noted earlier, scaffolding has been found to play a role in the acquisition of other linguistic behaviors such as reference and requesting (Bruner, 1983).

Finally, context-sensitivity was another key feature of the maternal language observed here, and this feature, as the others, has implications for instruction. Mothers introduced displaced speech selectively, not randomly. They engaged in such talk in the contexts that were highly familiar to their children. Mothers, like clinicians, have an opportunity in familiar situational activities to move beyond the here-and-now uses of language, because organization of the ongoing scene is already established and understood through the event representation.

There is evidence to suggest that the acquisition of many linguistic behaviors occurs in a contextually constrained way, with forms acquired in specific contexts, and their use restricted to those contexts before being generalized. For example, this occurs with the acquisition of first words (see Nelson & Lucariello, 1985, for review), relational terms (French, 1986), and many lexical items and constructions pertaining to the reading of picture-books

(Snow & Goldfield, 1983). If language acquisition proceeds in a contextually bound way, then to the extent that instruction is context-sensitive, it will facilitate acquisition and use. Hence, an attunement is required between training and the contexts in which training occurs. For example, in the case of language skills on the verge of emergence, a good match might consist in training in contexts where the to-be-learned items are most likely to appear, hence facilitating acquisition. Once a skill has made a breakthrough, however, training might better be undertaken in contexts where the newly learned items have not yet appeared, hence facilitating generalization.

•   •   •

Talk about the nonpresent, or TD speech, is one of the most important features of linguistic communication. The present research showed TD talk to have a cognitive basis, in that event knowledge had an effect on where such talk occurred and what it was about. TD talk occurred in routine, familiar contexts and was often about routine, familiar activities. Such talk was also found to have a social-interactive basis. How it occurred was a result of maternal scaffolding. Mothers' speech was found to be structured, to model appropriate linguistic forms, and to focus the child's attention.

The results showing context-dependency in the occurrence of TD speech have important implications for assessment. Context-sensitivity may be a significant feature of accurate assessment. The findings describing the properties of maternal speech have import for assessment and intervention. Maternal speech served to lead the child into TD speech, and this finding points to the importance of dynamic measures in assessing intellectual functioning (i.e., measures that take into account what the child can do with more competent others). Moreover, the scaffolded quality of maternal speech may represent, at least in part, the properties that characterize successful intervention.

## REFERENCES

Brown, A., & Ferrara, R. (1985). Diagnosing zones of proximal development. In J. Wertsch (Ed.), *Culture, communication, and cognition: Vygotskian perspectives*. Cambridge, England: Cambridge University Press.

Bruner, J. (1978). The role of dialogue in language acquisition. In A. Sinclair, R. Jarvella, & W. Levelt (Eds.), *The child's conception of language*. New York, NY: Springer-Verlag.

Bruner, J. (1983). *Child's talk*. New York, NY: Norton.

Donaldson, M. (1978). *Children's minds*. New York, NY: Norton.

Eisenberg, A. (1985). Learning to describe past experiences in conversation. *Discourse Processes, 8*, 177–204.

Fein, G. (1981). Pretend play in childhood: An integrative review. *Child Development, 52*, 1095–1118.

French, L. (1986). The language of events. In K. Nelson (Ed.), *Event knowledge: Structure and function in development*. Hillsdale, NJ: Erlbaum.

Lucariello, J., Kyratzis, A., & Engel, S. (1986). Event representations, context, and language. In K. Nelson (Ed.), *Event knowledge: Structure and function in development*. Hillsdale, NJ: Erlbaum.

Nelson, K., Fivush, R., Hudson, J., & Lucariello, J. (1983). Scripts and the development of memory. In M. Chi (Ed.), J.A. Meacham (Series Ed.), *Contributions to Human Development. Vol. 9 Trends in Memory Development Research*. Basel, Switzerland: Karger.

Nelson, K., & Gruendel, J. (1981). Generalized event representations: Basic building blocks of cognitive development. In A. Brown & M. Lamb (Eds.), *Advances in developmental psychology* (Vol. 1). Hillsdale, NJ: Erlbaum.

Nelson, K., & Lucariello, J. (1985). The development of meaning in first words. In M. Barrett (Ed.), *Children's single-word speech*. Chichester, England: Wiley.

Palincsar, A., & Brown, A. (1984). Reciprocal teaching of comprehension-fostering and monitoring activities. *Cognition and instruction*. Hillsdale, NJ: Erlbaum.

Sachs, J. (1983). Talking about the there and then: The emergence of displaced reference in parent-child discourse. In K. Nelson (Ed.), *Children's language* (Vol. 4). Hillsdale, NJ: Erlbaum.

Shatz, M. (1978). The relationship between cognitive processes and the development of communication skills. In C.B. Keasey (Ed.), *Nebraska symposium on motivation* (Vol. 25). Lincoln, NE: University of Nebraska Press.

Shatz, M. (1983). Communication. In J.H. Flavell & E.M. Markman (Eds.), P.H. Mussen (Series Ed.), *Handbook of child psychology: Vol. 3. Cognitive Development* (4th ed.). New York: Wiley.

Snow, C., & Goldfield, B. (1983). Turn the page please: Situation-specific language acquisition. *Journal of Child Language, 10*, 551–569.

Vygotsky, L. (1978). *Mind in society*. Cambridge, MA: Harvard University Press.

# Language sampling for repeated measures with language-impaired preschoolers: Comparison of two procedures

**Barbara A. Bain, PhD**
Professor
Department of Speech Pathology and
    Audiology
Idaho State University
Pocatello, Idaho

**Lesley B. Olswang, PhD**
Professor
Department of Speech and Hearing
    Sciences
University of Washington

**Glenn A. Johnson, MA**
Research Assistant
Department of Speech and Hearing
    Sciences
University of Washington
Seattle, Washington

## INTRODUCTION

The focus of this article is on sampling the language of young children enrolled in intervention for the purposes of documenting behavior change and evaluating treatment efficacy over time. Limitations of standardized assessment procedures are significant and lead to the conclusion that although they may be useful for documenting global change in behavior, they are not the best tools for obtaining frequent, repeated measurements regarding the effects of intervention (Bain & Dollaghan, 1991; McCauley & Swisher, 1984). Consequently, speech-language pathologists (SLPs) typically utilize conversational sampling to quantify language-impaired children's performance of specific language behaviors over time. This article will focus on sampling early semantic productions.

This article was supported in part by the NINCD Grant R29-DC00431 "Predicting the Benefits of Treatment." The authors wish to thank Pamela Crooke for her design of the graphs.

Top Lang Disord, 1992,12(2),13–27

Language sampling may appear to be a relatively straightforward task, but it is not. The complexity lies in the need to ensure adequate sampling of language behaviors over time. The goal is to obtain a rich enough sample of a child's language to determine whether growth has occurred. This goal requires that the language-measurement task ensure opportunities for sampling a variety of behaviors that are representative of the language-impaired child's habitual performance while minimizing adult support and guidance. Further, because documenting behavior change and evaluating treatment efficacy require longitudinal sampling, the task must be one that can be repeated over time yet remain sensitive to differential changes in behavior that occur during the intervention process.

To evaluate the efficacy of intervention designed to alter specific behaviors, the sample must contain opportunities for observing both the treated (or target) behaviors and untreated behaviors. Untreated behaviors include those that are expected to change as a result of change in the target behavior (i.e., generalization behaviors), and those not expected to change (i.e., control behaviors) (Bain & Dollaghan, 1991; Fey, 1986). Documenting a differential performance in the acquisition of target and generalization behaviors versus control behaviors allows the SLP to begin attributing change to treatment rather than to maturation or other extraneous factors as noted elsewhere in this issue.

Creating an effective language-sampling task requires consideration of the influence of context on language performance. Considerable research exists describing the many ways in which context can influence young children's language performance. Setting (home vs. clinic), person (parents vs. clinicians), situation (structured vs. unstructured, predictable vs. unpredictable), and materials (familiar vs. unfamiliar) are but a few variables that have been documented as influencing language performance. (For reviews of this literature, see Coggins, 1990; Gallagher, 1983; Lund & Duchan, 1988.)

When considering the influence of context on sampling preschool children's early multi-word utterances, one variable of primary significance is the situation. Situation, in this case, will be defined by two particular parameters: (1) structure and (2) predictability. Structure refers to the amount of adult input guiding the manipulation of materials and evoking particular utterances from a child. Predictability refers to the familiarity of the tasks and materials.

If structure and predictability were considered on a continuum from high to low, the high end would consist of a context in which a set of familiar materials are presented by the SLP in a specified, routine, predictable order, evoking particular verbal and nonverbal behaviors from the child. Materials and their manipulation are familiar. They may comprise a joint action routine (JAR; Snyder-McLean, Solomonson, McLean, & Sack 1984) between the child and the adult. Snyder-McLean et al. (1984) defined JAR as "a ritualized interaction pattern, involving joint action, unified by a specific theme or goal, which follows a logical sequence, including a clear beginning point, and in which each participant plays a recognized role, with specific response expectancies, that is essential to the successful completion of that sequence" (p. 214). The lower end of the continuum would include contexts in which the SLP exerts less direct control over materials and child behaviors. The SLP might remain in charge of introducing materials, but allow the child to dictate the pacing and manipulation. In this type of situation, the child is "more in charge;" the adult maintains some order, but clearly follows the child's lead. Materials might change each session, and neither the child nor adult have particular expectations about what materials will be used or the ways in which the materials will be manipulated. Any theme that develops in the manipulation of the toys is dictated by the child's play behaviors.

When designing a conversational language-sampling measurement task to document behavior change and evaluate treatment efficacy, the structure and predictability of the situation can be manipulated in a variety of ways along the continuum in order to obtain an adequate sample with a sufficient quantity and diversity of productions. Quantity refers to the frequency of occurrence of behaviors, and diversity refers to the variety of these behaviors.

The influence of situational structure on sampling young children's production of the possessor + possession semantic relation was examined by Landa and Olswang (1988). In the structured condition, the clinician evoked the target semantic relation using elicitation questions (e.g., *Whose is this?*) and sentence completion tasks (e.g., *This is Bob's hat and this is _____[Mary's coat].*). The unstructured condition contained naturalistic opportunities to sample the target semantic relation; the clinician followed the child's lead

rather than setting up preplanned opportunities for particular productions. The results indicated that the children produced a greater quantity and diversity of possessive constructions in the structured condition than in the unstructured condition, with no difference occurring between the two elicitation procedures in the structured condition. These findings are consistent with other research on young children's productions of semantic relations and communicative intentions, suggesting that the amount of situational structure can differentially influence verbal output (Coggins, Olswang, & Guthrie, 1987; Scott, Palin, & Davidson, 1979).

Predictability of the sampling situation may also influence young children's verbal output. Data on normal language development suggest that children use new forms in structured, highly predictable contexts before using them in less predictable contexts (Nelson, 1986; Ratner & Bruner, 1978; Snyder-McLean et al., 1984). This might be explained from a resource allocation perspective, in which the child is seen as having more resources for the verbal/linguistic task because of the relative ease of processing the familiar nonverbal context.

As part of a larger research project designed to examine the benefits of treatment for specific language-impaired (SLI) children who are learning to produce two-word utterances, language behaviors have been sampled under two conditions reflecting varying amounts of structure and predictability. The question of interest is as follows: Is there a significant difference between two sampling techniques for the production of semantic relations by SLI preschool children? Clinicians are clearly advised not to rely on the chance occurrence of opportunities for behaviors to be sampled, but how far do they need to go in their planning of the sampling situation?

## METHODS

### Subjects

Subjects were 6 children, ages 31 to 35 months who had been referred by parents, SLPs, physicians, and other health-related professionals in the Seattle, Washington, area because of concerns regarding their language development. All 6 children, 4 boys and 2 girls, were diagnosed as having specific language impairments by a certified SLP and met the following criteria: Normal motor, adaptive, and personal-social development (Boyd Developmental Scale, Boyd, 1974); normal intelligence (between plus and minus 1 standard deviation of the mean for children of a comparable chronological age on the Stanford-Binet Test of Intelligence-Fourth Edition, Thorndike, Hagen, & Sattler, 1986, and the Kaufman Assessment Battery for Children, Kaufman & Kaufman, 1983); normal hearing acuity (responding to puretone threshold testing consisting of pure tones presented at 500, 1k, 2k, and 4k at 20 dB HL or better, and to speech presented at 20 dB HL or better, in both ears); adequate oral structures and functions; phonological repertoires of a variety of vowels and at least 10 different consonants; and normal receptive skills [Sequenced Inventory of Communication Development (SICD), Hedrick, Prather, & Tobin, 1984, or the Peabody Picture Vocabulary Test-Revised (PPVT), Dunn & Dunn, 1981]. On the SICD, all subjects obtained an expressive communication age (ECA) approximately 1 year delayed of chronological age (CA) and demonstrated a receptive–expressive language gap of at least 6 months. In addition, all subjects demonstrated expressive language abilities primarily at the one-word level by having mean lengths of utterances in morphemes (MLUs) between 1 and 1.5, producing at least 50 different single words and producing no two-word semantic relations in a 30-minute language sample. Some subjects produced two-word functional relations, but none of the subjects produced any of the two-word semantic relations listed and defined in Table 1. Table 2 contains descriptive information on each subject.

### Procedures

The experiment had three phases: (1) baseline, (2) treatment, and (3) withdrawal. The first phase consisted of baseline in which language performance was monitored once a week prior to the initiation of treatment for a 3-week period. The second phase consisted of a treatment phase in which language performance was monitored once a week for a 3-week period while the children received individual therapy. The third phase consisted of a withdrawal phase in which the children's expressive language continued to be monitored weekly for 3 weeks after treatment had been terminated.

During the treatment phase, the subjects received individual therapy with an American Speech-Language-Hearing Association (ASHA)-certified SLP targeting a specific two-word semantic relation, either agent + action or possessor + possession. Targets were randomly assigned to each subject. Each child received three 30 to

**Table 1.**  Definition of semantic relations

| Semantic relations | Definition | Example |
|---|---|---|
| Agent + action | Typically marks an animate instigator of an action; "someone or something which is perceived to have its own motivating force and to cause an action or process" (Brown, 1973, p. 193). Action involves observed movement, but can also refer to attention as initiated by an animate being and includes verbs of notice. | *Mommy eat* *Chair fly* |
| Action + object | Marks an object as defined by Brown (1973) as "someone or something (usually something inanimate) either suffering a change of state or simply receiving the force of an action" . . . (p. 193) also refer to attention to a person, object or event, using a verb of notice. | *Push car* *See sock* |
| Possessor + possession | Associates persons with the things they habitually wear, use, etc. (Edwards, 1974) | *Daddy coat* |
| Entity + attribute | Specifies some attribute of an entity that could not be known from the class characteristics alone. | *Big dog* *Yellow bird* |
| Entity + locative | Marks the spatial position or orientation of an object | *Ball table* *Baby bed* |
| Action + locative | Marks the spatial orientation of an action, referring to movement of an object or person toward or away from a particular position. | *Where go* *Fly air* |

45-minute, individual therapy sessions each week over a 3-week period for a total of nine therapy sessions. Treatment consisted of providing each subject with 40 to 60 opportunities to produce the target behavior in a JAR that had been devised especially for treatment. Two JARs for each target were developed that supported the production of the targeted semantic relation. The same JARs were provided to subjects with the same semantic-relation targets.

In order to measure treatment efficacy, the subjects were also seen once a week, on a nontreatment day, by a second ASHA-certified clinician who was different from the clinician who provided therapy. During this weekly session, two different sampling procedures, a free-play situation and a JAR, which differed from the one used in treatment, were utilized to monitor the children's production of multiword utterances in conversational speech over time. These two procedures were employed throughout the baseline, treatment, and withdrawal phases of the experiment. The order of presentation for administering the two sampling procedures was counterbalanced across the 9 weeks. The clinician had been trained in criteria for implementing the two sampling procedures.

Both the free-play and the JAR sampling procedures were designed to provide the subjects with a minimum of 10 opportunities to produce each of six different semantic relations, agent + action (AGAC), action + object (ACO), possessor + possession (PP), entity + attribute (EA), entity + locative (EL), and action + locative (AL), for a total of 60 different opportunities. These relations are defined in Table 1. The six semantic relations were

**Table 2.** Subject description

| Subject | Chronological age months | Sex | PPVT* Percentile | KABC† Percentile | SICD‡ | | MLU¶ |
| | | | | | RCA§ months | ECA‖ months | |
|---|---|---|---|---|---|---|---|
| 1 | 32 | M | 66 | 61 | 36 | 20 | 1.00 |
| 2 | 32 | M | 78 | 73 | 36 | 20 | 1.01 |
| 3 | 35 | M | 24 | 55 | 32 | 20 | 1.07 |
| 4 | 31 | F | 48 | 45 | 32 | 20 | 1.02 |
| 5 | 31 | M | 60 | 61 | 32 | 20 | 1.07 |
| 6 | 32 | F | 87 | 98 | 40 | 24 | 1.13 |

*PPVT = Peabody Picture Vocabulary Test: revised (Form L).
†KABC = Kaufman Assessment Battery for Children—composite score.
‡SICD = Sequenced Inventory of Communication Development.
§RCA = receptive communication age.
‖ECA = expressive communication age.
¶MLU = mean length of utterance in morphemes.

grouped into two categories for analytical purposes, based on their apparent logical relationships. Each category consisted of one of the two semantic relations (AGAC, PP) alternated across subjects as the treatment target, and two generalization categories. Logically, action relations consisted of AGAC, ACO, and ACL. Static relations consisted of PP, EA, and EL. Therefore, when AGAC was the targeted semantic relation, ACL and ACO were considered generalization categories. When PP was targeted, EA and EL were used as generalization categories. Thus, for each child, three categories served as the treatment semantic relations (one target and two generalization categories), and the three remaining semantic relations served as controls.

### Free-play procedure

The free-play sampling procedure was designed to be relatively low with regard to structure and predictability. The clini-cian was to follow the subject's interest in materials and activities. The free-play procedure was designed to provide 10 opportunities for each of the six semantic relations in approximately 25 to 30 minutes. Opportunities were judged to have occurred if a subject or the clinician manipulated toys and objects supportive of a specific linguistic structure. For example, if a subject walked a horse, an opportunity for agent + action (horse walk) was assumed to have occurred. In addition, a subject's spontaneous productions were counted as opportunities.

The free-play procedure was designed to be low with regard to predictability in at least two ways. First, because the clinician primarily followed the subject's lead, activities varied from session to session. Second, a different box of toys and materials was used each session, although every box contained materials that supported 10 opportunities for the production of the six semantic relations. Corresponding to the different materials used each session, the opportunities consisted of different lexical items each session. Thus, the subjects could not predict from one session to the next which activities or materials would be employed to provide the opportunities for the different semantic relations.

### JAR procedure

In contrast to the free-play procedure, the JAR sampling procedure was designed to be highly structured and predictable. A routine designed to make/build an animal was devised that supported 10 opportunities for each of the six semantic relations. Prior to obtaining a language sample using the JAR procedure during baseline, the clinician assessed comprehension of the lexical items that occurred during the making/building JAR. Items that were apparently not known by the subject were taught. Consistent lexical items for the specific opportunities occurred during all nine sessions. For example, 1 of the 10 opportunities for action + object was *button shirt*, and the subjects encountered this same opportunity during each of the nine measurement sessions. All 60 opportunities for production of the semantic relations were specified with regard to the way the context was manipulated and for lexical items to be produced.

The JAR was constructed such that three core routines or general episodes occurred each session. The first episode involved the clinician and subject "getting ready" to make the animal. The subject and the clinician took materials and supplies from the cabinet, put on their art garments, and so forth. During the second episode, they made an animal. The specific

animal differed each week; for example, a turtle was constructed 1 week, and a lion was constructed during another week. The third episode consisted of playing with the animal in a set format by having the animal dance, laugh, and so forth as the clinician and subject cleaned up and put materials away.

The JAR was considered to be highly structured because the same general activities occurred each week. This resulted in a highly predictable situation for the subjects with regard to the activities that occurred and the materials used during the session. For example, each week the clinician and subject gathered materials from a cabinet, cut paper, glued paper to make an animal, put trash in the garbage, and washed their hands. Table 3 contains a few of the core episodes and specific semantic opportunities that occurred in the sampling JAR.

As would be expected, the clinician assumed an active role during the JAR. Although the clinician varied the antecedents across the measurement sessions, a minimum of one cue was provided for each specific linguistic structure opportunity unless the subject spontaneously produced the target item. Attending to an opportunity was an important part of the JAR. Attending was defined as both the subject and the clinician looking at the appropriate objects, pictures, activity, and so forth. If the subject was distracted, the clinician refocused the subject's attention and presented another cue to provide an additional opportunity to produce the linguistic structure. Up to three cues could be presented for each opportunity.

The clinician's role during both sampling procedures was to provide realistic

**Table 3.** Segment from joint action routine

| Context | Episode | Acts | Goal act |
|---|---|---|---|
| Making/building | Setting up | Child hangs up coat and sits | Coat on hook, EL |
| | | | Child sits in chair, AL |
| | | | Buckle backpack, AO |
| | | Child gets bear out of box | Bear eye, PP |
| | | | (Bear) walk to chair, AL |
| | | | Bear jumps, AA |
| | | Child gets Bert out of box | (Bert) knocks on door, AL |
| | | | Closet's door, PP |
| | | | Look in closet, AL |
| | | Child gets out materials from closet | Paper on shelf, EL |

*Note.* PP = possessor + possession; EA = entity + attribute; EL = entity + locative; AA = agent + action; AL = action + locative; AO = action + object.

interactional opportunities that promoted the subjects' production of target and control linguistic structures in a naturalistic manner. Both procedures had similarities. When implementing the two procedures, the clinician provided a variety of antecedents to provide the opportunities for target responses: general attention (e.g., *Oh lookit*), elicitation question (e.g., *What is going to happen?*), cloze procedure or sentence completion (e.g., *This is _____[Ernie's shirt]*), and setting up of the context (e.g., *It's time to go. Tell me what to do.* [Open door.]). The clinician did not model two-word semantic relations during either procedure and was discouraged from modeling target words used in therapy. If the subject produced multiword utterances, the examiner acknowledged the response but did not reinforce or expand the production.

### Data reduction and coding

In order to complete data analysis, all sessions were video recorded. The clinician conducting the free-play and JAR sampling procedures transcribed the subjects' utterances orthographically from the videotape and entered them into a computer. Adult utterances were also entered to provide context to aid in coding. Each child utterance was then coded according to the semantic relation expressed. Utterances of more than two words were coded for all of the semantic relations that were expressed. For example, if the subject said *big boy hit*, the utterance was coded as consisting of the semantic relations entity + attribute and agent + action. Utterances that the clinician was unable to understand or code were designated as being "deviant" and later viewed with a second observer to resolve glossing and coding. Transcripts were searched for all nonimitated types (different two-word combinations) and tokens (total two-word combinations) for semantic relations using Systematic Analysis of Language Transcript (SALT) searches (Miller & Chapman, 1984). The semantic relations included agent + action, action + object, possessor + possession, entity + attribute, entity + locative, and action + locative in addition to others (Brown, 1973).

### Reliability

One third of the subjects (2) and one third of the sessions were randomly selected, with the restriction that a session must be selected from the baseline, treatment, and withdrawal phases to assess interobserver reliability. Measurement reliability was conducted for two tasks: (1) segmenting/glossing the utterances and (2) coding the utterances. A Cohen's Kappa (Cohen, 1960) was calculated for segmenting/glossing utterances into one-, two-, and three- or more word utterances and for coding the semantic relations. Kappas for segmenting/glossing ranged from .7 to .89 for the six JAR conditions and ranged from .91 to .98 for the six free-play conditions. The Kappas for coding the semantic relations ranged from .88 to 1.0 for the six sessions in the JAR and from .8 to .9 in the free-play condition. Thus, interobserver reliability for glossing/segmenting and coding was judged to be acceptable, because Kappas met the criterion of .7 or better as established by Bowers and Courtright (1984).

### Data analysis

The dependent measures consisted of the tokens and types of each child's production of semantic relations, in the two elicitation contexts (free play vs. JAR) during baseline, treatment, and withdrawal phases of this study. Data were analyzed in terms of frequency counts. Data for group analysis were obtained from the JAR and free-play sampling conditions at three different points in time:

during Week 3 of baseline (BL/3), during Week 3 of treatment (Tx/3), and during Week 3 of withdrawal (WD/3). These were selected for analysis because they represented each child's most productive and habituated use of language under the baseline and treatment conditions, and most represented habitual productivity after withdrawal of treatment. Data for the individual analysis were based on 3 individual subjects who responded differentially to treatment. The 3 subjects selected were representative of children in the larger study who showed limited (Subject 2), moderate (Subject 3), and large (Subject 4) treatment effects. These data, number of different multiword combinations, were collected weekly across the three experimental phases: three during baseline, three during treatment, and three during withdrawal.

## RESULTS

The results will be presented in two sections, (1) group data and (2) individual data. Both types of analyses addressed the research question of interest: Is there a difference between free-play and JAR sampling techniques for the production of semantic relations by SLI preschool children over time?

### Group analysis

The first group analysis examined the production of tokens (total number of occurrences) of semantic relations produced during each of the two sampling conditions, free play and JARs. The data are presented in Figure 1. The graph includes the total number of tokens for

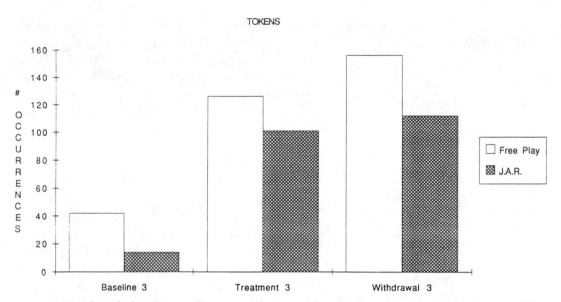

**Figure 1.** Number of token two-word semantic relations produced in free-play and joint action routine (JAR) sampling contexts by 6 children during the third week of baseline, the third week of treatment, and the third week of withdrawal from treatment.

multiword semantic relations for all 6 subjects produced during BL/3, during Tx/3, and during WD/3. The results indicate subjects consistently produced more tokens of semantic relations in the free-play sampling condition than in the JAR sampling condition at the three time periods. Further, the number of occurrences in both sampling conditions increased over the three time periods with the least frequent production of semantic relations occurring during baseline and the most frequent production occurring during the withdrawal phase.

The second group analysis examined the production of types (number of different occurrences) of semantic relations in multiword utterances in the two sampling conditions. These data are presented in Figure 2. The graph includes the total number of different types of multiword semantic relations for all 6 subjects during

the three time periods. As with the tokens, the subjects consistently produced more types of semantic relations in the free-play sampling condition than in the JAR sampling condition at BL/3, Tx/3, and WD/3. Further, the number of occurrences for types of semantic relations in both sampling conditions increased over the three time periods with the least frequent production of semantic relations occurring during baseline and the most frequent production occurring during the withdrawal phase.

### Individual analysis

Figure 3 contains data from 3 individual children who responded differentially to treatment. The data presented in Figure 3 represent the number of different semantic relations in multiword utterances produced by 3 of the 6 subjects reported above; these are labeled in Figure 3 as

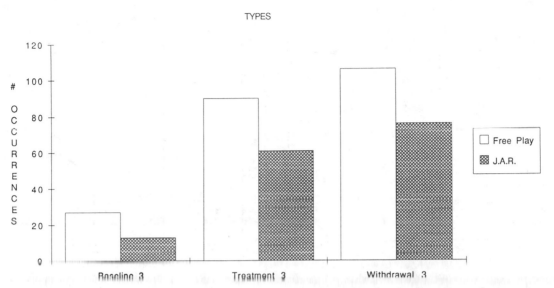

**Figure 2.** Number of types (different) of two-word semantic relations produced in free-play and joint action routine (JAR) sampling contexts by 6 children during the third week of baseline, the third week of treatment, and the third week of withdrawal from treatment.

two-word combinations. The 3 subjects selected were representative of children in the larger study who showed limited (Subject 2), moderate (Subject 3) and large (Subject 4) treatment effects. The different responses to treatment are evident in the treatment and withdrawal phases. All 3 subjects demonstrated relatively stable performance during the baseline periods, although a slight upward trend was noted for Subject 3. Furthermore, the production of different two-word semantic relations in multiword utterances was consistent across both sampling procedures (JAR and free play) during the baseline phase.

Subject 2 showed limited response to treatment, as the production of different two-word combinations returned to the baseline level during the withdrawal phase. Although he produced a slightly greater number of different two-word combinations in the free-play context than in the JAR context during the treatment phase,

the difference between the two conditions was judged to be clinically insignificant.

Subject 3 showed a moderate response to treatment, as the production of different two-word combinations increased slightly during treatment and continued to increase slightly during the withdrawal phase. Subject 3 produced a greater number of different two-word combinations in the JAR than in the free-play condition during the treatment and withdrawal phases.

Subject 4 appeared to be very responsive to treatment, as an increase in different two-word combinations was noted during the treatment phase, and the production of two-word combinations continued to increase after treatment was withdrawn. Subject 4 produced a greater number of two-word combinations during the free-play procedure than during the JAR, especially during the withdrawal phase.

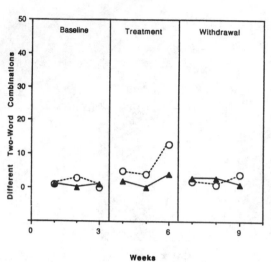

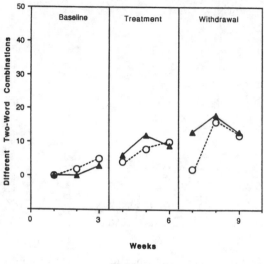

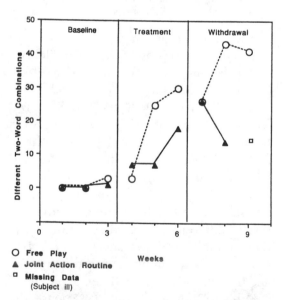

**Figure 3.** Number of types (different) of two-word combinations produced in free-play and joint action routine (JAR) sampling contexts by 3 children who showed limited (Subject 2), moderate (Subject 3), and large (Subject 4) treatment effects.

In summary, the detailed presentation of the production of two-word combinations for 3 subjects in the free-play and JAR conditions indicated slightly different profiles during the treatment and withdrawal phases. None of the subjects produced more two-word utterances in either

sampling condition during the baseline phase.

## DISCUSSION

The results of this investigation suggest that SLI preschool children produce a greater frequency and diversity of multi-word utterances in the free-play sampling situation than in the JAR sampling situation. These findings clearly cast in a new light the hypothesis that new forms would emerge first in the structured, predictable JAR situation, at least for the SLI population. Although the data presented a clear and consistent trend across the three time periods, they are considered preliminary in that statistical significance is unknown.

There are several possible explanations for these results. First, the two sampling situations may not have been as perceptibly different as they were intended to be. Although the free-play situation was composed of materials not presented in order by the clinician, each box contained not only unrelated items, but also items that could be manipulated in a thematic way (e.g., tea set, doll house, school house, hospital, farm, etc.). Thus, each box of materials allowed for the creation of a theme, or routine, if desired by the child. The clinician's involvement each session included initially offering the child a box of toys, controlling the flow of objects during the 30 minutes while providing the 60 opportunities for two-word productions, and replacing the toys in the box at the end of the allotted time. Therefore, the free-play condition may have contained a somewhat routinized sequence of events, including the child's thematic play and the clinician's structure. Thus, the real differences between the two conditions may have been the variety of materials (more in the free play than in the JAR) and the specific way in which the materials were manipulated (unpredictable in the free play and highly predictable in the JAR). For these 6 children, these differences

may have been sufficient to encourage them to produce a greater frequency and diversity of multiword semantic relations in the free-play situation over time.

A second possible explanation for the greater production in the free-play condition concerns the variability in the children's involvement in the JAR. Anecdotally, the children appeared differentially interested in the JAR. Although they all clearly participated in the entire routine, they seemed to show preferences and varying degrees of involvement in the different episodes and specific activities (e.g., cutting, pasting, painting, coloring, cleaning up, etc.). Thus, the JAR situation may not have been as appealing *overall* as the free play.

A third issue that may be of significance in explaining the results addresses the pragmatic differences inherent in the two contexts. By definition, the repeated JAR develops over time, resulting in familiar topics of conversation between the child and adult. The semantics and the pragmatics of the situation remain constant, and speaker/listener knowledge about the content is common. In such a context, a child, particularly one with limited resource allocation in terms of language abilities, may be able to assume that a great deal of situational information is known by the adult listener, and does not need to be encoded. By contrast, the free-play situation is defined by unplanned manipulation of novel materials each week. Assumptions about topics and specific content cannot be made by the child. Encoding information to elicit the involvement of the adult may become more of a necessity. Thus, in terms of an "informativeness principle," time may play against a particular JAR in terms of the child's need to encode linguistically his or her activities, ideas, and/or messages.

The present results suggest that in sampling the language of SLI preschool children to document treatment effects, it is important to impose enough structure on the context to ensure sufficient sampling of the behaviors of interest. However, extraordinary efforts to impose structure and familiarity may not be necessary. Methodologically, the free-play situation in this study was structured, in that a specified number of opportunities was provided for each two-word utterance of interest. Opportunities included not only nonlinguistic situational cues (i.e., manipulation of materials), but also linguistic cues (i.e., *Oh lookit* or *What's going to happen?*) to evoke

verbal responses from the child. An ideal language-sampling context appears to be one that allows a sufficient number of such opportunities for a child to produce the behaviors of interest. Although predictability may be less important to manipulate, the clinician must be cognizant of the materials that are available and the ways in which they can be manipulated to provide opportunities for verbalization. Clinicians need not focus on creating special events and episodes, but rather on providing enough interesting materials to ensure opportunities will arise for language behaviors of interest. This seems to be clinically feasible and an effective way to monitor productive language change over time.

## REFERENCES

Bain, B., & Dollaghan, C. (1991). Treatment effectiveness: The notion of clinically significant change. *Language, Speech & Hearing Services in Schools, 22,* 264–70.

Bowers, J.W., & Courtright, J.A. (1984). *Communication research methods.* Glenview, IL: Scott, Foresman.

Boyd, R.D. (1974). *The Boyd Developmental Progress Scale.* San Bernadino, CA: Inland Counties Regional Center, Inc.

Brown, R. (1973). *A first language.* Cambridge, MA: Harvard University Press.

Coggins, T. (1990). Bringing context back into assessment. *Topics in Language Disorders, 11*(4), 43–54.

Coggins, T., Olswang, L., & Guthrie, J. (1987). Assessing communicative intents in young children: Low structured observation or elicitation tasks. *Journal of Speech and Hearing Disorders, 52,* 44–49.

Cohen, H. (1960). A coefficient of agreement for nominal scales. *Educational and Psychological Measurements, 20,* 37–46.

Dunn, L., & Dunn, L. (1981). *Peabody Picture Vocabulary Test* (rev.). Circle Pines, MN: American Guidance Service.

Edwards, D. (1974). Sensory–motor intelligence and semantic relations in early child grammar. *Cognition, 4,* 395–434.

Fey, M.E. (1986). *Language intervention with young children.* San Diego, CA: College-Hill.

Gallagher, T. (1983). Pre-assessment: A procedure for accommodating language variability. In T. Gallaher & C. Prutting (Eds.), *Pragmatic assessment and intervention issues in language.* San Diego, CA: College Hill.

Hedrick, D.L., Prather, E.M., & Tobin, A.R. (1984). *Sequenced Inventory of Communication Development* (rev. ed.). Seattle, WA: University of Washington Press.

Kaufman, A., & Kaufman, N. (1983). *The Kaufman Assessment Battery for Children.* Circle Pines, MN: American Guidance Service.

Landa, R., & Olswang, L. (1988). Effectiveness of language elicitation tasks with two-year-olds. *Child Language Teaching and Therapy, 4,* 170–192.

Lund, N., & Duchan, J. (1988). *Assessing children's language in naturalistic contexts.* Englewood Cliffs, NJ: Prentice Hall.

McCauley, R., & Swisher, L. (1984). Use and misuse of norm-referenced tests in clinical assessment: A hypothetical case. *Journal of Speech and Hearing Disorders, 49,* 338–348.

Miller, J., Chapman, R. (1984). Systematic analysis of language transcripts. Madison, Wisconsin: University of Wisconsin.

Nelson, K. (1986). *Event knowledge: Structure and function in development*. Hillsdale, NJ: Erlbaum.

Ratner, N., & Bruner, J. (1978). Games, social exchange and the acquisition of language. *Journal of Child Language, 5*, 391–401.

Scott, C., Palin, S., & Davidson, A., (Nov. 1979). *Semantic and pragmatic coding of early child language: Methodological and sampling issues*. Paper presented at the convention of the American Speech-Language-Hearing Association Annual Convention, Atlanta, GA.

Snyder-McLean, L., Solomonson, B., McLean, J., & Sack, M. (1984). Structuring joint action routines: A strategy for facilitating communication and language development in the classroom. *Seminars in Speech and Language, 3*, 213–225.

Thorndike, R.L., Hagen, E.P., & Sattler, J.J. (1986). *Stanford-Binet Test of Intelligence*. 4th Ed. Riverside, CA: The Riverside Publishing Co.

# Normal and disordered phonology in two-year-olds

**Carol Stoel-Gammon, PhD**
*Associate Professor*
*Department of Speech and Hearing*
*   Sciences*
*University of Washington*
*Seattle, Washington*

A MAJOR DIFFICULTY in describing and assessing early linguistic development results from tremendous individual variation in the early stages of development. Normal infants begin to babble as early as 6 months or as late as 9 months, and first words appear anywhere from 10 to 15 months. As children grow older, the amount of individual variation tends to decrease in areas such as vocabulary size and phonology, making it easier to identify atypical development. Thus, evaluation of prelinguistic and early linguistic development from babbling to first words and then to word combinations must be broad with an emphasis on the entire communicative system, rather than specific parts such as individual phonemes, grammatical morphemes, or sentence types.

The broad range of intersubject varia-

*This research was supported in part by the National Institutes of Health: NIDCD #5PO1DC00520. The author would like to thank Judith Stone and the anonymous reviewers for comments on an earlier draft.*

*Top Lang Disord*, 1991,11(4),21–32

tion at 24 months makes it difficult to formulate strict clinical norms for toddlers. It is, however, possible to classify subjects into three groups based on their vocal and verbal behaviors. The first group is composed of the majority of children, for whom there are no concerns; all aspects of linguistic development are within normal range. The second group includes those toddlers whose development is slow, but who evidence no major deviations from patterns of normal acquisition; this is the group of "late talkers" who should be monitored to see if they are going to catch up with their peers. The third group consists of those children for whom clinical concerns can be identified at 24 months or even earlier; these are children whose developmental patterns deviate substantially from the norms, even the broadest norms, in terms of order of acquisition or achievement of certain milestones (e.g., onset of meaningful speech). The second and third groups comprise approximately 15% of the population at 24 months. Some of these will have joined the "normal" group by age 3; others will be in need of treatment for speech-language problems (Rescorla, 1989; see also this issue).

The focus of this article is to review recent research on phonological development in 2-year-olds with particular attention to the course of normal development and the characteristics associated with delay. One way to think about early phonological development is to liken it to a road down which each child walks—a path leading to the adult phonological system. The road is broad, and children move along it at varying speeds and using various gaits; however, it is not as though

"anything goes." It is highly unusual, for instance, for a child to walk only on his or her tiptoes or to spend much time hopping on one foot. Some will advance rather methodically, step by step, down the middle, whereas others may skip or jump at times, switching from one edge of the path to the other, even circling back at particular places before moving ahead again. Many children will walk on the shoulder of the road for a brief time, but will return to the main path before long.

There are three important aspects of this analogy. First, the course of phonological development is broad; children can travel on the left side, on the right side, or down the middle. In each case, they arrive at their goal (the adult phonology). Second, the rate at which a child moves down the road is not fixed; although there may be something like a minimum speed limit for normal development—those traveling more slowly fall behind their peers in terms of their acquisition process. Finally, although the road is wide, it is flanked by shoulders and, beyond that, by ditches. A child who spends too much time on the shoulder of the road, who moves at a peculiar gait, or who travels too slowly would be considered atypical.

Within the framework of this analogy, the following discussion focuses on three components of early phonological development: (1) general patterns of acquisition (the main path), (2) commonalities and individual differences in the normally developing child (the width of the road, possible variations in gait), and (3) characteristics associated with atypical development.

## NORMAL DEVELOPMENT: THE CENTER OF THE ROAD

In the early stages of acquisition, it is not possible to separate measures of phonological development from early lexical development. Descriptions of a child's phonological system are based on analysis of the sounds used in the production of meaningful speech, and if the child is a late talker and has only a few words, his or her phonology will be simpler than that of a peer with a large vocabulary. Thus, any description of early phonological development in an individual child, particularly a child who seems to be delayed in other aspects of language acquisition, must include a statement of lexicon size.

This section is devoted to describing the "middle-of-road" child, age 24 to 36 months, whose vocabulary size and phonological system are well within normal limits. This profile of the typical toddler is based not on a particular child, but represents a composite derived from the average performance across a number of measures. The section below begins with a brief consideration of general aspects of early development and then presents a picture of the phonological system of the typical 2-year-old.

### General patterns of development

According to a recent report by Dale and Thal (1989), the average toddler at 24 months has a productive vocabulary of slightly over 300 words, a finding similar to those of previous researchers (Smith, 1926; Wehrabian, 1970). Typical 2-year-olds communicate primarily using content words (nouns, verbs, adjectives) and some functor words that can be combined in short phrases and sentences. According to parental report, about half of what the 2-year-old says can be understood by a stranger (Coplan & Gleason, 1988). A year later, at age 3, the linguistic system has advanced considerably, with an average vocabulary of around 1,000 words (Wehrabian, 1970), a mean length of utterance (MLU) of 3.1 morphemes (Miller, 1981), and the presence of a range of sentence types. At this stage, about 75% of a child's speech can be understood by a stranger (Coplan & Gleason, 1988).

The child's phonological system changes considerably between 2 and 3 years, with marked increases in the number of different sounds produced, the types of syllable and word shapes that occur, and the accuracy of production. All of these contribute to the increase in overall intelligibility noted by Coplan and Gleason. The following sections describe the normally developing phonological system from 24 to 36 months, using the framework of independent and relational analyses adopted by Stoel-Gammon and Dunn (1985).

### Phonological development: Independent analysis

An independent analysis describes the child's phonological system independent of the adult model. The focus here is not on what is right and what is wrong because the child's pronunciations are not compared with the target form of a word; rather, this type of analysis focuses on the sound types and syllable structures the child produces independent of the adult target. Stoel-Gammon (1987) presented findings from an independent analysis of the productions of 33 children, age 24 months, whose spontaneous speech samples were analyzed to determine the inventories of initial and final consonants, and the range of syllable and word shapes that occurred. She reported that at least half the 2-year-olds in her sample evidenced the following:

- An inventory of 9 to 10 different consonants in word-initial position, including phones at the three major places of articulation (i.e., labial, alveolar, velar), and the manner classes of stop, nasal, fricative, and glide. Phones occurring in the inventories of at least 50% of the subjects were [b, t, d, k, g, m, n, h, w, f, s].
- An inventory of five to six different consonantal phones in word-final position including stops at all three places of articulation, a nasal, a fricative, and often a liquid. Consonants occurring in 50% of the inventories included [p, t, k, n, s, r].
- Syllables and words of the form CV, consonant (C) vowel (V), occurred in all samples and CVC syllables in all but one (i.e., in 97% of the samples). Words of the form CVCV (e.g., baby, doggie) were found in 79% of the samples and CVCVC words (e.g., pocket, chicken) occurred in over 65%. In addition, 58% of the subjects produced at least two words with initial consonant clusters (i.e., CCV-), and 48% produced two words with final clusters (-VCC).

These findings indicate that the normally developing 2-year-old is capable of producing a variety of word and syllable

shapes and articulating consonantal sounds with a range of place and manner features. Although the consonantal repertoire is by no means complete, 2-year-olds are well on their way toward the full repertoire of the adult system.

From 24 to 36 months, the inventory of speech sounds and syllable and word shapes expands considerably as children begin to fill in the gaps in the system. Dyson's (1988) quasi-longitudinal investigation of 20 subjects between 24 and 39 months of age revealed that the repertoires of the older children (39 months) contained a wide range of sound types, including the palatal consonants [ʃ] and [ʧ], the voiced fricatives [v, z], and the two liquids [l, r]. The greatest changes in profile occurred in the size of the repertoire of consonants in word-final position. Stoel-Gammon's subjects (1985, 1987) evidenced a marked difference in the size of initial and final consonantal inventories with an average of 9.5 consonants in initial position and 5.7 in final. Ingram (1981) reported a comparable initial:final ratio in his summary of the inventories of 15 children, age 15 to 26 months. In contrast, Dyson's data showed that, at 39 months, the average size of initial and final inventories was the same, with 15 phones in each.

There was also a substantial increase in the number of different consonant clusters produced by the 24- and 39-month-old subjects. Stoel-Gammon's subjects evidenced a mean of 2.2 different clusters in initial position and 1.7 in final. In contrast, Dyson's 39-month-old subjects produced 10.7 different clusters in initial position and 7.7 in final position.

## Relational analysis

### Correct production

Relational analyses compare the child's pronunciation of a word with the adult form and identify what is right (i.e., matches between the two forms) and what is in error (mismatches). The first type of relational analysis reported here focuses on what is right in the child's productions, that is, on the consonantal sounds of the child's form that match those of the adult model. There are two ways to analyze accuracy of pronunciation, and each provides a different perspective on the child's phonological system. One approach is to obtain a general measure by examining an entire sample and calculating the overall percentage of consonants produced correctly (Shriberg & Kwiatkowski, 1982); this is the measure used by Stoel-Gammon in her analysis of the samples from the 2-year-olds in her study (1987; also Olswang, Stoel-Gammon, Coggins, & Carpenter, 1987). An alternative approach is to assess the accuracy of individual phonemes; this is the method adopted by most studies designed to provide norms on phoneme acquisition (e.g., Prather, Hedrick, & Kern, 1975; Templin, 1957).

Stoel-Gammon's analysis of general accuracy in conversational samples showed that the subjects' productions were quite accurate, the limitations on phonetic inventories not withstanding, and the mean percentage of consonants produced correctly was 70% (range 41% to 90%). It should be remembered that this number is based on analysis of intelligible utterances only, because accuracy can only be calculated when an item has an identifiable adult model.

Paynter and Petty (1974) used a phoneme-by-phoneme type of analysis in their study of imitated productions of a group of 24-month-old children. Despite differences in methods of data collection and analysis, the findings were quite similar to those of Stoel-Gammon cited above. Phonemes produced correctly by at least 51% of the children included voiced and voiceless stops at all three places of articulation, the glides /h, w/, the nasals /m, n/, and the fricative /f/. Similar results were reported by Prather et al. (1975) and Wellman, Case, Mengert, and Bradbury (1931) in their normative studies.

The findings of Sander (1972) and Prather et al. (1975) provide a picture of the changes in correct production from 2 to 3 years. By 3 years, at least half the children evidence customary production (defined roughly as the age at which half the subjects produced the phoneme correctly at least half the time) of 16 to 20 consonantal phonemes of English (of a total of 24). The only consonants not listed as customarily produced at age 3 in both studies were the fricatives /v, θ, ð, z, ʒ/; in addition, the palatals /ʃ, tʃ, dʒ/ were absent in Sander's data.

### Error patterns

The second way to examine the relation between the adult target and the child's production is to focus on the mismatches (i.e., errors) that occur. In the past decade, this type of analysis has resulted in descriptions of errors in terms of phonological processes, error patterns that affect sound classes (e.g., liquids) or syllable shapes (e.g., closed syllables). Once the phonological processes in a child's speech have been identified, the relative strength of each phonological process is computed by comparing the number of actual occurrences of the process with the number of possible occurrences and calculating the percentage of occurrence. Within this framework, Preisser, Hodson, and Paden (1988) examined the elicited productions of 20 children, age 22 to 25 months, describing the errors in 24 "assessment words" in terms of a small set of phonological processes. The only processes that appeared with an average occurrence greater than 40% were

- *cluster reduction,* with a mean occurrence of 76% (clusters were typically reduced by the omission of one of the members);
- *liquid deviation,* with an average occurrence of 75% (liquids were deleted, particularly in clusters, or were substituted by vowels or glides); and
- *stridency deletion,* with an average of 41% (strident consonants in clusters were generally omitted; singleton strident consonants were substituted by nonstrident phones).

None of the other processes examined had a mean percentage of occurrence greater than 25%. Among an older group of subjects, age 26 to 29 months, only two processes evidenced a mean occurrence greater than 25%: (1) cluster reduction, with a mean of 51% and (2) liquid deviation, with a mean of 64%.

Although the classification of phonological processes differed somewhat from those in the Preisser et al. study, Dyson and Paden's (1983) longitudinal investigation of errors in the elicited single-word productions of 40 children yielded similar findings. At the beginning of data collection, when the subjects were 23 to 35 months old, only the processes of gliding of liquids and cluster reduction were frequent, with mean occurrences of 54% and 50% respectively. Other processes occurred, on average, in fewer than 16% of the possible opportunities. When the same set of words was elicited from the subjects 6 months later (age range: 29 to 41 months), the mean occurrence of cluster reduction had decreased substantially to 30%; in contrast, only a slight decline occurred in the frequency of gliding, from 54% at the first testing to 48% at the second. The mean percentage of occurrence of other processes at this age period was less than 10%.

These studies, as well that of Haelsig and Madison (1986), show that children in the third year of life tend to have relatively few persistent error patterns. In terms of syllable shape, the main difficulty lies in the production of sequences of consonants as evidenced by the high proportion of the process of cluster reduction; in terms of sound classes, the most common errors are in the production of liquids and stridents (i.e., /f, v, s, z, ʃ, ʒ, tʃ, dʒ/).

## Summary of analyses

Although the three types of analysis presented above provide different perspectives on the phonologies of young children, they are in close agreement as to the areas of difficulties. The independent analysis showed that clusters were just emerging in the speech of 2-year-olds and the error analysis showed a high rate of cluster reduction. The independent analysis showed a lack of fricatives and affricates, and the error analysis showed a high percentage of occurrence of stridency deletion. The inventories showed a lack of liquids, and the error analyses showed the presence of the processes of gliding and liquid deviation.

A close tie can also be found between phonetic inventories and correct production. Those consonants that appear early in the repertoire of a 2-year-old, typically stops, nasals, and glides, are those that evidence early mastery in the normative studies. In other words, young children seem to use their repertoires appropriately—if a sound is in their repertoire, they tend to use it to match the appropriate adult sounds. This relationship between phonetic repertoire and correct production may seem obvious, but it has been noted that some phonologically disordered children have relatively complete phonetic inventories (i.e., they can produce a wide variety of sounds), but they have difficulties using those sounds to match the sounds of the target word (see Stoel-Gammon & Dunn, 1985; Stoel-Gammon & Herrington, 1990, for examples of this phenomenon).

### Acquisition of vowels

The discussion to this point has centered exclusively around consonants, but vowels must also be considered. To date, research on the acquisition of vowels is limited. Many researchers pay no attention to vowels or treat them as an aside in a discussion of consonants. This approach has been justified, in part, by the fact that vowels are mastered earlier than consonants and, even at young ages, tend to evidence fewer errors. At the same time, vowels cannot be entirely ignored, espe-

cially in a discussion of delayed or disordered phonological development (Stoel-Gammon, 1990). The limited data available indicate that at 24 months, overall vowel accuracy exceeds 75%, with some vowels above 90% correct (Hare, 1983; Wellman et al., 1931). At 3 years, normative data indicate that, on average, 93.3% of the vowel phonemes are produced correctly (Templin, 1957). The only targets that are often in error after age 3 are the r-colored phonemes /ʒ/ and /ɚ/.

## INDIVIDUAL DIFFERENCES

Clinically, the critical question related to individual variation is, what are the limits of normal variation? To return to the analogy introduced at the outset, we need to determine the following: the width of the road that leads to the adult phonological system; the amount of time a child can spend on the shoulders of the road (i.e., deviating from the main path); and the rate at which a child must move down the road to be within normal limits.

As noted earlier, the age at which children achieve particular stages of early linguistic and phonological development varies substantially during the first 2 years, but the range of variability declines between 24 and 36 months, making it easier to identify the child whose development is not normal. A recent study of vocabulary development (Fensen, Dale, Reznick, Hartung, & Burgess, 1990), for example, showed that at 18 months, the average lexicon size was 109.7 words, with a standard deviation of 111.4, which is larger than the mean. At 24 months, the average vocabulary was 311.6 words, standard deviation, 176.3; at 30 months, the average had risen to 546.1 words, whereas the standard deviation had dropped to 97.0. Thus, the standard deviation, expressed as a proportion of the mean, declined from 102% at 18 months to 18% at 30 months.

In terms of phonological development, certain measures evidence considerable variability, but strong uniformity is found in others. Among the 34 subjects in Stoel-Gammon's study of consonantal inventories, for example, the size of the initial inventory at 24 months ranged from a low of 3 to a high of 16; in final position, the comparable numbers were 0 and 11 (Stoel-Gammon, 1985, 1989a). In spite of this range in inventory size, a common pattern was noted; across the 34 subjects, the number of consonants in the final inventory never exceeded the number in the initial inventory. Thus, the slowest child in the group, with an initial inventory of only three consonants, had no consonants in her final inventory; in contrast, one of her peers, a more precocious subject with 16 consonants in the inventory of initial sounds (the highest in the group) had 11 consonants in the final inventory (again the highest).

Examination of the specific consonants in the individual inventories also revealed considerable intersubject variation, even when inventory size was held constant. For example, the sets of consonants for 3 subjects with average-sized initial inventories (9 to 10 phones) were as follows: Subject JJ: [b, d, k, g, m, n, w, f, l, r]; Subject NC: [b, t, d, m, h, w, f, s, l]; and Subject MS: [b, t, d, k, g, m, n, h, w]. Although these inventories exhibit some overlap in specific sounds (all three contain [b, d, m, w]), there are also clear differences. If, however, the inventories

are analyzed in terms of sound classes rather than specific sounds, the picture is much more uniform. All 3 subjects had inventories that included front stops, at least one nasal ([m] or [n]), and one glide ([w] or [h]). In addition, one or more fricatives and one or more liquids appeared in two inventories.

These inventories illustrate the common patterns observed in Stoel-Gammon's (1985) longitudinal analysis from onset of meaningful speech to 24 months. Developmentally, there was a strong tendency for stops, nasals, and glides to appear before fricatives, liquids, and affricates, and for front (i.e., labial, alveolar) consonants to appear before back ones. Thus, the slower developing subjects, those with small inventories, would typically have only front stops, nasals, and glides, whereas subjects with larger inventories might have representatives from all place and manner classes. No subject exhibited an inventory that included liquids and fricatives, but lacked stops and nasals. To a certain extent, then, the nature rather than the size of a phonetic inventory may be used as an index of normalcy.

Further examination of the data from the 34 subjects (Stoel-Gammon, 1989b) revealed the presence of a marked synchrony among different aspects of the developing linguistic system. Statistical analyses of the 24-month data revealed strong correlations between the following measures:

- number of consonants in the initial inventory and number in the final inventory ($r = .74, p < .001$);
- number of consonants in the initial inventory and lexicon size as measured by the number of different

words produced in 100 intelligible or partially intelligible utterances ($r = .79, p < .001$); and

- number of consonants in the final inventory and lexicon size ($r = .85, p < .001$).

These correlations suggest that in spite of intersubject variability on phonetic measures, phonetic inventory is linked to lexicon size. In addition, lexicon size and size of phonetic inventory were highly correlated with age of onset of meaningful speech ($p < .001$); as would be expected, this was a negative correlation indicating that an early onset of speech was tied to a larger lexicon and larger phonetic inventories at 24 months.

The basic picture that emerges from this perspective of individual differences is that although children may proceed at different rates down the path of phonological development, each child's phonological system exhibits a set of common characteristics:

- stops, nasals, and glides appear before liquids, affricates, and fricatives;
- the inventory of initial consonants tends to be larger than the inventory of final consonants;
- the number of different sounds in the child's phonetic inventory is correlated with lexicon size; and
- age at onset of meaningful speech is correlated (negatively) with the size of the lexicon and the phonetic inventory at 24 months.

## ATYPICAL DEVELOPMENT

The outline of normal development and discussion of individual differences presented above provide a basis for the prelim-inary identification of atypical development. It is not possible, or even desirable, to describe a phonological disorder in a 2-year-old in terms of specific sounds; however, particular phonological patterns would constitute reasons for concern. These will be discussed in four sections: (1) order of acquisition, (2) unusual error patterns, (3) asynchronous development between phonology and other aspects of language, and (4) rate of acquisition.

### Order of acquisition

The research on normal development has shown that despite considerable differences in rate of phonological development, there is a regular and predictable order of acquisition of syllable types and sound classes, and major deviations from this pattern would be considered atypical. Such deviations indicate that the child is spending too much time traveling on the shoulder of the road rather than adhering to the main path. The most basic phonetic unit in speech production, the consonant-vowel (CV) syllable with a supraglottal consonant (i.e., any consonant but [?] or [h]), typically appears before 10 months (Oller & Eilers, 1988) and is essential to subsequent phonological development. Lack of such syllables at 24 months would be a clear signal of a phonological disorder; to use the road analogy, a child who did not produce these syllables would be off the road, in the ditch. For children who produce CV syllables, the following patterns would be considered atypical by virtue of the fact that they violate the normal order of acquisition: an inventory of final consonants larger than the inventory of initial consonants; a phonetic inventory composed of liquids, fricatives, and affricates, but lacking stops, nasals, and glides; velar (i.e., back) consonants but no labial or alveolar consonants.

## Atypical error patterns

The literature on phonological development documents the wide variety of error patterns that occur in the normally developing child, making it unwise to attempt to formulate a list of atypical phonological processes that serve as a clear signal of a disorder. Rather than distinguishing normal from disordered processes on the basis of particular types of errors, the distinction should be based on differences in the use of various processes. In normal subjects, atypical errors tend to occur for a relatively short period of time, are applied to a limited set of words, and are abandoned as the child moves closer to the adult system (Stoel-Gammon & Dunn, 1985). In the disordered child, the error pattern is more consistent and occurs for an extended period. With these caveats in mind, the following represents a list of red flags, that is, errors that would be cause for concern if they were persistent and widespread:

- numerous vowel errors; at 24 months, it is not unexpected for a child to exhibit some vowel errors, but by 3 years, most vowels (except the r-colored phonemes) should be produced correctly;
- widespread deletion of initial consonants; at 24 months, the child should produce CV syllables with 3 to 4 different consonantal types; at 36 months, the inventory of initial consonants should be considerably larger;
- substitution of glottal consonants [ʔ] or [h] for a variety of target consonants;
- substitution of back consonants for front ones, particularly velars for alveolars, in the absence of assimilatory contexts; and
- deletion of final consonants; at 24 months, lack of final consonants in the productions of a child with a limited phonetic inventory and relatively small lexicon would not necessarily be a concern, but at 36 months, all children should be producing some CVC syllables.

## Lexicon–phonology interface

As mentioned earlier, there is a strong tendency for synchrony between the development of the lexicon and the phonological system. At one end of the continuum, we find the child with a small phonetic repertoire who tends to have relatively few words; at the other end is the child with a large vocabulary and a relatively complete phonetic repertoire (Stoel-Gammon, 1990). If a child has a limited set of speech sounds at his or her disposal and attempts to produce a large number of different words, he or she simply does not have enough sound types to distinguish among these words and ends up producing many homonymous forms. To illustrate, consider the child with no final consonants and only voiced stops and nasals in his or her inventory of initial consonants; for such a child, words as disparate as "bead, beet, beep, peep, peek, please, Pete, peas, peel," among others, would all be pronounced [bi]. Given the lack of differentiation among target words, the speech of this child would be difficult to understand. Although some toddlers seem to tolerate the presence of many homonymous forms, others try to avoid it by using atypical errors to signal word differences (Leonard, 1985). In either case, the mismatch between phonetic inventory and lexicon size creates pressures on the system that may lead to atypical patterns of acquisition.

### Rate of acquisition

Given the extent of variability in speech and language development in the first 2 years of life, this is probably the hardest area in which to provide clinical guidelines. The crucial question regarding rate of acquisition is what is the minimum rate at which a child must be progressing to be considered normal? The research summarized in this article suggests that, at 24 months, a child with a vocabulary smaller than 50 words or a phonetic inventory with only 4 to 5 consonants and limited variety of vowels would be viewed as a late talker who would be placed in the "needs to be monitored" category assuming other aspects of development (e.g., order of acquisition, error types) were unremarkable. By 30 months, the decrease in intersubject variability would provide a firmer database for clinical decisions regarding normalcy and the possible need for therapy.

•   •   •

As noted early on, at 24 months, children could be divided into three groups based on their linguistic profile: (1) a normal group, (2) a slow group, and (3) a disordered group. In view of the wide path of normal development, the major problem for the speech-language pathologist is to determine which toddlers to place in the latter two categories. This article has emphasized that normal phonological development cannot be determined by comparing the child's performance with a set of speech-sound norms like those used to evaluate older children. Examination of subparts of the phonological system is not enough; the focus must be on the interrelationships among various parts, including age at onset of meaningful speech, lexicon size, size and nature of the phonetic inventory, correct productions, error types, and overall intelligibility. If the child's system is viewed as a whole, not as a conglomeration of parts, atypical patterns of development can be identified and appropriate types of intervention implemented. The aim of therapy, then, will be to bring the child back toward the middle of the road traveled by the normal child; the road leading to the adult phonological system.

## REFERENCES

Coplan, J., & Gleason, J. (1988). Unclear speech: Recognition and significance of unintelligible speech in preschool children. *Pediatrics, 82,* 447–452.

Dale, P., & Thal, D. (1989). *Assessment of language in infants and toddlers using parent report.* A short course presented at the annual meeting of the American Speech-Language-Hearing Association, St. Louis, Missouri.

Dyson, A. (1988). Phonetic inventories of 2- and 3-year-old children. *Journal of Speech and Hearing Disorders, 53,* 89–93.

Dyson, A., & Paden, E. (1983). Some phonological acquisi-

tion strategies used by two-year-olds. *Journal of Childhood Communication Disorders, 7,* 6–18.

Fensen, L., Dale, P., Reznick, S., Hartung, J., & Burgess, S. (1990). *Norms for the MacArthur communicative development inventories.* Poster presented at the International Conference on Infant Studies, Montreal, Quebec.

Haelsig, P., & Madison, C. (1986). A study of phonological processes exhibited by 3-, 4-, and 5-year-old children. *Language, Speech and Hearing Services in Schools, 17,* 107–114.

Hare, G. (1983). Development at 2 years. In J.V. Irwin &

S.P. Wong (Eds.), *Phonological development in children: 18–72 months.* Carbondale, IL: Southern Illinois University Press.

Ingram, D. (1981). *Procedures for the phonological analysis of children's language.* Austin, TX: Pro-Ed.

Leonard, L.B. (1985). Unusual and subtle phonological behavior in the speech of phonologically disordered children. *Journal of Speech and Hearing Disorders, 50,* 4–13.

Miller, J. (1981). *Assessing language production in children.* Austin, TX: Pro-Ed.

Oller, D.K., & Eilers, R. (1988). The role of audition in babbling. *Child Development, 59,* 523–549.

Olswang, L.B., Stoel-Gammon, C., Coggins, T.E., & Carpenter, R.L. (1987). *Assessing prelinguistic and early linguistic behaviors in developmentally young children.* Seattle, WA: University of Washington Press.

Paynter, E., & Petty, N. (1974). Articulatory sound: Acquisition of two-year-old children. *Perceptual and Motor Skills, 39,* 1079–1085.

Prather, E., Hedrick, D., & Kern, D. (1975). Articulation development in children aged two to four years. *Journal of Speech and Hearing Disorders, 40,* 179–191.

Preisser, D., Hodson, B., & Paden, E. (1988). Developmental phonology: 18–29 months. *Journal of Speech and Hearing Disorders, 53,* 125–130.

Rescorla, L. (1989). The language development survey: A screening tool for delayed language in toddlers. *Journal of Speech and Hearing Disorders, 54,* 587–599.

Sander, E. (1972). When are speech sounds learned? *Journal of Speech and Hearing Disorders, 37,* 55–63.

Shriberg, L., & Kwiatkowski, J. (1982). Phonological disorders III: A procedure for assessing severity of involvement. *Journal of Speech and Hearing Disorders, 47,* 256–270.

Smith, M.E. (1926). An investigation of the development of the sentence and the extent of vocabulary in young children. *University of Iowa Studies in Child Welfare, 3,* 5.

Stoel-Gammon, C. (1985). Phonetic inventories, 15–24 months: A longitudinal study. *Journal of Speech and Hearing Research, 28,* 506–512.

Stoel-Gammon, C. (1987). The phonological skills of two-year-olds. *Language, Speech, and Hearing Services in Schools, 18,* 323–329.

Stoel-Gammon, C. (1989a). Prespeech and early speech development of two late talkers. *First Language, 9,* 207–224.

Stoel-Gammon, C. (1989b). *From babbling to speech: Some new evidence.* Paper presented at the Child Phonology Conference, Evanston, IL.

Stoel-Gammon, C. (1990). Issues in phonological development and disorders. In J. Miller (Ed.), *Research on child language disorders.* Austin, TX: Pro-Ed.

Stoel-Gammon, C., & Dunn, C. (1985). *Normal and disordered phonology in children.* Austin, TX: Pro-Ed.

Stoel-Gammon, C., & Herrington, P. (1990). Vowel systems of normally-developing and phonologically disordered children. *Clinical Linguistics and Phonetics, 4,* 145–160.

Templin, M.C. (1957). Certain language skills in children: Their development and interrelationships. *Institute of Child Welfare Monographs, 26,* Minneapolis, MN: University of Minnesota Press.

Wehrabian, A. (1970). Measures of vocabulary and grammatical skills for children up to age six. *Developmental Psychology, 2,* 439–446.

Wellman, B.L., Case, I.M., Mengert, I.B., & Bradbury, D.E. (1931). Speech sounds of young children. *University of Iowa Studies in Child Welfare, 2,* 5.

# Early assessment and intervention with emotional and behavioral disorders and communication disorders

**Geraldine Theadore, MS**
*Speech–Language Pathologist*
*Department of Communicative*
*Disorders*
*University of Rhode Island*
*Kingston, Rhode Island*

**Suzanne R. Maher, MS**
*Speech–Language Pathologist*
*Communication Disorders Department*
*Bradley Hospital*

**Barry M. Prizant, PhD**
*Director, Communication Disorders*
*Department*
*Bradley Hospital*
*Associate Professor of Psychiatry and*
*Human Behavior*
*Division of Child and Adolescent*
*Psychiatry*
*Brown University Program in Medicine*
*East Providence, Rhode Island*

A S FULL implementation of Public Law (PL) 99-457, the Early Intervention Program for Infants and Toddlers with Handicaps (1989), draws near, speech–language pathologists are placing greater emphasis on serving children aged 0 to 3 years and their families. PL 99-457 mandates that by 1992, children who have developmental delays or who are biologically or environmentally at risk for developmental delays be served within a family focus. This article addresses issues related to providing services to a subgroup of this population and their families—young children identified as having both communication disorders and emotional and behavioral disorders and those at risk for developing these disorders.

While many young children with communication disorders do not present with significant emotional or behavioral symptomatology, a significant number demonstrate symptoms of sufficient severity to warrant professional attention (Prizant et al., 1990). These young children may dem-

*Top Lang Disord*, 1990,10(4),42–56
© 1990 Aspen Publishers, Inc.

onstrate a number of behavioral difficulties including overactivity, impulsivity, low tolerance for frustration, aggression, and, in general, difficulty in behavioral control and regulation of emotional arousal (Greenspan, 1988). Emotional difficulties may be demonstrated by symptoms such as severe separation anxiety, fearfulness of new situations, and avoidance or withdrawal from interactions.

Research also has demonstrated that a child's communication development and socioemotional well-being are highly dependent on a history of positive caregiver–child interactions that meet the emotional and instrumental needs of both children and their caregivers (Dunst, Lowe, & Bartholomew, 1990). Caregivers, in turn, must have the necessary fiscal, social, and emotional supports to enable them to develop relationships and interactive styles with their children that facilitate their children's development while meeting their own emotional needs as parents. Thus, a family focus is defined, in part, as services that view a child's needs in the context of relationships and communicative interactions with caregivers. Other aspects of family-focused intervention, which are beyond the scope of this discussion, address the family's fiscal, social, and emotional support systems (Dunst et al., 1990 provide further information).

In this article a number of themes are emphasized. First, assessment and intervention must occur within the context of caregiver–child interactions and relationships. Thus, assessment entails documenting both the child's emerging communicative competence and the characteristics of caregiver–child interaction. Intervention goals focus on enhancing child abilities through modification of caregiver–child interaction. Second, the interrelationships between children's communication ability and the ability to regulate emotional states is of primary significance. Finally, caregivers are viewed as partners and primary change agents, since the caregiver–child relationship is the primary socioemotional context in which communication develops (MacDonald, 1989; Prizant & Wetherby, "Toward an integrated view of early language and communication development and socioemotional development," this issue).

## RISK FACTORS

In considering a young child's development of communicative competence and social and emotional well-being, speech-language pathologists need to consider within-child factors, transactional factors, and environmental factors. Within-child factors, such as very low birth weight and perinatal complications, place a child at risk for delays in a number of areas, including language and communication development (Klein & Briggs, 1987) and emotional and behavioral problems (Baker & Cantwell, 1987). In addition to developmental delays, within-child factors may result in limited attentional abilities and an impulsive learning style, which may further exacerbate difficult caregiver–child social and communicative interactions (Greenspan, 1988).

Transactional factors are those that arise in the context of interactions. For example, patterns of caregiver interaction with high-risk and developmentally delayed infants have been found to be different from those of normally developing infants

(Dunst, 1983; Field, 1987; Mahoney & Powell, 1988). Clark and Seifer (1983) found that developmentally delayed infants often do not develop a clear system of prelinguistic signaling, leaving caregivers frustrated in their attempts to interpret their children's needs. Caregiver behavior may become intrusive and overcontrolling as the caregiver works harder at making the interaction successful. Unclear signals from the infant leave the caregiver confused about how to respond and may result in more inappropriate and noncontingent responses. Once this transactional pattern is established, the child is at risk not only for significant communication difficulties, but also for the development of emotional and behavioral problems (Field, 1987).

In addition to the difficulties that result from delays or disabilities, other distal factors affecting caregivers also must be considered as they indirectly influence a child's development (Sameroff & Fiese, 1990). Environmental and family factors such as limited caregiver education, stressful life events, caregiver mental illness, and history of family difficulties including alcohol and drug abuse may place caregivers at risk for developing maladaptive caregiving styles that result in disturbed interactional experiences with their children (Field, 1987). Clearly, no single factor is responsible for the developmental outcome of a child. Within-child, environmental, and transactional factors are highly interrelated, and, in fact, it may be impossible to distinguish among these factors when considering a child's development over time. A cumulative risk model best helps to predict developmental outcomes in children (Sameroff & Fiese, 1990). This model states that developmental outcomes are multiply determined, with different factors having differential degrees of influence at different points in time (Kochanek, Kabacoff, & Lipsitt, 1990).

## CONSIDERATIONS IN ASSESSMENT

Traditionally, communication assessment tools used with very young children have focused on developmental milestones or within-child factors. That is, communication within the context of social transaction with caregivers was rarely considered (Prizant & Wetherby, 1988). More recently, greater emphasis has been placed on observing children in more natural social interactions, with consideration of child factors, caregiver behavior, and transactional patterns (Rossetti, 1990).

### Assessing children's abilities

As the focus of assessment has shifted from developmental milestones and skills acquisition to social and communicative competence, a child's effectiveness in using communicative behaviors to regulate interactions has become a major consideration. Some abilities identified as crucial to children's social and communicative com-

*As the focus of assessment has shifted from developmental milestones and skills acquisition to social and communicative competence, a child's effectiveness in using communicative behaviors to regulate interactions has become a major consideration.*

petence include the ability to express intentions through the use of conventional and readable signals, to participate actively in reciprocal interactions, to repair communicative breakdowns, and to signal emotional states (Dunst & Lowe, 1986; Greenspan, 1988; Prizant & Wetherby, 1988).

Dunst et al. (1990) presented a classification scheme designed to identify a young child's primary level of communication. Seven levels ranging from *behavior state communication* (0–3 months) to *verbal communication* (18–30 months) are delineated by the presence or absence of distinctive features (e.g., intentionality, goal-directedness, rule-governedness). The classification scheme is based on the premise that communication encompasses "any overt conventional or nonconventional behavior, whether used intentionally or not, that has the effect of arousing in an onlooker a belief that a child is attempting to convey a message, make a demand, request, etc." (p. 42). This system allows for precise delineation of the level of a child's expressive communication whether intentional or not.

Wetherby and Prizant (1990) presented a framework and series of procedures for analyzing spontaneous communicative behavior and related cognitive and social-affective abilities in children functioning from early intentional stages of communication to early language stages (i.e., 8–24 months developmental). This framework includes an analysis of gestural communicative means (e.g., conventional and distal gestures), complexity of vocal communicative means, coordination of gestures and vocalizations, and use of early language forms.

Functions of preverbal and early verbal communicative acts are analyzed along a continuum of sociability ranging from acts used to serve behavioral regulation functions (e.g., requests, protests) through acts used for social interaction (e.g., requesting comfort, social routines) to acts used for joint attention (e.g., commenting, requesting information). Social-affective signaling (i.e., positive affect, negative affect, gaze shifts for social referencing), reciprocity (i.e., rate, responsive acts, communicative repairs), language comprehension, and nonverbal symbolic behavior (i.e., symbolic play, combinatorial play) are profiled along with expressive communicative means in order to document relative strengths and weaknesses in a child's communicative, symbolic, and social-affective functioning.

Consideration is also given a child's ability to clearly signal his or her emotional state to a communicative partner, since the child's competence in this area will have a strong impact on how each partner's emotional needs will be met within interactions (Tronick, 1989). A critical aspect of a child's expression of emotional states is whether affective signals are directed to or shared with the caregiver through vocalization, facial expression, or bodily movements. For example, a child who has mastered a task such as completing a puzzle may share his pleasure by showing the completed project to or looking at the caregiver and smiling. On the other hand, a child with social-affective impairments may stare at the completed project and vocalize excitedly, but not share this positive affective experience by looking toward an adult.

Expression of negative affective states must also be considered. A child who has been hurt may approach his or her mother for comfort, signaling recognition that the mother can help the child to cope in a stressful situation. A child who cannot be comforted by a caregiver may be difficult to console, and may experience extreme diffuse states of emotional arousal (e.g., distress, fear), leaving caregivers feeling helpless and confused (Bristol & Schopler, 1984). Thus, the ability of a caregiver to console or comfort a child, as well as a child's responsiveness to such efforts, needs to be considered. Specific strategies used successfully by caregivers (e.g., a soft voice, tactile stimulation) should also be documented.

### Assessment contexts

Both familiar routines and less familiar and less structured activities should be observed to obtain information about a young child's communicative competence. Observation of certain predictable and consistent routines that occur in everyday activities, such as caregiving activities, sharing a snack, engaging in simple social games, and playing with favorite toys, allows for assessment of the child's highest level of social-communicative functioning. Situations that are less predictable or familiar, and thus more stressful and challenging, also are important to observe. For example, free-play situations, transitions from one activity to another, and unexpected events such as spilling a drink or breaking a toy provide information on how a child engages in interactions, repairs breakdowns in interactions, and expresses emotional states such as distress, frustration, or joy to others. Caregivers

should be asked which situations tend to be most difficult, with attempts made to observe these circumstances. Through observations in both highly familiar and less familiar situations, as well as less and more stressful situations, hypotheses may be developed about a child's strengths and weaknesses in communicating his or her physical, social, and emotional needs to a communicative partner.

### Assessing caregiver–child interaction

As the focus of assessment shifts to observing interaction within a family context, consideration must be given to identifying the strategies a caregiver uses to facilitate and support interactions. One informal tool developed to identify caregiver strategies is the Observation of Communicative Interactions (OCI) Scale (Klein & Briggs, 1987). This scale was designed to measure caregiver responsivity to infant's cues. It comprises ten categories that represent a continuum ranging from basic caregiving responses to more sophisticated behavior used to facilitate language and conceptual development. The OCI has been used to guide professionals' observations of caregiver–infant interactions, to provide qualitative measures of mothers' interactions with their infants, and to identify relative strengths and weaknesses in maternal interaction patterns (Klein & Briggs, 1987).

Another scale, the Parent Infant Interaction Scale (Clark & Seifer, 1983), provides information about caregiver interaction behaviors, caregiver and child social referencing, reciprocity, and caregiver affect. This scale was designed to provide a systematic approach to the assessment and enhancement of caregiver–child interactions. One part of the scale focuses specifically on the caregiver's style of interaction, using a hierarchy of caregiver behaviors ranging from those least sensitive to the infant's cues (i.e., highly intrusive) to those most sensitive (i.e., highly responsive) to the infant's cues. An example of a highly intrusive behavior is forcing or physically coercing a child to respond, such as turning a child's head or restraining a child's movements. Ratings on this dimension are based on the frequency and intensity of these behaviors and whether the caregiver ceases to use them when they are upsetting to the child. On the other end of the continuum are more responsive behaviors such as expansion or elaboration of a child's behavior when, for example, a parent follows a child's focus of attention and comments on what he or she is observing.

Finally, for children who are beginning to understand language, specific attention should be given to language adjustments made by caregivers relative to a child's developmental level (Tiegerman & Siperstein, 1984) and emotional state (Greenspan, 1988). The use of language by a caregiver to resolve emotional conflicts or to console a child should be observed for effectiveness. Emotive tone, volume, and accompanying nonverbal and paralinguistic features should be noted.

By obtaining information on these dimensions of caregiver–child interaction patterns, each partner's behavior may be analyzed as to its relative contribution and influence on social-affective exchange. Thus, in planning intervention, language specialists and caregivers can work together in investigating ways to make inter-actions more successful and emotionally satisfying for all involved.

## TRANSACTIONAL APPROACH TO EARLY INTERVENTION

Sameroff (1987) indicated that transactional developmental processes involving the interplay between young children and their caregiving environments must be considered in targeting intervention programs. Approaches to working with young children and their families should thus be transactional in nature; that is, the mutual ongoing influences between a child and his or her social or nonsocial world must be considered.

### Intervention principles

Recent research and literature on working with caregivers and their young children have espoused a consistent set of principles for guiding intervention efforts (Dunst et al., 1990; MacDonald, 1989; Mahoney & Powell, 1988; Sameroff & Fiese, 1990). These principles are relevant for children who have or are at risk for developing communication disorders and emotional behavioral disorders and their caregivers.

First, intervention efforts must be individualized and based on assessment of child strengths and weaknesses, caregiver–child interaction patterns, family strengths and weaknesses, and the family's stated needs. Sameroff and Fiese (1990) noted that a unique set of risk factors is associated with each family situation, requiring a unique set of intervention strategies. The use of an Individual Family Service Plan as stipulated by PL 99-457 ensures such individualization.

Second, to the extent possible, intervention efforts should occur within the context of naturally occurring routines and play situations (Dunst et al., 1990; MacDonald, 1989). This will ensure that caregivers can apply facilitative strategies and observe progress in communicative interactions in real-life settings. It also allows for targeting more difficult and stressful situations such as mealtime, getting dressed, and other necessary activities.

Third, intervention should focus on helping caregivers to develop a responsive, child-centered style when interacting with their children; research has demonstrated that some caregivers of at-risk children are highly directive and controlling (Dunst et al., 1990). MacDonald (1989) noted that characteristics of a responsive approach include being a partner with children, matching their developmental level, responding sensitively and being nondirective, and building emotional attachments.

*Being a partner* with children refers to the importance of developing reciprocity, that is, recognizing that both partners contribute actively to making interactions work. Reciprocal turntaking and a pace of interaction conducive to active participation by caregiver and child is exemplary of strategies leading to a partnership.

*Matching* refers to interacting with a child at developmentally appropriate levels, taking into account the complexity of language or signals used, the appropriateness of tasks or activities, and a child's interests and focus of attention. Mahoney and Powell (1988) found that matching strategies were easily learned by caregivers and were significantly related to developmental gains made by children they studied.

> *Being a partner with children refers to the importance of developing reciprocity, that is, recognizing that both partners contribute actively to making interactions work.*

*Responding sensitively* and *being nondirective* refer to following a child's lead and interpreting and responding to a child's subtle communicative signals. The general goal is to help a child develop a sense of control. For a behaviorally challenging child, frequent protesting may be a response to an overcontrolling and directive caregiver style, especially when adult and child agendas are in conflict. Both MacDonald (1989) and Dunst et al. (1990) cite a number of studies supporting the positive effect of caregivers' developing facilitative or nondirective styles.

Finally, *building emotional attachments* refers to caregivers' sensitive attuning to their children's emotional states and needs. Greenspan (1988) noted that delayed or at-risk children face a number of barriers to emotional growth due to developmental limitations and maladaptive caregiver interactive styles. With a growing sense of mutual efficacy and active involvement in interactions, caregivers and children are more likely to develop deeper emotional ties (Dunst et al., 1990; MacDonald, 1989). Additionally, successful interactions may help some caregivers modify their attributions of their child as being "difficult" or "bad."

The importance of developing positive caregiver–child experiences cannot be overestimated. Tronick (1989) noted that through successful early caregiver–child interactions, a young child develops mutual and self-regulatory capacities that support emotional development (see Prizant & Wetherby, "Toward an integrated view of early language and communication development and socioemotional development," this issue).

**Intervention strategies**

Sameroff and Fiese (1990) noted that a transactional approach to early intervention is based on three general intervention strategies: remediation, redefinition, and reeducation. These strategies are not mutually exclusive and should be selected based on child and caregiver needs.

*Remediation* focuses on helping delayed or disabled children develop skills that more closely approximate behavior expected at a given chronological age within their cultural system. For example, an important goal in working with young children with communication disorders and emotional and behavioral problems is providing them with socially acceptable means of expressing their needs. Thus, in remediation, the focus is on a child's behavior, with efforts toward enhancing abilities using a developmental model.

*Redefinition* occurs when professionals enable caregivers to redefine their perception of their child's abilities by helping them to evaluate their child's developmental strengths and weaknesses. Professionals also must help caregivers recognize the potential for positive change (Wetherby, Prizant, & Kublin, 1989). Redefinition also focuses on helping caregivers identify and develop interactive strategies that facilitate their child's development. Children with disabilities often require special pat-

terns of care to enable them to progress through stages of social and emotional development (Greenspan, 1988). In working with families of children with identified communication disorders, professionals must recognize that caregivers may have strong parenting skills; however, the caregivers often need support and guidance in recognizing their child's strengths and weaknesses and in modifying their own interactive style to support their child's development (MacDonald, 1989; Mahoney & Powell, 1988).

*Reeducation* is defined as "teaching parents how to raise children" (Sameroff, 1987, p. 287). Through reeducation, professionals provide more direct instruction so that caregivers better understand their children's developmental needs. This strategy is particularly relevant when environmental risk factors are operative. For example, speech language pathologists may become involved in programs for adolescent mothers that focus on increasing the mothers' understanding of language and communication development and helping them develop skills to facilitate their child's development (Maher, Prizant, & Gjording, 1990).

**PROVIDING SERVICES TO CAREGIVERS AND CHILDREN**

Speech–language pathologists must be aware of complexities of interactions and the amount of stress experienced by families when a child has significant emotional and behavioral factors that coexist with a communication impairment. Young children who experience both communication problems and emotional and behavioral problems have significant difficulties participating in interactions. They have been found to be less persistent when breakdowns occur in interaction (Wetherby, et al., 1989). In addition, such children are more likely to develop socially unacceptable means of communicating, including other-directed behaviors such as aggression and, in more rare instances, self-directed behaviors such as self-abuse (Donnellan, Mirenda, Mesaros, & Fassbender, 1984). There may be an extensive history of interactional disturbances in the families of such children accompanied by the development of maladaptive response strategies by caregivers (e.g., overly controlling, disengaged) (Clark & Seifer, 1985). The intervention strategies of remediation and redefinition are particularly well-suited to working with families of children with identified disabilities (Sameroff & Fiese, 1990).

## Remediation strategies

Bristol and Schopler (1984) documented a number of stressors reported by families of preschool children with identified social-communicative disorders. These stressors included the child's lack of an effective communication system, the child's lack of response to family members, and the caregiver's difficulty in managing the child's behavior. To address these stress factors, the first aspect of remediation should be aiding caregivers in understanding the child's emotional and behavioral difficulties in specific reference to developmental and communicative limitations (Prizant & Wetherby, in press). This strategy may help caregivers to redefine their perceptions of their child in light of his or her difficulties.

A second important aspect of remediation is helping the child develop a clear and socially appropriate system for signaling intentions. A child who stands in front of a shelf and cries may be signaling that he or she wants something that cannot be reached. A speech-language pathologist and a caregiver may first work together to develop an understanding of a child's system of communicative signaling and then work directly with the child to develop a more readable signal, such as taking the caregiver by the hand to the shelf and reaching or pointing to a desired object. A child who throws his or her food on the floor to signal that he or she has finished eating may need help in developing a more socially appropriate signal, such as pushing his or her plate away, gesturing, or saying "all done."

A third aspect of remediation involves helping young children develop the ability to persist and to modify signals to repair communication breakdowns. For example, joint activity routines (Snyder-McLean, Solomonson, McLean, & Sack, 1984) such as rolling the child on a large ball may be developed. Initially, this routine may be facilitated by helping caregivers interpret and impute intent to subtle behavior, such as the child rocking back and forth and to respond as if such behavior were a request for continuation. As the routine becomes familiar to the child, the adults may violate the routine or delay responding in order to encourage the child to persist by repeating the signal or modifying the signal (e.g., pairing body movements with vocalization or eye contact). More sophisticated signals can then be modeled and prompted (MacDonald, 1989, provides an in-depth presentation of therapeutic strategies).

### Redefinition strategies

When focusing on redefinition, speech–language pathologists address caregiver's concerns about their child's lack of responsiveness by helping caregivers look more closely at successes and breakdowns in interactions. The major purpose is to help caregivers adjust or modify perceptions or attributions of their child's behavior, with an emphasis on emerging competence and potential for change. As with remediation, this process involves helping caregivers

---

*The major purpose is to help caregivers adjust or modify perceptions or attributions of their child's behavior, with an emphasis on emerging competence and potential for change.*

---

identify the subtle ways in which the child may be communicating, such as gaze shifting, proximity, physical manipulation, and vocalization. In addition to identifying the means the child is using to communicate, the caregivers may need assistance in recognizing the communicative function that a behavior is serving. For example, a child may use the verbalization *bye bye* to request cessation of an activity. The caregiver and speech–language pathologist may need to look closely at the situations in which this behavior occurs to be certain that the communication is requesting the end of an activity rather than requesting to leave the session.

Attention also must be given to the response strategies the caregiver is using. Strategies used successfully by a caregiver to keep the child engaged in interaction need to be identified. For example, the caregiver may notice that by using exaggerated intonation patterns and positive affect, he or she can keep the child focused on a social routine for longer periods of time. Caregivers also are assisted in looking at their nonfacilitative responses and exploring alternative responses. For example, caregivers may experience a great deal of frustration when trying to get their child to follow simple verbal directions (e.g., retrieve an object) and may assume that the child is being noncompliant. In exploring alternative responses, the caregiver may find that the child follows simple directions when he or she is already attending to the object or when the request is paired with demonstration of the desired response, and this discovery can alleviate frustration for both the child and the caregiver.

The importance of predictable and consistent routines for children also needs to be emphasized when working with caregivers. Predictable routines help children develop self-regulatory capacities leading to anticipation and planning. Children gain a better sense of self in time and space when the environment is routine and predictable. They then become more able to plan actions and predict consequences, allowing for more control over the environment. For example, when transitional objects are used to signal routine events (e.g., showing a child a cup to signal meal time), the child gradually comes to associate the object with the event. When the child can anticipate the event, he or she frequently has less difficulty in the transition from one activity to another and has more success in planning his or her actions. Clinical experiences suggest that such strategies help to preclude or mitigate behavioral problems.

## PROVIDING SERVICES TO ENVIRONMENTALLY AT-RISK CHILDREN

### Reeducation strategies

Within a family-focused intervention, emphasis should be placed on the caregiver's role in understanding and fostering the child's development. When circumstances such as relationship disturbances (e.g., separation anxiety, abuse, neglect) create situations that interrupt healthful child-rearing practices, patterns of dysfunctional interactions may be established, leaving caregivers and children feeling frustrated and upset (Field, 1987). Parents may lose sight of or abandon positive child-rearing patterns of behavior. Thus, when caregivers are deficient in skills necessary for optimal parenting, reeducation is a primary intervention approach (Sameroff & Fiese, 1990). Early intervention efforts with these families focus on helping the caregivers get back on track by educating the caregivers in facilitating positive interactional experiences. The family will not be able to get back on track, however, unless its members' psychosocial needs are addressed through other support services (Dunst et al., 1990).

In working with families where interactional or relationship disturbances increase the risk of communication prob-

lems, reeducation can be implemented in various ways. Direct instruction is provided in the areas of child development and appropriate child-rearing techniques. Speech–language pathologists play an important role as part of the team in the reeducation process. They may educate caregivers about the interrelationship between language development, socioemotional development, play, cognition, and interactional skills. They may assist caregivers in recognizing their child's levels of functioning and in developing appropriate expectations for their child. Parents are supported as they gain confidence in their abilities to facilitate their child's development.

When working with families with children at risk for communication disorders and emotional and behavioral disorders, another important aspect of treatment is increasing caregivers' flexibility and improving their self-evaluation skills. Caregivers are taught the importance of recognizing their child's skills and specific interests and adjusting the activity or interaction appropriately. Focus here is often on increasing the caregiver's ability to develop a responsive style and to follow the child's lead and abandon their own agenda when necessary (Manolson, 1985). Increasing the caregivers' skills, along with increasing positive interactional experience, aids the caregivers in becoming appropriate language facilitators and in modifying their perceptions of their children.

### Treating interactional disturbances

A speech–language pathologist may use coaching strategies in working with caregiver–child interactional or relationship disturbances (Field, 1982; McDonough, 1989). The work of Clark and Seifer (1985) provides strategies that have been found useful. For a caregiver who frequently is observed to be disengaged or uninvolved in interaction, as is often seen with depressed mothers (Tronick, 1989), professionals may work with caregivers to help them become more aware of the child's attempts to communicate and to acknowledge these attempts through various behaviors such as nodding, smiling, and moving closer to the child (Clark & Seifer, 1985). Emphasis is placed on how the caregiver's behavior affects the child. In this case, a mother's disengagement suggests that she is emotionally unavailable for her child. When a child's attempts to communicate go unacknowledged, the child's behaviors may then resemble that of depression or withdrawal, or the child's behavior may escalate negatively to hitting, screaming, or throwing tantrums. When the caregiver is better able to recognize the child's subtle attempts to communicate or interact, he or she is encouraged to start imitating. As greater comfort is experienced in responding contingently to the child's vocal and play behaviors, the caregiver is encouraged to expand on these behaviors during interactions.

Another dysfunctional interactional pattern may be observed when a caregiver consistently forces his or her own agenda on the child during play. Here speech–language pathologists may help the caregiver realize when the child moves away or disengages from the caregiver because of the caregiver's overly intrusive style. The professional should highlight when the caregiver's more facilitative, less overriding approach results in a successful interaction. The focus here is on flexibility during interaction and the development of the child's mutual regulatory skills, such as negotiating in stressful situations and using others to help solve problems. When parents override, children are not given the opportunity to develop mutual regulatory skills. Caregivers may be encouraged to wait and observe their child's attempts to engage the caregiver, acknowledge and respond contingently, then imitate and expand (Clark & Seifer, 1983; Manolson, 1985).

When disturbed interactional patterns appear to be deeply rooted in dysfunctional caregiver behavior related to extremely stressful life circumstances, speech–language pathologists must work closely with mental health professionals to ensure that other emotional and social supports are addressed (Prizant et al., 1990). In fact, progress with a caregiver and child will be minimal unless the family context is of primary concern (Dunst et al., 1990).

## SERVICE DELIVERY OPTIONS

A number of service delivery options may be used when addressing goals for young children and their families. One option is caregiver–child therapy sessions. An important aspect of caregiver–child sessions is interactive coaching or guidance that facilitates successful caregiver–child interaction (Field, 1982; Mahoney & Powell, 1988; McDonough, 1989). The focus of the caregiver–child sessions is on helping caregivers to develop appropriate styles of interaction in light of the child's level of social-communicative competence and specific communicative profile

(MacDonald, 1989; Snow, Midkiff-Borunda, Small, & Proctor, 1984). Another goal is to give parents the confidence and skills to overcome feelings of helplessness and hopelessness in raising children who may be difficult to interact with (McDonough, 1989).

Caregiver–toddler groups are another service delivery option for meeting the goals of education and facilitation of interaction. Caregiver–toddler groups may be staffed by interdisciplinary or transdisciplinary team members such as speech-language pathologists, child psychologists or psychiatrists, and social workers or special educators. Within the caregiver-toddler groups, the professionals engage in coaching and modeling strategies to assist caregivers in becoming more aware of successes and breakdowns in interaction and to provide them with a repertoire of strategies to improve interactions with their children.

Another option for service provision is educational support programs for caregivers that focus on helping caregivers understand principles of communication development and the caregivers' role in facilitating their child's development of social-communicative competence. This service delivery option may be used in conjunction with individual or group caregiver–child sessions.

The Hanen Early Language Parent Program (Manolson, 1985) is an example of a program designed to help caregivers develop the skills to become more effective language facilitators. The program uses a group format and adult learning principles to help parents develop a mindset for active problem solving in relation to facilitation of language and social-communica-tive competence. The content of the program is divided into two parts. The first part focuses on identifying a child's communicative strategies and the caregivers' responses, emphasizing the importance of recognizing, acknowledging, and expanding on a child's attempts to communicate. The second part assists caregivers in increasing opportunities for communication within a child's daily experiences. Weekly evening sessions are conducted over a 3-month period and include center-based meetings and home visits. A mutually supportive atmosphere allows caregivers to share their successes and challenges with other caregivers (Manolson, 1985).

In both caregiver–child therapy sessions and educational support programs, the use of videotapes to review and discuss interactive successes and breakdowns is becoming more prevalent. Videotape allows for more objective discussion of child abilities and caregiver interactive styles and has proved to be an effective teaching tool (Mahoney & Powell, 1988; Manolson, 1985; McDonough, 1989).

Finally, caregiver support groups may be used in conjunction with caregiver–child therapy sessions and caregiver educational programs. These groups may deal with caregiver and family issues that affect relationships between caregivers and children (e.g., marital discord, social support, caregiver feelings about raising their child). These groups also may be helpful in looking at the family's history and typical family patterns of interaction, which may provide information as to why caregivers may find interactions with their children so difficult.

The speech–language pathologist's role in such groups is dependent on a number of factors, including the focus of the group as determined by the families' stated needs, the professional's training relative to the focus of the group, and the availability of other professionals to address families' emotional needs, particularly mental health professionals. For speech–language pathologists who become involved in caregiver support groups, it is important to recognize professional roles and limitations. For example, most speech–language pathologists would be more prepared to comment on aspects of caregiver–child interaction and communication than on marital issues or strategies for coping with stress related to raising a child with challenging behavior. In settings where mental health professionals and speech–language pathologists work as part of a team, the two types of professionals may consider working together as cotherapists for a caregiver support group. For speech–language pathologists who are not working within a treatment team model, developing contacts with a network of mental health professionals with expertise in family dynamics and family systems is crucial. Mental health professionals are a valuable resource in helping to provide appropriate support services for caregivers.

• • •

The challenge of providing family-focused intervention to young children with both communication disorders and emotional and behavioral disorders requires that speech–language pathologists be aware of the impact these coexisting conditions have on a child's development and the family's functioning. Active caregiver involvement and the development of positive interactional experiences are important aspects of treatment with these children. Appropriate treatment should increase caregivers' competence and confidence and reduce the level of stress experienced by caregivers and children. By precluding the development of maladaptive patterns of interaction and thereby fostering mutually satisfying interactions and relationships, further problems in both communication development and emotional and behavioral development may be prevented or alleviated.

## REFERENCES

Baker, L., & Cantwell, D. (1987). Comparison of well, emotionally disordered and behaviorally disordered children with linguistic problems. *Journal of the American Academy of Child and Adolescent Psychiatry, 26,* 193–196.

Bristol, M., & Schopler, E. (1984). A developmental perspective on stress and coping in families of autistic children. In J. Blacher (Ed.), *Families of severely handicapped children.* New York, NY: Academic Press.

Clark, G., & Seifer, R. (1983). Facilitating mother–infant communications. A treatment model for high-risk and developmentally delayed infants. *Infant Mental Health Journal, 4,* 67–82.

Clark, G.N., & Seifer, R. (1985). Assessment of parent's interactions with their developmentally delayed infants. *Infant Mental Health Journal, 6,* (4), 214–225.

Donnellan, A., Mirenda, P., Mesaros, R., & Fassbender, L. (1984). Analyzing the communicative functions of aberrant behavior. *Journal of the Association for Persons with Severe Handicaps, 9,* 201–212.

Dunst, C. (1983). Communicative competence and deficits: Effects on early social interactions. In E. McDonald & D. Gallagher (Eds.), *Facilitating social-emotional development in the young multiply handicapped child.* Philadelphia, PA: Home of Merciful Saviour Press.

Dunst, C., & Lowe, L. (1986). From reflex to symbol: Describing, explaining, and fostering communication competence. *Augmentative and Alternative Communication, 2,* 11–18.

Dunst, C., Lowe, L., & Bartholomew, P. (1990). Contingent social responsiveness, family ecology and infant communicative competence. *National Student Speech Language and Hearing Association Journal, 17,* 39–49.

Early Intervention Program for Infants and Toddlers with Handicaps: Final regulations. (1989). *Federal Register, 54,* 26306–26348.

Field, T. (1982). Interaction coaching for high-risk infants and their parents. In H. Moss, R. Hess, & C. Swift (Eds.), *Early intervention programs for infants.* Binghamton, NY: Haworth Press.

Field, T. (1987). Affective and interactive disturbances in infants. In J. Osofsky (Ed.), *Handbook of infant development* (2nd ed.). New York, NY: Wiley.

Greenspan, S. (1988). Fostering emotional and social development in infants with disabilities. *Zero to Three, 8,* 8–18.

Klein, M.D., & Briggs, M.H. (1987). Facilitating mother–infant communicative interaction in mothers and high-risk infants. *Journal of Communication Disorders, 10,* 95–106.

Kochanek, T., Kabacoff, R., & Lipsitt, L. (1990). Early identification of developmentally disabled and at-risk preschool children. *Exceptional Children, 56,* 528–538.

MacDonald, J. (1989). *Becoming partners with children: From play to conversation.* San Antonio, TX: Special Press.

Maher, S., Prizant, B., & Gjording, L. (1990). *The Hanen Early Language Parent Program: A modification for adolescent mothers.* Unpublished manuscript.

Mahoney, G., & Powell, A. (1988). Modifying parent–child interaction: Enhancing the development of handicapped children. *Journal of Special Education, 22,* 82–96.

Manolson, A. (1985). *It takes two to talk: Hanen early language parent guidebook.* Toronto, Canada: Hanen Resource Centre.

McDonough, S. (1989, April). *Interaction guidance: Treatment of early relationship disturbances.* Paper presented at Child Psychiatry Grand Rounds, Bradley Hospital, East Providence, RI.

Prizant, B.M., Audet, L., Burke, G., Hummel, L., Maher, S., & Theadore, G. (1990). Communication disorders and emotional/behavioral disorders in children. *Journal of Speech and Hearing Disorders, 55,* 179–192.

Prizant, B., & Wetherby, A. (1988, October). *Toward early detection of communication problems in infants and toddlers.* Paper presented at the International Association of Infant Mental Health, Providence, RI.

Prizant, B., & Wetherby, A. (in press). Communication in preschool autistic children. In E. Schopler, M. Van Bourgandien, & M. Bristol (Eds.), *Preschool issues in autism.* New York, NY: Plenum.

Rossetti, L.M. (1990). *Infant-toddler assessment: An interdisciplinary approach.* Boston, MA: College-Hill.

Sameroff, A. (1987). The social context of development. In N. Eisenburg (Ed.), *Contemporary topics in development.* New York, NY: Wiley.

Sameroff, A., & Fiese, B. (1990). Transactional regulation and early intervention. In S. Meisels & P. Shonkoff (Eds.), *Early intervention: A handbook of theory, practice and analysis.* New York, NY: Cambridge University Press.

Snow, C., Midkiff-Borunda, S., Small, A., & Proctor, A. (1984). Therapy as social interaction: Analyzing the contexts for language remediation. *Topics in Language Disorders, 4* (4), 72–85.

Snyder-McLean, L., Solomonson, B., McLean, J., & Sack, S. (1984). Structuring joint action routines: A strategy for facilitating communication and language development in the classroom. *Seminars in Speech and Language, 5,* 213–228.

Tiegerman, E., & Siperstein, M. (1984). Individual patterns of interaction in the mother-child dyad: Implications for parent intervention. *Topics in Language Disorders, 4* (4), 50–61.

Tronick, E. (1989). Emotions and emotional communication in infancy. *American Psychologist, 44,* 112–119.

Wetherby, A.M., & Prizant, B.M. (1990). *Communication and symbolic behavior scales—experimental edition.* San Antonio, TX: Special Press.

Wetherby, A., Prizant B., & Kublin, K. (1989, November). *Assessing infants and toddlers with an eye towards intervention.* Short course presented at Annual Convention of American Speech-Language-Hearing Association, St. Louis, MO.

# Bringing context back into assessment

*Truman E. Coggins, PhD*
Associate Professor
Department of Speech and Hearing
    Sciences
University of Washington
Seattle, Washington

OVER THE PAST two decades, speech-language clinicians have developed a deeper understanding of the relationship between language and the social context in which it occurs. They now appreciate that besides word meanings, children must also acquire knowledge about the conditions and rules that govern how they use language for communicative purposes. The implications of such information for the assessment and intervention of developmentally delayed infants, or infants at risk for developmental delays, are beginning to be recognized.

A review of the literature that has examined the communicative basis of language reveals two important themes. First, children are successful in using a variety of intentional behaviors at a time when their expressive language is characterized by few, if any, words. By the time children begin to produce their first multiword utterances, they have developed strategies for "here and now communication in the here-and-now of the situation" (Brether-

*Top Lang Disord*, 1991,11(4),43–54

ton, 1988, p. 245). In fact, during the first 18 months, a child's development may be manifest more by the number of communicative intentions used than by either lexical or structural advances (Ingram, 1974). Second, speech-language pathologists are beginning to appreciate the dramatic effect of context on language learning. What children say, why and when they say it, and how they interpret what others say to them, is conditioned by or contingent on the context. Prutting (1982) argued that understanding communicative interactions and meaning is tantamount to understanding context. Because the context in which communication takes place is dynamic, complex, and often elusive, its effect "cannot be predicted for an individual child" (Gallagher, 1983, p. 12). Thus, individual differences in children's social use of language are expected.

Although language specialists have become more aware of the effect of context on communication, they still behave as if context is not all that important with respect to assessment. Generally speaking, the lion's share of time devoted to clinical assessment revolves around selecting and administering particular diagnostic measures, recording and transcribing protocols, and analyzing and interpreting the data. Precious little time is set aside to consider the ways in which contextual variables may influence or determine children's communicative interactions and the meanings they express. Therefore, the purpose behind this article is to examine how various dimensions of the context may affect the clinical assessment of communicative intentions in developmentally young children.

## THE IMPORTANCE OF COMMUNICATIVE INTENTIONS

By the time most children developing language normally celebrate their first birthday, they are able to communicate intentionally through gestures or gestures paired with vocalizations. Intention refers to "the deliberate pursuit of a goal by means of instrumental behaviors subordinated to that goal" (Dore, 1975, p. 36). During the next few months (i.e., 12 to 15 months), gestural communicative acts decrease substantially while words or phonetically consistent forms show a steady increase (Carpenter, Mastergeorge, & Coggins, 1983). By the end of the sensorimotor period, communication has become a predominately verbal enterprise with children often using word combinations to express their intentions during social interactions.

A significant accomplishment of this preverbal period is the child's ability to influence purposefully the actions of their communicative partners. Even though these children are at the threshold of verbal language, they are quite capable of making their wants and needs known (Coggins & Carpenter, 1981). Because communicative intent may be regarded as a necessary precursor for the acquisition of subsequent conversational (i.e., dialogue) skills, this period holds special significance for researchers attempting to show continuity between preverbal communicative intent and subsequent linguistic and communicative skills. Further, as Wetherby, Cain, Yoṇclas, and Walker (1988) have aptly noted, the frequency and type of communicative intentions may serve as a harbinger of later linguistic difficulties. Thus, communicative intentions have become an important, if not essential, component of clinical assessment for children who do not use language or children at-risk for language delays.

## PATTERNS OF PERFORMANCE IN CLINICAL POPULATIONS

Over the past 10 years, numerous studies have examined communicative intentions in different clinical populations. A review of the literature reveals communicative profiles for children identified as specifically language impaired (Fey, Leonard, Fey, & O'Connor, 1978; Leonard, Camarata, Rowan, & Chapman, 1982; Rom & Bliss, 1981; Snyder, 1978), autistic (Wetherby, 1986; Wetherby & Prutting, 1984), Down syndrome (Coggins, Carpenter, & Owings, 1983; Greenwald & Leonard, 1979; Smith & vonTetzchner, 1986), and most recently, "late talkers" (Paul, 1989). Most investigators who examined and described the intentional communicative behaviors in these populations have tended to focus on diversity of use and mode of expression. Recently, Wetherby and colleagues (1988; Wetherby, Yonclas, & Bryan, 1989) have explored the usefulness of rate of communicative intents as an important clinical measure for children functioning in the preverbal and earliest stages of linguistic development.

### Diversity of use

Several studies have examined whether language-impaired children exhibit delays in their intentional use of language that go beyond their level of delay in cognitive and/or linguistic development (Blank, Gessner, & Esposito, 1979; Coggins et al., 1983; Greenwald & Leonard, 1979; Snyder, 1978). The underlying assumption is that communicatively impaired children use language differently in communicative contexts from children developing language normally. The data that have accumulated over the last 10 years reveal variation within and between handicapping conditions.

The results from several independent investigations reveal language-impaired children and children developing language normally use communicative intents similarly during the earliest stages of language learning (i.e., the first 2 years of life). To illustrate, when matched for general linguistic abilities, some children with Down syndrome, specific language impairment, or delayed onset of language have demonstrated interpersonal communicative behaviors that are generally commensurate with their overall linguistic level. Moreover, their ability to communicate intentionally is consistent with what one might expect from children developing language normally.

The findings from other experimental studies, however, reveal quite a different profile of abilities. Investigators have identified delays or differences in the acquisition of communicative intents in children with specific language impairments (Wetherby et al., 1989), children diagnosed as autistic (Wetherby, 1986; Wetherby & Prutting, 1984; Wetherby et al., 1989), and developmentally delayed adolescents functioning below the age of 2 (Cirrin & Rowland, 1985).

## Mode of expression

A second issue of interest has centered on the mode children use to encode intentional communicative acts. Because communicatively impaired children are at risk for delayed onset of language, it has been suggested that they may rely heavily on gestures or gestural/vocal sequences to encode their communicative intents during the early stages of development. Not surprisingly, children who are language impaired or are at risk for language impairments have been found to produce fewer vocalizations and verbalizations and more gestures or gestural sequences to encode their communicative intents (Greenwald & Leonard, 1979; Rowan, Leonard, Chapman, & Weiss, 1983; Snyder, 1978; Wetherby & Prutting, 1984). It has even been suggested that the dependency on gestures may be a typical pattern of infants and toddlers with communicative impairments (Wetherby et al., 1989).

## Rate of communicative intentions

The frequency of communicative acts may prove to be a useful clinical measure. Wetherby and colleagues (1988) found that the rate of intentional communication in children developing language normally increased substantially with age. The communicative behavior of their 15 subjects was assessed at three stages of development over a 12-month period: prelinguistic stage, one-word stage, and multiword stage. Data were collected at each of the three target ages in both an unstructured and structured context. During the prelinguistic stage, subjects expressed an average of one communicative act per minute.

By the time the subjects were in the one-word stage of development, they were encoding nearly two acts per minute. Subjects expressed roughly five intentional acts by the time they reached stage 2 of linguistic development (i.e., mean length of utterance/morphemes $\geq$ 2.15).

Recently, Wetherby et al. (1989) compared the communicative profiles of children with Down syndrome, specific language impairments, and autism with those of the 15 normal children summarized above. The investigators reported that the rate with which the handicapped subjects used intentional communicative acts was not contingent on linguistic advances. Thus, Wetherby and colleagues proposed that communicative rate may prove to be an effective means of predicting communicative impairments in preverbal children.

While the Wetherby data regarding rate are encouraging, they are also variable. For example, a 30-minute sample of communicative behavior was obtained for 2 children diagnosed as specifically language impaired (SLI). The 2 children were the same age (29 months), had the same expressive and receptive communication age (16 months and 24 months, respectively), and had equivalent mental ages (26 months and 25 months). Despite these similarities, 1 SLI child used 234 communicative acts in 30 minutes whereas the second used 89.

The range of variability between these two children presents a dilemma for professionals who are assessing the communicative intentions of developmentally delayed children or children at risk for future delays. In short, little is known about the range of expected variability in children at this stage of development. Because contextual variables are known to contribute to individual differences in children's social use of language, it seems essential for speech-language clinicians to consider the ways in which context might influence patterns of performance during clinical assessment.

## VARIABILITY AND CONTEXT

Much of the research devoted to the analysis of children's communicative intents has centered on assessment taxonomies. Numerous classification systems representing a variety of philosophical viewpoints, have been constructed over the last 10 years (for a detailed summary, see Chapman, 1981; Wetherby & Prizant, 1989). These protocols have yielded considerable information about the early stages of normal communicative development and, as noted above, a growing body of knowledge regarding the intentional communicative behavior of children with language impairments.

Although considerable time and energy has gone into observing and coding intentional communicative behavior, little attention has been paid to the ways in which contextual variables may influence a child's behavior. Ervin-Tripp (1978) has aptly stated that context is most everything that clinicians and experimenters used to disregard when they analyzed language (Ervin-Tripp, 1978). For many investigators, controlling context has meant observing a child in a free-play situation, with a standard set of toys, where the adult (usually the mother) has been instructed to "play with your child as you usually do." The

implicit assumption underlying these instructions is that context exerts a consistent influence across children. However, following a comprehensive and critical review of the literature in normal and language-impaired children, Gallagher (1983) concluded that language use varies substantially depending on the context. Trying to use one clinical context to measure a child's ability or potential no longer appears to be a realistic goal of assessment.

McCabe (1989) recently has presented a conceptual model that illustrates how linguistic and nonlinguistic contextual factors may influence a child's rate and style of development. With respect to context, she writes the following:

... it is important that we not lose sight of the fundamental interactive nature of language and the context in which it occurs. As an interactive system, both parent and child influence the content as well as the form of communication. In considering the context of language interaction we must recognize that the child has a host of characteristics in addition to that of being a language learner, and each of these characteristics is a potential influence on the form and content of communication. (p. 6)

The reason young children select particular communicative intentions is a function of their experience and the multifaceted aspects of the context, as they perceive it. Thus, it is necessary to account for important and influential aspects of context if we expect to generate meaningful assessment data and effective intervention programs.

The following section reviews selected experimental research to demonstrate the context-dependent nature of communication. The summary focuses on important contextual variables that have the potential to influence substantially the performance of infants and young children. The article concludes with a discussion regarding how the speech-language pathologist can manipulate these variables in order to increase the likelihood of obtaining a child's optimal level of performance during clinical assessment.

## CONTEXTUAL VARIABLES

### Task characteristics

The purpose of a particular activity may exert a notable influence on a child's communicative use of language. Jones and Adamson (1987) observed 32 mother–child dyads during a book-reading activity and free play. They found that children's use of referential speech (i.e., utterances that focused the listener's attention on specific objects and/or attributes) was far more frequent during free play. However, during the book-reading activity, children were much more likely to request information than to produce contingent utterances.

O'Brien and Nagel (1987) have examined the influence that different types of eliciting stimuli exert on parents' use of language. In contrast to earlier reports, the investigators found that parents systematically adjusted their speech to the materials at hand rather than to the sex of the child. For example, when parents played with dolls, they commented frequently, asked many questions, produced a variety of lexical items, and, perhaps most importantly, encouraged verbalizations from their children. In contrast, when parents played with cars and trucks, they typically resorted to "imaginative sounds" rather than engaging their children in conversational interactions. In a related study, Conti-Ramsden and Friel-Patti (1987) also demonstrated that stimulus materials may influence the number and length of conversational interactions.

The collective findings from these three studies underscore the context-dependent nature of communication. Children are likely to receive different opportunities for using intentional communicative behaviors as a result of the distinctive patterns of adult language that accompanies different play contexts. Speech-language clinicians must begin to monitor the materials and opportunities available to adult–child dyads during free play or low-structured activities in order to obtain representative assessment data.

### Opportunities

Language use has been found to vary substantially as a function of context, and this variability appears difficult to control (Gallagher, 1983). For example, Bates, Camaioni, and Volterra (1975) report protesting to be one of their subjects' earliest communicative intentions. Yet, other researchers have observed few intentional protests in their sensorimotor subjects (Carpenter, et al., 1983; Dore, 1975). In attempting to account for these differences, Carpenter et al. (1983) suggested that mothers become increasingly adept at predicting which activities their children will reject or decline to perform and frequently removed potential sources of conflict. Thus, protesting may be observed infrequently in a particular situation because the child has insufficient opportunities to use the intention.

Elicitation procedures may be considered when opportunities for communicative intents are limited in naturalistic interactions or specific intents are to be analyzed. Carpenter et al. (1983) created specific tasks for mothers to elicit intentional communicative behaviors from their children. The tasks provided contexts in which the behavior of interest could be readily identified, and created some type of activity that involved the mutual participation of the mother and child. The specific tasks were administered as appropriate opportunities arose during the assessment rather than in a predetermined order. Wetherby and Prutting (1984) used clinicians to structure "communicative temptations" in which the child is likely to emit the desired intention. For example, in order to elicit an intentional request, the clinician would open a jar of bubbles, blow several in the direction of the child, then screw the cap tightly on the bubbles and hand the jar to the child.

While an elicitation task provides specific opportunities for a child to produce a desired behavior, it does not guarantee a response. In fact, a single assessment method is unlikely to produce a representative sample of children's intentional communication. For example, Coggins, Olswang, and Guthrie (1987) demonstrated that structured elicitation tasks were effective in sampling intentional requests in children as young as 15 months. However, the investigators were largely unsuccessful in their attempts to elicit intentional comments from these same children until late in the second year (i.e., 21 months).

This discrepancy appears to be the result of two contextual factors. First, children generally comment on objects or events that they find interesting. Because stimuli are controlled and directed by the examiners during elicitation tasks, children seem far less likely to comment. Second, early comments are most often used in familiar and supportive environments about familiar topics or events. Thus, infants and young children tend to share information with familiar and responsive adults (i.e., their parents) in spontaneously occurring events rather than with strangers (i.e., examiners) during contrived elicitation tasks. These findings suggest that accurate and reliable information regarding children's early communication may require more than just sufficient opportunities to encode intentions. Clinicians must judiciously evaluate the effect that contextual variables exert on different assessment techniques with children at different developmental levels.

**Event context**

Routine events provide an important context in which communicative intents may be mutually understood and conventionalized (Ninio & Wheeler, 1983). In a real sense, parents create order in their children's world that helps them to acquire new social and experiential knowledge (Vygotsky, 1978). Children rely on this order and parental cuing to produce situationally appropriate behaviors while they are learning what to do or how to perform.

Platt and Coggins (1990) have recently examined the effect of adult structure on the social-action game participation of 29 children from 9 to 15 months of age. By design, the mothers of the children were obligated to elicit two social-action games (e.g., peek-a-boo, patty cake) using the least amount of cuing possible. If, however, the child did not participate in the game, the mothers were instructed to provide additional cues or physical prompts to facilitate responding. The results revealed that children rely on parental cuing to produce situationally appropriate behaviors while their understanding of communication games are being formed. Moreover, the children used a significantly greater number of behaviors typically associated with the games when their parents paired gestural and physical cues with verbal requests. The results were interpreted as support for the notion that structuring an event may optimize a child's level of performance.

Children's use of language in predictable or routine events is closely aligned with the notion of "scripts" (see Nelson, 1986). A script is a framework for organizing real-world events that are temporally and causally related. Conti-Ramsden and Friel-Patti (1987) have explored the effects of scripts on situational variables. The investigators discovered that when children were confronted with a new toy, their communicative interactions contained few routine interaction patterns. Because their communicative attempts were not temporally and causally organized, semantic contingency was remarkably low. In contrast, when mothers and their children were observed playing with a variety of *familiar* toys, semantic contingency was quite high. That is, in "low-script" contexts, the subjects generated fewer topics and fewer contingent utterances; however, during "high-script" contexts, children demonstrated more complex conversational competence.

Routine events appear to reduce the amount of effort children need to expend in order to understand messages or participate in social interactions. It would not be unreasonable, therefore, to expect that the frequency with which a child uses communicative intents would be enhanced if the eliciting context contained familiar and predictable scripts or structured events.

## Maintaining joint attention

During episodes of joint attention, children participate in extended conversations and are best able to determine the meanings or intentions of the adult's language (Snow, Perlmann, & Nathan, 1987; Tomasello & Farrar, 1986; Tomasello & Todd, 1983). Maintaining joint attentional episodes is best accomplished by following the child's lead and talking about people, objects, and events on which the child is focused. Clinicians or caretakers who are controlling and directing during social interactions may hinder joint focus and restrict discourse episodes that act to confirm, extend, or expand children's communicative attempts.

## Responsivity

The timing of verbal responses may affect the quantity and quality of communicative interactions. Adults who respond to children's vocalizations in a timely fashion may actually facilitate communication. Prompt and consistent verbal responses may contribute to the infant's understanding of how and when to use language.

Roth (1987) examined the communicative interactions of mothers and their 12-month-old children. She observed 6 dyads in their respective homes for 30 minutes during unstructured play. The findings led Roth to conclude that mothers who provide relevant information within an optimal temporal interval may facilitate the infant's acquisition. According to Roth, a 1-second interval is the time window in which children are readily able to perceive the contingency of their partner's utterance.

## INFLUENCE OF CONTEXT ON ASSESSMENT

Based on the literature reviewed, it seems reasonable to argue that the frequency, the diversity, and even the mode with which communicative intents are expressed may vary considerably depending on the context. Because the effects of contextual variables "cannot be predicted for an individual nor can they be assumed to be consistent across children (Gallagher, 1983, p. 12), speech-language clinicians cannot automatically assume that a sample obtained under one set of conditions will yield the same information for different children. Consider, for example, two hypothetical 30-month-old children with delayed expressive language development. The communicative intentions of both children are assessed by an examiner during a naturalistic interaction with their respective mothers. If one child was observed under a set of conditions that optimized performance (e.g., responsive adult, routine or predictable social interactions, familiar toys, specific communicative opportunities), whereas the other child was observed under less favorable conditions (e.g., directive adult, low "scriptedness," novel objects, restricted communicative opportunities), differences in outcome could be a function of performance variables rather than communica-

tive competence. In order to obtain representative samples of performance from different children, the examiner will need to configure a variety of contextual variables during the assessment. Only in this way will the clinician be able to reconcile variability in children's use of language (Coggins & Olswang, 1987).

Developmentally young children use intentional nonverbal gestures and vocalizations as well as words during communicative interactions. Thus, a clinical evaluation should determine the mode, meanings, and intentions an at-risk child is capable of understanding and producing. To meet this assessment goal, the clinician must use techniques for determining the conditions under which different communicative intentions can be used in their most sophisticated, conventional form. The focus of this type of clinical assessment is on a child's best performance when varying amounts of contextual support are provided. This dynamic approach to assessment can provide clinicians with crucial information regarding which contextual variables influence performance and provide some insight into a child's potential for change (see Coggins & Olswang, 1987; Olswang, Bain, & Johnson, 1990).

In order to assess a child's optimal performance, both nonlinguistic and linguistic variables must be skillfully managed. Nonlinguistic factors include many of the contextual variables summarized above: purpose/type of activity; nature of stimulus materials; responsivity of listeners; and familiar, routine events. Linguistic variables, also discussed earlier, focus on the adult's verbalizations. Skillful management involves the systematic manipulation of these variables along a continuum

Table 1.  Manipulating contextual variables that influence performance

| Variable | Minimal contextual support | Maximal contextual support |
|---|---|---|
| *Nonlinguistic* | | |
| Interaction | Naturalistic | Contrived tasks |
| Materials | No toys or props | Familiar and thematic |
| Interactor | Clinician | Mother/caregiver |
| Activities | Novel | Event routines |
| *Linguistic* | | |
| Cuing | Indirect model | Elicited imitation |

that varies from minimal amounts of support to maximum amounts of cuing. If performance improves when nonlinguistic and linguistic factors are more explicit, the child shows the potential for change—a crucial piece of knowledge in designing intervention programs. No change, however, raises a question regarding the modifiability of performance and the child's immediate potential for change. A summary of these important contextual variables is presented in Table 1.

Gallagher (1983) developed a preassessment interview to "individualize language sampling contexts by systematically obtaining information from parents and/or adult caretakers who may be knowledgeable about the child's language use" (p. 13). Information gathered through this type of interview may allow for a more effective

assessment of the contextual variables in Table 1. In fact, the knowledge clinicians gain through a preassessment interview allows them to individualize relevant contextual variables, raising the possibility that a child's best performance may actually be obtained in the clinical setting.

• • •

Because communicative intents are acquired in context-dependent situations, communication and context stand as essential variables to manipulate during the assessments of developmentally young children. Clearly, the only way in which speech-language clinicians will ultimately attain a complete and satisfying understanding of a handicapped child's social use of language is to bring context back into the assessment process.

## REFERENCES

Bates, E., Camaioni, L., & Volterra, V. (1975). The acquisition of performatives prior to speech. *Merrill-Palmer Quarterly, 21,* 205–226.

Blank, M., Gessner, M., & Esposito, A. (1979). Language without communication: A case study. *Journal of Child Language, 6,* 329–352.

Bretherton, I. (1988). How to do things with one word: The ontogenesis of intentional message making in infancy.

In M. Smith & J. Locke (Eds.), *The emergent lexicon: The child's development of a linguistic vocabulary.* New York, NY: Academic Press.

Carpenter, R., Mastergeorge, A., & Coggins, T. (1983). The acquisition of communicative intentions in infants eight to fifteen months of age. *Language and Speech, 26,* 101–116.

Chapman, R. (1981). Exploring intentional communication. In J. Miller (Ed.), *Assessing language production in children*. Baltimore, MD: University Park Press.

Cirrin, F., & Rowland, C. (1985). Communicative assessment of nonverbal youths with severe/profound mental retardation. *Mental Retardation, 23*, 52–62.

Coggins, T., & Carpenter, R. (1981). The communicative intention inventory: A system for observing and coding children's early intentional communication. *Applied Psycholinguistics, 2*, 235–251.

Coggins, T., Carpenter, R., & Owings, N. (1983). Examining early intentional communicative behaviors in Down's syndrome and non-retarded children. *British Journal of Disorders of Communication, 18*, 99–167.

Coggins, T., & Olswang, L. (1987). The pragmatics of generalization. *Seminars in Speech and Language, 8*, 283–302.

Coggins, T., Olswang, L., & Guthrie, J. (1987). Assessing communicative intents in young children: Low structured observation or elicitation tasks? *Journal of Speech and Hearing Disorders, 52*, 44–49.

Conti-Ramsden, & Friel-Patti, S. (1987). Situational variability in mother-child conversations. In K.E. Nelson (Ed.), *Children's language (Vol. 6)*. Hillsdale, NJ: Erlbaum.

Dore, J. (1975). Holophrases, speech acts, and language universals. *Journal of Child Language, 2*, 21–40.

Ervin-Tripp, S. (1978). [Conference discussion.] Stanford Child Language Forum, Stanford University, Palo Alto, CA.

Fey, M., Leonard, L., Fey, S., & O'Connor, K. (1978). *The intent to communicate in language-impaired children*. Paper presented at the Third Annual Boston University Conference on Language Development, Boston, MA.

Gallagher, T. (1983). Pre-assessment: A procedure for accommodating language variability. In T. Gallagher & C. Prutting (Eds.), *Pragmatic assessment and intervention issues in language*. San Diego, CA: College-Hill Press.

Greenwald, C., & Leonard, L. (1979). Communicative and sensorimotor development of Down's syndrome children. *American Journal of Mental Deficiency, 84*, 296–303.

Ingram, D. (1974). *Stages in the development of one-word utterances*. Paper presented at the Child Language Research Forum, Palo Alto, CA.

Jones, C., & Adamson, L. (1987). Language used in mother-child and mother-child-sibling interactions. *Child Development, 58*, 356–366.

Leonard, L., Camarata, S., Rowan, L., & Chapman, C. (1982). The communicative functions of lexical usage by language impaired children. *Applied Psycholinguistics, 3*, 109–127.

McCabe, A. (1989). Differential language learning styles in young children: The importance of context. *Developmental Review, 9*, 1–20.

Nelson, K. (1986). *Making sense: The acquisition of shared meaning*. Orlando, FL: Academic Press.

Ninio, A., & Wheeler, P. (1983). Functions of speech in mother infant interaction. In L. Feagans, C. Garvey, & R. Golinoff (Eds.), *The origins and growth of communication*. Norwood, NJ: Ablex.

O'Brien, M., & Nagel, K. (1987). Parents' speech to toddlers: The effect of play context. *Journal of Child Language, 14*, 269–279.

Olswang, L., Bain, B., & Johnson, G. (1990). Using dynamic assessment with children with language disorders. In S. Warren and J. Reichle (Eds.), *Causes and effects of communication and language intervention*. Baltimore, MD: Paul H. Brookes.

Paul, R. (1989). *Outcomes of delayed expressive language development: Age three*. Paper presented to the 10th annual Conference of Child Language Disorders, Madison, WI.

Platt, J., & Coggins, T. (1990). Comprehension of social-action games in prelinguistic children. *Journal of Speech and Hearing Disorders, 55*, 315–326.

Prutting, C. (1982). Pragmatics of social competence. *Journal of Speech and Hearing Disorders, 47*, 123–133.

Rom, A., & Bliss, L. (1981). A comparison of verbal communicative skills of language impaired and normal speaking children. *Journal of Communication Disorders, 14*, 133–140.

Roth, P. (1987). Temporal characteristics of maternal verbal styles. In K.E. Nelson and A. vanKleeck (Eds.), *Children's Language Volume 6*. Hillsdale, NJ: Erlbaum.

Rowan, L., Leonard, L., Chapman, C., & Weiss, A. (1983). Performative and presuppositional skills in language-disordered and normal children. *Journal of Speech and Hearing Research, 26*, 97–106.

Smith, L., & vonTetzchner, S. (1986). Communicative, sensorimotor, and language skills of young children with Down syndrome. *American Journal of Mental Deficiency, 91*, 57–66.

Snow, C., Perlmann, R., & Nathan, D. (1987). Why routines are different: Toward a multiple-factors model of the relation between input and language acquisition. In K.E. Nelson and A. vanKleeck (Eds.), *Children's language (Vol. 6)*. Hillsdale, NJ: Erlbaum.

Snyder, L. (1978). Communicative and cognitive abilities and disabilities in the sensorimotor period. *Merrill-Palmer Quarterly, 24*, 161–180.

Tomasello, M., & Farrar, M. (1986). Joint attention and early language. *Child Development, 57*, 1454–1463.

Tomasello, M., & Todd, M. (1983). Joint attention and lexical acquisition style. *First Language, 4*, 197–212.

Vygotsky, L. (1978). *Mind in society: The development of psychological processes.* Cambridge, MA: Harvard University Press.

Wetherby, A. (1986). Ontogeny of communicative functions in autism. *Journal of Autism and Developmental Disorders, 16,* 295–316.

Wetherby, A., Cain, D., Yonclas, D., & Walker, V. (1988). Analysis of intentional communication of normal children from prelinguistic to the multi-word stage. *Journal of Speech and Hearing Research, 31,* 240–252.

Wetherby, A., & Prizant, B. (1989). The expression of communicative intent: Assessment guidelines. *Seminars in Speech and Language, 10,* 77–94.

Wetherby, A., & Prutting, C. (1984). Profiles of communicative and cognitive-social abilities in autistic children. *Journal of Speech and Hearing Research, 27,* 364–377.

Wetherby, A., Yonclas, D., & Bryan, A. (1989). Communicative profiles of preschool children with handicaps: Implications for early identification. *Journal of Speech and Hearing Disorders, 54,* 148–158.

# The role of world knowledge in language comprehension and language intervention

*Linda M. Milosky, PhD*
*Assistant Professor*
*Communication Sciences and Disorders*
*Syracuse University*
*Syracuse, New York*

THE GOAL OF this introductory article is to provide a clinically relevant explication of what world knowledge is and how it should be considered in the intervention process. The clinical applications suggested are derived from a theoretical model about language comprehension and from empirical studies of normal development. As such, they are tentative and are intended to provoke thought about the assumptions on which intervention is based.

## WHAT IS WORLD KNOWLEDGE?

World knowledge, in its totality, is the knowledge gained from experience, from interacting with others and with the objects, events, and situations in life. Upon examination, the role of world knowledge in language learning seems at the same time both obvious and completely overwhelming. Indeed, what cannot be characterized as "world knowledge," given that

*Top Lang Disord*, 1990,10(3),1–13
© 1990 Aspen Publishers, Inc.

anything termed knowledge is likely to have been gained as a result of interactions in and with the world? Yet, clinicians and researchers need to characterize and account for the wealth of information individuals bring to the communication process as a result of their experiences. Clinicians may see children who seem to lack relevant experience or who seem not to connect an ongoing activity or discussion to what they already know about the topic. Thus, experience-based knowledge of the world is crucial to a theory of language processing and in the practice of language intervention. However, often such knowledge is delineated only vaguely.

As models of language processing have been modified and reconceptualized by the pragmatic revolution, the importance of "background knowledge," shared information, and contextualization of talk has been the subject of much discussion. Language clinicians who have long focused on specifying syntactic and semantic target structures more recently have specified pragmatic targets as a focus of therapy. However, often as a result of didactic tradition, syntax, semantics, and pragmatics are considered separate areas of language intervention (see Lund & Duchan's 1988 discussion of "sensemaking" for a notable exception). What follows is a brief description of a model of language comprehension embedded in, and hence inseparable from, context; a listing of the various elements of context and background knowledge; and selected illustrations of how these aspects have been determined to affect comprehension of language. Clinical implications are suggested within the discussion of each element. The literature has not been exhaustively reviewed for each aspect; rather, the concepts have been illustrated.

## COMPREHENSION: DECODING OR INTERPRETATION?

Many models of language comprehension that have been used to explain language disorders have relied on the notion of sentence decoding (ASHA Committee, 1980; Bernstein & Tiegerman, 1989; Nation & Aram, 1984). In defining language disorders, they have spoken of a disruption in the linguistic code for representing ideas. In this view, then, comprehension of language is presented as a process in which the listener uses syntactic and semantic codes to determine meaning. In fact, in discussing language learning, one often sees references to children "cracking the code." According to a decoding model, word meanings are accessed from a mental dictionary, sentences are divided into syntactic structures by a parser, relations between word meanings are determined by the nature of the parsing (by the syntactic structures contained in the sentence), and the meaning of the sentence is determined by the interaction of sentence structure and word meanings (Cairns, 1983; Ford, Bresnan, & Kaplan, 1982; Tanenhaus, Carlson, & Seidenberg, 1985). After this linguistic meaning is achieved, the sentence is then related to what is broadly termed "context," and meaning is enhanced by placing the sentence in context. In this view, sentence syntax and semantics are seen as being deterministic—that is, as generating a finite and generally small number of alternative sentence meanings. The comprehender then selects from among these possible meanings.

Language, however, is filled with potential ambiguities—syntactic, semantic, pragmatic, and phonological. One might be inclined to assume that most words have one, perhaps two, or at most three meanings. But there are often many more meanings. The many possible meanings or senses of words can be combined with the senses of other words in different ways, resulting in a very large number of potential meanings for any one sentence. For example, the Box delineates the possible meanings of the words "approach" and "bugs" in the sentence "Jane approached the man looking for bugs." If listeners created various combinations of those meanings, a very large number of potential sentence meanings would result. Given

this large number of potential interpretations for a sentence, a model in which all possible meanings are generated for each sentence and then are compared with the context seems less plausible.

How, then, is successful communication achieved? An alternative model (Clark, 1983; Garrod & Sanford, 1983; Marslen-Wilson & Tyler, 1980; Waltz & Pollack, 1985) would suggest that we activate only relevant senses of words and information and attempt to make incoming information relevant to what we already know. For example, if listeners first heard "Jane was a school nurse. She was concerned about an outbreak of lice among the teachers and children in the elementary school. Her next patient was the fourth grade teacher.", this context would help them activate relevant information. The relevant information, or world knowledge, that is accessed and activated is based on experience, and it is selectively activated. In the process of comprehending, what gets activated is, in part, determined by what knowledge is relevant given the speaker, the physical environment, the social occasion, the goals of the interaction, the affective variables, and the prior discussion. These all enable a listener to determine rapidly and selectively what a speaker is saying.

The implications of such a world-knowledge–driven model are considerable for the clinician. Therapy stimuli or targets cannot be considered as merely words or language, but must be considered as packets of information about the world. Although language is often described as being abstract and arbitrary, its use in the real world is far from that. In conveying meaning and in creating a representation

---

### Possible Meanings of "Bugs" and "Approach"

**Bugs**

Vermin
Insects
Electronic surveillance devices
Bugs Bunny
Bugs Malone (gangster)
Annoys (i.e., "He really bugs me.")
Computer glitches
Hobgoblin (dialectical or literary)
Defects or difficulty (i.e., "I still need to work the bugs out.")

**Approach**

To come near or nearer to
To come near to in quality, character, time, or condition
To begin work on (to approach a problem)
To bring near to something
To make advances or a proposal to
To approximate (a fair approach to accuracy)
To prepare to ask about

Source: Barnhart, Co. (Editor in Chief) (1968). *The American College Dictionary*. New York, NY.: Random House.

> **Therapy stimuli or targets cannot be considered as merely words or language, but must be considered as packets of information about the world.**

of that meaning in a listener's mind, language processing incorporates physical context, knowledge of the speaker, event context, prior experience, and affective states of the interactants; most often, it is firmly tied to everyday experience. Given that orientation, therapy goals, stimuli, materials, and tasks need to be reconceptualized. The goals of therapy are not how to teach a child a set of words or a set of structures, but rather how to teach a child to call up relevant knowledge and to use language in order to interact and add to that knowledge in some coherent fashion. Therefore, the following sections will provide brief examples of how different aspects of context may affect processing of language.

## LINGUISTIC CONTEXT

When interpreting any given utterance, listeners rely on their knowledge of what has come before in the discourse. Understanding of an utterance does not occur in isolation, but rather by interpreting the utterance in relation to the already established topic. In fact, temporary communication breakdowns are likely to occur when listeners cannot make a new utterance fit into their representation of the content of the conversation. A striking example of this occurred when the author

was shopping for computer hardware and software with a colleague at the campus bookstore. After investigating the price of several items, the author remarked "Now all I have to decide is if I want a cookie." (The bookstore, in addition to purveying textbooks, featured a large assortment of cookies, candies, and chips of the edible variety.) My colleague remarked "I don't know what that is." Because he and I had often laughed about our mutual tendency to go to the bookstore in the middle of long afternoons to buy a snack, I was surprised by this remark and repeated, "A cookie—you know." Again, he reiterated, somewhat defensively, "No, I really don't know what that is." It finally dawned on me that he had thought I was referring to some esoteric piece of computer hardware. This example illustrates how the listener is driven to use prior discussion and nonverbal context to call up the appropriate meanings of words and relevant experiences so that images can be created from language. When current topics are not consistent with prior context, a listener may go so far as to reject common meanings of words.

Without knowledge of a topic, a listener may find a well-constructed piece of discourse almost meaningless. For example, read the following passage about a familiar activity, taken from a study by Bransford and Johnson (1972):

A newspaper is better than a magazine. A seashore is a better place than the street. At first it is better to run than to walk. You may have to try several times. It takes some skill but it's easy to learn. Even young children can enjoy it. Once successful, complications are minimal. Birds seldom get too close. Rain, however, soaks in very fast. Too many people doing the same thing can also cause problems.

One needs lots of room. If there are not complications, it can be very peaceful. A rock will serve as an anchor. If things break loose from it, however, you will not get a second chance (p. 722).

The words are understandable, the sentences grammatical, and yet you would have great difficulty remembering the details. However, if you had been told that a passage about flying a kite was to follow, the entire passage not only makes sense but also becomes much easier to remember as Bransford and Johnson (1972) have shown. When listeners/readers know that flying a kite is the topic, they bring up their relevant personal experience with flying kites and seeing them flown. If language-impaired children are unable to call up relevant senses of words and relevant experiences, then their experience may be much like ours in reading the above passage without knowing the topic.

In assessing and treating language-impaired children, pragmatic theory dictates embedding language in a meaningful context, but at times specification of the nature of that context has been lacking. Typically, the degree and type of contextualization have not been characterized as part of clinical goals. Instead, context often has been relegated to the realm of the therapy activity, the relatively unimportant vehicle for presenting target stimuli. However, research suggests context should not be equated with activity. Crais (see "World knowledge to word knowledge," this issue) has shown how embedding novel words in familiar story contexts allows children to learn about the words very rapidly. However, children may need to be taught how to use contextual information. Sternberg (1987) has demonstrated that even adults benefit from training on how to use contextual cues to figure out the meanings of novel words in paragraphs. Such metalinguistic training would seem particularly beneficial to school-aged children, and yet such comprehension instruction may not occur very often. Anderson (1984) cites a study by Durkin (1978–79), who observed 18,000 minutes of elementary school reading and social studies periods and found that less than 1% of that time consisted of comprehension instruction. The category of comprehension instruction was defined as "teacher doing or saying something that would help a child figure out the meaning of a unit of language larger than a word" (pp. 9–10). Linguistic context is a vital source of information for comprehending further language, and as such should be carefully structured and incorporated into therapeutic goals.

## PHYSICAL CONTEXT

Interpretation of utterances also is affected in a variety of ways by physical surroundings. For example, knowledge of the physical surroundings in which interaction occurs is required to be able to assign exact meaning to deictic terms (i.e., verbal pointers of time, place, or person, e.g., *That's* the book *I* want. *Yesterday, you* couldn't find it.). As individuals interact and make reference to the physical surroundings and objects present during ordinary conversation, processing demands may be lower than when those objects are not present. When relevant objects, people, or surroundings are absent, that information must be mentioned in the conversation, it must be activated in the minds of speaker and listener, and shared meaning must be determined for communication to be successful. If interactants are referring to physically present objects, much less description may be necessary, and the shared meaning may be obvious.

The difficulties inherent in communicating when one does not have access to common physical surroundings have been explored in depth in the referential communication literature (see Dickson, 1982 for review). When interactants cannot rely on the physical surrounding to help support their meaning, they must take their communication partner's perspective in order to produce and comprehend utterances effectively. The effects of physical support on conversations have been examined in younger children's play. French, Lucariello, Seidman, and Nelson (1985) have shown that preschool children's play conversations were much more elaborate, with a better developed story line, when realistic props were provided than when they engaged in pretend play on a Jungle Gym. French et al. attributed the greater sophistication to the fact that children provided with realistic props did not need to define objects explicitly (e.g., "Pretend this is the car.") and remember the designations. Asquith and French (1989) reported that a model-kitchen setting resulted in more fantasy talk between peers ranging in age from 2-½ to 3-½-years than did an assortment of various toys. However, when children can engage readily in role and meaning negotiation, then less realistic props may encourage them to do so. Pellegrini and Galda (see "Children's play, language, and early literacy," this issue) concluded from their research that older preschool children are more likely to exhibit imaginative language when using functionally ambiguous toys such as blocks, whereas younger children (2-½ to 3-½-years) were more likely to do so with functionally explicit props such as kitchen toys. These authors demonstrate that such imaginative language has many commonalities with the language of school and early literacy.

The above findings suggest that clinicians need to observe the effects of various physical contexts on children's play and the language embedded within that play. Shatz (1977, 1985) has applied Kahneman's (1973) notion of limited capacity processing to children's communication development, and she illustrates the trade-offs that occur in language performance as one or another aspect of a task is changed. If clinicians wish to encourage more sophisticated narrative play themes in younger preschool children, then providing explicit theme-related toys is indicated to enhance children's performance in both the speaker and listener roles. If clinicians wish to encourage children to designate meanings more explicitly, then selectively removing aspects of physical context may be appropriate. Use of objects and manipulation of physical surroundings should be done in a meaningful naturalistic fashion, replicating or extending children's real world interactions. Bunce (1989) demonstrated that children may be trained using barrier games of the sort used in referential communication studies to improve their referencing abilities. However, barrier games are not usually encountered as a part of everyday interaction, whereas talking on the telephone or talking to someone in another room is an everyday activity that provides the same lack of shared physical context. Warren-Leubecker and Tate (as cited in Warren-Leubecker & Bohannon, 1989) have compared the face-to-face conversations and telephone conversations of preschool children and found that although children were less likely to respond to their partner's queries, they did adapt their communication by using fewer gestures and fewer deictic terms (e.g., here, this). Thus, manipulation of physical context can result in language changes, suggesting that such manipulation be included as part of the specification of therapeutic goals.

## KNOWLEDGE OF THE SPEAKER

Knowledge of the speaker is generally recognized as aiding in the comprehension process. Certainly a familiar speaker will presume that the listener will call on shared knowledge in interpreting the speaker's utterances. Speaker knowledge also helps the listener to perceive correctly a speaker's intentions. That is, a listener must determine the point of a speaker's remark and experience with, or knowledge of, the speaker helps to do so. The majority of work on correctly perceiving intention is found in the literature on indirect requests. Studies of comprehension of indirect requests reveal that children use an action strategy when the situation suggests an action is necessary or appropriate and possible (Shatz & McCloskey, 1984), except perhaps during the time around 3 years of age when they are likely to answer requests of the form "Why don't you . . ." with "because." These requests are also likely to be coming from adults, a factor that undoubtedly adds to the adoption of an action strategy.

Knowledge about the speaker and the speaker's state of mind also is required for understanding later-developing communicative intents. Take, for example, the woman who is asked about her blind date and says "He had nice shoes." Her statement may be literally true, but her intention is clearly not to communicate something about how her date was shod. In this example of irony, which Winner (1988) attributes to Hiram Brownell, the listener makes sense of the utterance by making inferences about the speaker's state of mind. It is the violation of the Gricean cooperative principle (i.e., the assumption that speakers will be clear, truthful, relevant, and informative [Grice, 1975]) that drives the listener to make the inference. Winner (1988) examines the difference between two types of nonliteral language comprehension, metaphor and irony, and she compares the skills required. She argues that both require an awareness that what is said and what is meant may be quite different. However, metaphor comprehension requires conceptual development, whereas irony comprehension requires social cognitive development. In comprehending irony, one must infer the state of the speaker's mind, and one must have a sense of the knowledge shared by speaker and listener. Not surprisingly, developmental studies of the comprehension of irony suggest that irony may not be understood until the later elementary school years. Younger children, in explaining a potentially ironic remark occurring in a story, may either change the facts of the story to fit the remark or they may report that the speaker is lying. However, the tasks that have been used to assess comprehension of irony have not typically provided the listener with a potential reason for ironic intent. For example, Ackerman (1983) uses the following stimulus story in a study of comprehension of irony:

It was a nice spring day. Ralph didn't get one right on the test in school that day. He went over to sharpen his pencil. His teacher, Mrs. Smith, said, 'You really did well this time, didn't you?' (p.492).

Listeners are not given a reason for a teacher making what seems like an inordinately critical remark, and listeners may not expect stories in which teachers speak to their students in this way. If listeners were given the information that Ralph had been goofing off despite his teacher's repeated efforts to help him, the likelihood of children understanding ironic intent might be greater. Hence, my current research examines children's ability to comprehend irony when they are given sufficient social background. Given that one of the requisite skills for understanding irony is knowing the speaker's state of mind, further studies may find that children do, in fact, understand ironic intent when the speaker is someone they know well and the circumstances are familiar to them. Certainly, anecdotal evidence exists of children producing ironic remarks at much younger ages. A graduate student recently reported on a 5-year-old sitting next to another child who was vigorously banging away on a peg-hammering toy. The 5-year-old turned to the future carpenter and said in an annoyed tone of voice, "Who gave you a noise license?"

Green and Chapman (1986) have investigated development of comprehension of another, later developing intention that also requires the listener to make inferences about the speaker's state of mind:

evasion for the sake of politeness. This may occur when one is asked to evaluate something that one does not like, but feels the need to be polite. For example, if someone asks, "How do you like my new suit?", and if the listener does not like the suit, he or she can avoid being rude by saying, "It certainly is gray." Green and Chapman presented stories to 7-, 10-, and 13-year-old children that contained either evasive but polite answers, or direct (and hence informative) but impolite answers. They found that whereas 7- and 10-year-olds recognized violations of politeness, only 13-year-olds recognized and were able to infer correctly that violations of informativeness meant that the speaker was feeling negative about the entity being discussed, but was seeking to be polite. Children have expectations, based on their general knowledge of speakers, that speakers will make remarks that are truthful and relevant. Thus, the skill that children are acquiring is one of recognizing violations of cooperative conversation and realizing the implications that those violations have for inferring the speaker's state of mind, and hence, communicative intention.

As clinicians seek to improve the communicative interactions of older children, they need to include utterances that are increasingly indirect, requiring varying types of nonliteral interpretations. In the course of such work, it is necessary to focus less on linguistic elements alone, and more on what can be inferred from knowledge of the speaker, what the speaker's goals might be, and hence how the message should be interpreted. For example, an important social skill is recognizing when a speaker is jesting or serious. With older

> *As clinicians seek to improve the communicative interactions of older children, they need to include utterances that are increasingly indirect, requiring varying types of nonliteral interpretations.*

children, metacommunicative training might employ videos of familiar television shows, given that children have the opportunity over repeated episodes to develop knowledge of speakers. They could be asked to identify and explain instances of various indirect speech acts or utterances in which nonliteral interpretation is intended, using their knowledge of the speaker and the speaker's goals.

## GOALS AND LEVEL OF INVOLVEMENT

When individuals interact, they have reasons for doing so. Interactions may be directed toward receiving information, being entertained, figuring out how to be helpful, or being wooed. Most often, speakers and listeners are likely to have multiple goals. Cognitive psychologists have identified the importance of goal structure in accounting for how and what people remember of events and narratives (Trabasso, Secco, & Van Den Broek, 1984; Trabasso & Stein, 1981; Trabasso & Van Den Broek, 1985). Clinically, this suggests presenting tasks to be accomplished in a situation that is meaningful for the child. For example, recently a student clinician reported having great difficulty getting her client to generate or retell narratives.

The child had begun to complain about coming to therapy and often was inattentive during sessions. When asked how she was eliciting the narratives, she indicated that she had been instructing the child to tell her a story or had been telling the child a story and asking him to retell it. However, she was not providing the child with a reason to tell a story. The child could achieve no goal in telling a story other than to obtain the clinician's approval. It was suggested that she give the child a reason for telling a story—for example, have the child go on an adventure with the clinician somewhere in the building housing the clinic, and then return to the clinic and tell his mother about the adventure. In order to promote the child's narrative abilities and to reduce the chance of an unsophisticated list-like recall of occurrences, it was suggested that a "problem" could arise requiring the trip around the building, with complications and resolutions arising during the course of the trip. Providing the child with a goal of telling a naive audience about an unusual occurrence resulted in a dramatic increase in the degree of cohesiveness and the degree of detail in the child's stories, and attention problems abated.

The above example illustrates that closely related to goal is our level of involvement in a situation. As we speak about words having a history, it is only natural to ask how one's level of involvement affects memory for, and comprehension of, the words and the situation. A new and rapidly developing body of literature examines the relation between cognition and affect. Lehnert and Vine (1987) and Miall (1989) have argued that emotional responses to typical situations guide comprehension in narrative processing. Bower (1978) found that when individuals read stories, the meaning that readers obtained for a story depended on the characters with which they identified. When readers identified with a character, they were more likely to remember the thoughts of the character, describe events from that character's point of view, and interpret that character's actions sympathetically. Also, the mood of readers affected the choice of character with which individuals identified. Subjects were induced into either happy or sad moods via posthypnotic suggestion, and it was found that they chose the character with the mood similar to their own as the central focus of the story; that was the character about whom they remembered the most.

Degree of involvement influences a listener's memory for conversations as well as narratives. Keenan, MacWhinney, and Mayhew (1977) recorded a conversation among a group of academic psycholinguists and then selected utterances that were judged to be of high versus low involvement (utterances in which the speaker made fun of some portion of his experiment versus utterances that focused solely on the content). Individuals who had been listeners in the conversation were much more able to recall exact wording of high involvement interpersonal statements than low involvement expository statements. This experimental evidence supports the intuitive expectation that emotional involvement affects memory for exact wording.

The investigations of involvement reaffirm clinical practice that emphasizes communication being taught in a pleasurable interactive context. Nelson (1988) emphasized the importance of engagement in children's language learning, citing "hot spots" that are determined by cognitive, affective, and social factors as crucial learning times. However, in the course of planning and executing multiple therapy sessions per day, the clinician's attention to the child's level of emotional involvement may wane. It is argued that keeping children highly engaged in therapeutic interactions is not just a luxury, but rather a necessity for effective teaching and learning. Pellegrini and Galda (1982) compared kindergarten, first-, and second-grade children's comprehension and retention of a story following dramatic reenactment of it, drawing a picture about it, and discussing it. They found that kindergarten and first-grade children who had reenacted the story performed better on a comprehension test than those who had drawn a picture or discussed the story. Children in the dramatic play condition also recalled more events and in a more accurate sequence when retelling the story than the children in the other conditions. Dramatic play differs in a number of ways from drawing or discussing a story; a primary difference may be in the level of involvement each requires.

Recently, this author observed a clinician attempting to teach a 9-year-old how to provide adequate reference in his stories and how to edit his stories. The clinician had had the child bring a photograph album containing photos of a family vacation that had occurred 2 years previously, and they had been writing short stories about these photos for several sessions. As they began that part of the session, the child obviously was prepared to do his duty and talk about the photos. However, the clinician had briefly mentioned Halloween in passing and the child suddenly, very tentatively asked if they could possibly do a Halloween story instead. He then embarked on creating a sophisticated literary version of a haunted hay ride he had experienced, reflecting on his production, and editing it so rapidly that the clinician had difficulty performing her assigned role of scribe. The child proposed that they record the story and add sound effects so that he could play it for friends and scare them. In the course of this session, he took a great deal of initiative, and seemed almost to be directing the session, which the clinician very wisely allowed him to do. Hence, flexibility and a continual sensitivity to what is likely to cause a child to take the initiative are clinical tools that allow the clinician to take advantage of the affective bases of learning.

## EXPERIENCE WITH EVENTS

Comprehension in a given situation also is likely to be affected by the degree and type of experience listeners have with that situation. It is not surprising to find few studies dealing with the role of specific experiences in language comprehension, as control and quantification of experience is difficult at best. Ross and Berg (see "Individual differences in script reports," this issue) have carefully examined the nature of individual differences in event knowledge for two common events, a doctor's appointment and an airplane trip. They have found that idiosyncrasies in event knowledge may interfere with recall of stories in which the event description is not similar to the individual's event knowl-

edge. Ross and Berg elucidate the implications for assessment.

Anderson, Reynolds, Schallert, and Goetz (1977) tested the role of experience by presenting two passages to students majoring in either physical education or a music education. One passage could have been interpreted as being about either a prison break or a wrestling match, and the other could have been interpreted as being about either an evening of card playing or a rehearsal of a woodwind ensemble. After reading each passage, students were asked to recall it and then answer a series of multiple choice comprehension questions about it. The effects of background on interpretation were striking. Physical education majors understood the first passage to be about wrestling, whereas other individuals generally understood it to be about a prison escape. Music education majors understood the second passage to be about a woodwind ensemble, whereas others understood it to be about card playing. Thus, as the various aspects of a situation and the incoming language activate those aspects of experience that are relevant, that experience in turn strongly shapes expectations about what is yet to come in an interaction.

Children's use of experience-based expectations in interpreting language has been examined in the literature on comprehension strategies (see Paul, "Comprehension strategies," this issue). Lucariello (see "Freeing talk from the here-and-now," this issue) has found that parents seem to take advantage of familiarity with routines to introduce time-displaced talk, and Constable (1986) has discussed the benefits of both creating and violating routines in conducting treatment of language-impaired children. Thus, it is argued that the manipulation and specification of experience is as integral to language treatment as the manipulation and specification of linguistic targets.

•   •   •

As listeners comprehend language, the words and the sentence frames they are comprehending come with a history. As Chapman et al. (1989) and Anderson (1984) maintain, a complete history is not activated each time a word is mentioned. Rather, the situation activates the relevant aspects of the word and hence the relevant aspects of the word's history. Because of the inextricable relationship between words and their history, it is necessary to develop intervention and assessment goals that include the various aspects of world knowledge as an integral part of the goals, and not merely the therapy activities. Such goal development will provide exciting opportunities for teaching language in a truly communicative manner.

## REFERENCES

Ackerman, B. (1983). Form and function in children's understanding of ironic utterances. *Journal of Experimental Child Psychology, 35*, 487–508.

Anderson, R. (1984). Some reflections on the acquisition of knowledge. *Educational Researcher, 13*, 5–10.

Anderson, R., Reynolds, R., Schallert, D., & Goetz, E. (1977). Frameworks for comprehending discourse. *American Educational Research Journal, 14*, 367–381.

ASHA Committee on Language, Speech and Hearing Services in the Schools. (1980). Definitions for communicative disorders and differences. *ASHA, 22*, 317–318.

Asquith, P., & French, L. (1989). *Talking while playing: Fantasy in the kitchen.* Paper presented at the annual meeting of the American Educational Research Association, San Francisco, CA.

Barnhart, C. (Editor in Chief) (1968). *The American College Dictionary.* New York, NY: Random House.

Bernstein, D., & Tiegerman, E. (1989). *Language and communication disorders in children.* Columbus, OH: Merrill.

Bower, G. (1978). Experiments on story comprehension and recall. *Discourse Processes, 1*, 211–231.

Bransford, J., & Johnson, M. (1972). Contextual prerequisites for understanding: Some investigations of comprehension and recall. *Journal of Verbal Learning and Verbal Behavior, 11*, 717–726.

Bunce, B. (1989). Using a barrier game format to improve children's referential communication skills. *Journal of Speech and Hearing Disorders, 54*, 33–43.

Cairns, H. (1983). Research in language comprehension. In R. Naremore (Ed.), *Language science.* San Diego, CA: College Hill.

Chapman, R., Streim, N., Crais, E., Salmon, D., Strand, E., & Negri-Shoultz, N. (1989). *Child talk: Assumptions of a developmental process model for early language learning.* Unpublished manuscript.

Clark, H. (1983). Making sense of nonce sense. In G. Flores d'Arcais & R. Jarvella (Eds.), *The process of language understanding.* New York, NY: John Wiley and Sons.

Constable, C. (1986). The application of scripts in the organization of language intervention contexts. In K. Nelson (Ed.), *Event knowledge: Structure and function in development.* Hillsdale, NJ: Erlbaum.

Dickson, W.P. (1982). Two decades of referential communication research: A review and meta-analysis. In C.J. Brainerd & M. Pressley (Eds.), *Verbal processes in children.* New York, NY: Springer-Verlag.

Durkin, D. (1978–1979). What classroom observations reveal about reading comprehension instruction. *Reading Research Quarterly, 14*, 481–533.

Ford, M., Bresnan, J., & Kaplan, R. (1982). A competence-based theory of syntactic closure. In J. Bresnan (Ed.), *The mental representation of grammatical relations.* Cambridge, MA: MIT Press.

French, L., Lucariello, J., Seidman, S., & Nelson, K. (1985). The influences of discourse content and context on preschoolers' use of language. In L. Galda & A. Pellegrini (Eds.), *Play, language, and stories: The development of children's literate behavior.* Norwood, NJ: Ablex.

Garrod, S., & Sanford, A. (1983). Topic dependent effects in language processing. In G. Flores d'Arcais & R. Jarvella (Eds.), *The process of language understanding*. New York, NY: John Wiley and Sons.

Green, K., & Chapman, R.S. (1986). *When informativeness and politeness conventions conflict: A developmental study*. Unpublished manuscript.

Grice, H. (1975). Logic and conversation. In P. Cole & J. Morgan (Eds.), *Syntax and semantics: Volume 3*. New York, NY: Academic Press.

Kahneman, D. (1973). *Attention and effort*. Englewood Cliffs, NJ: Prentice-Hall.

Keenan, J., MacWhinney, B., & Mayhew, D. (1977). Pragmatics in memory: A study of natural conversation. *Journal of Verbal Learning and Verbal Behavior, 16,* 549–560.

Lehnert, W., & Vine, E. (1987). The role of affect in narrative structure. *Cognition and Emotion, 1,* 299–322.

Lund, N., & Duchan, J. (1988). *Assessing children's language in naturalistic contexts*. Englewood Cliffs, NJ: Prentice-Hall.

Marslen-Wilson, W., & Tyler, L. (1980). The temporal structure of spoken language understanding. *Cognition, 8,* 1–71.

Miall, D. (1989). Beyond the schema given: Affective comprehension of literary narratives. *Cognition and Emotion, 3,* 55–78.

Nation, J., & Aram, D. (1984). *Diagnosis of speech and language disorders*. San Diego, CA: College-Hill.

Nelson, K.E. (1988). Strategies for first language teaching. In M. Rice & R. Schiefelbusch (Eds.), *The teachability of language*. Baltimore, MD: Brookes.

Pellegrini, A., & Galda, L. (1982). The effect of thematic-fantasy play training on the development of children's story comprehension. *American Educational Research Journal, 19,* 443–452.

Shatz, M. (1977). The relationship between cognitive processes and the development of communication skills. In C. Keasey (Ed.), *Nebraska symposium on motivation*. Lincoln, NE: University of Nebraska Press.

Shatz, M. (1985). A song without music and other stories: How cognitive process constraints influence children's oral and written narratives. In D. Schiffrin (Ed.), *Georgetown University round table on language and linguistics: Meaning, form, and use in context: Linguistic applications*. Washington, DC: Georgetown University Press.

Shatz, M., & McCloskey, L. (1984). Answering appropriately: A developmental perspective on conversational knowledge. In S. Kuczaj (Ed.), *Discourse development: Progress in cognitive development research*. New York, NY: Springer-Verlag.

Sternberg, R. (1987). Most vocabulary is learned from context. In M. McKeown & M. Curtis (Eds.), *The nature of vocabulary acquisition*. Hillsdale, NJ: Erlbaum.

Tanenhaus, M., Carlson, G., & Seidenberg, M. (1985). Do listeners compute linguistic representations? In D. Dowty, L. Kartunnen, & A. Zwicky (Eds.), *Natural language parsing*. New York, NY: Cambridge University Press.

Trabasso, T., Secco, T., & Van Den Broek, P. (1984). Causal cohesion and story coherence. In H. Mandl, N. Stein, & T. Trabasso (Eds.), *Learning and comprehension in text*. Hillsdale, NJ: Erlbaum.

Trabasso, T., & Stein, N. (1981). Children's knowledge of events: A causal analysis of story structure. In G. Bower (Ed.), *The psychology of learning and motivation*. New York, NY: Academic Press.

Trabasso, T., & Van Den Broek, P. (1985). Causal thinking and the representation of narrative events. *Journal of Memory and Language, 24,* 612–630.

Waltz, D., & Pollack, J. (1985). Massively parallel parsing: A strongly interactive model of natural language interpretation. *Cognitive Science, 9,* 51–74.

Warren-Leubecker, A., & Bohannon, J. (1989). Pragmatics: Language in social contexts. In J. Gleason (Ed.), *The development of language*. Columbus, OH: Merrill.

Winner, E. (1988). *The point of words: Children's understanding of metaphor and irony*. Cambridge, MA: Harvard University Press.

# Intervention issues for toddlers with specific language impairments

**Lesley B. Olswang, PhD**
*Associate Professor*
*Department of Speech and Hearing*
*Sciences*
*University of Washington*
*Seattle, Washington*

**Barbara A. Bain, PhD**
*Associate Professor*
*Department of Speech Pathology and*
*Audiology*
*Idaho State University*
*Pocatello, Idaho*

**T**HIS ARTICLE focuses on intervention issues for toddlers who demonstrate a primary deficit in language acquisition as compared with other aspects of their development. They are not children who are generally low functioning, such as developmentally delayed children. Rather, these are children performing minus 1 standard deviation on standardized tests of language development, or who are functioning at least 6 months below their chronological age in language production and/or comprehension on criterion-referenced tests or developmental scales, but who are performing age appropriately in other aspects of development. These specific language impaired (SLI) toddlers range in age between approximately 18 and 36 months. The linguistic focus is therefore on the acquisition of single words, word combinations, early grammatical morphemes and simple syntactic construc-

*This article is supported in part by the NINCD Grant, R29-DC00431 "Predicting the Benefits of Treatment."*

*Top Lang Disord*, 1991,11(4),69–86
© 1991 Aspen Publishers, Inc.

tions, corresponding roughly to Brown's (1973) Stages I, II, and early III, that is, mean length of utterance (MLU) is between 1.0 and 3.5.

Intervention is defined as focused, intensive stimulation to alter specific behavior. Intervention is being contrasted with monitoring (i.e., the "wait and watch" disposition) and general stimulation (i.e., general suggestions provided to the parents to encourage communication). Intervention is viewed as targeted stimulation that can be provided individually or in groups by the speech-language clinician or by the parents or day-care providers, and focuses on the improvement of particular aspects of language. The intervention issues of interest in this article are those that relate to decisions regarding when and how best to intervene with the SLI toddler.

Deciding a toddler needs language intervention is based on the clinician's knowledge that the child's language performance is discrepant enough from normal development to warrant concern. Further, the clinician must have decided that extra environmental stimulation is necessary to bring about the desired change in language acquisition. Although the toddler's primary language learning environment (i.e., home, day care, etc) may appear to be appropriate for facilitating language growth, the child does not seem to benefit maximally from the language input. Something about the toddler's learning style, an organismic variable(s), seems to be preventing him or her from learning language naturally. Thus, intervention is recommended to better match environmental input with the child's processing abilities

with the goal of improving language performance.

In this article, the focus of intervention will be on the child (i.e., the organismic variables), addressing the clinical questions of when and how to intervene. As such, the main issue will be in what ways intervention can change the language acquisition process for toddlers who are growing and changing; they are intact children who are developing normally except in language. These are children whose motor, social, and cognitive abilities are sustaining their development, as is their primary language learning environment, and yet they exhibit significant deficits in their language acquisition. With intervention designed to focus on changing the child, two main questions emerge: (1) How does intervention interface with maturation, and (2) what role can we expect intervention to play in the growth process?

## GOALS OF INTERVENTION

A clinician's intervention should directly reflect his or her assumptions about the mechanism of change and the dimensions that are relevant or possible to change in the impaired child (Johnston, 1983). A very basic question arises: What can we teach SLI toddlers? As clinicians, we must consider which organismic variables can actually be changed, and thus determine the ways the language acquisition process can be altered. Three rather broad intervention goals are apparent; they are designed to

1. change or alleviate the underlying deficit (i.e., the "basic"/"underlying" language deficiency); thus making

the child a normal language learner who will not need intervention in the future;

2. change the disorder; thus normalizing the child on a discrete aspect of language by teaching him or her particular linguistic behaviors, corresponding to underlying linguistic rules, making the child more proficient at that point, but not suggesting the child is "cured" forever; and

3. provide the child with compensatory strategies for his/her language learning and communicative functioning; thus providing the child with tools for using the most sophisticated and conventional behaviors possible given the child's abilities and limitations.

The ultimate accomplishment, in an ideal world of speech-language pathology, would be to strive for and achieve goal 1, but is that always possible? The literature reflects that for many SLI preschoolers, deficits last throughout their lives. At least throughout the school years, language-impaired children are at risk for academic failure (Aram, Ekelman & Nation, 1984; Aram & Nation, 1980; Bishop & Edmundson, 1987; Hall & Tomblin, 1978; Kamhi & Catts, 1989; Wallach & Butler, 1984). The learning deficit remains, although symptoms or behaviors change over time. Early difficulty learning language seems to herald future problems in learning, particularly in areas related to literacy. Although we might (and should) strive to alleviate the underlying language learning deficit, given the state of the art, we must be realistic about the possibility of falling short of reaching that goal. Further, intervention for toddlers hardly, if ever, is

designed to teach compensatory strategies (goal 3), for such a goal requires metacognitive and metalinguistic skills beyond the capabilities of this age population. Rather, clinicians focus their efforts on teaching toddlers specific language behaviors, whether expressive or receptive form, content or use (goal 2). The targeted behaviors are assumed to be those that reflect underlying linguistic rules. The expectation is to bring children's language skills up to the level of their abilities in other developmental areas, and, when this goal is reached, to terminate treatment and monitor future growth. The assumption is that should the children's language skills once again fall behind their performance in other areas, treatment will be reinstituted, but with new language behaviors or rules as targets.

The clinician's task is to identify language behaviors that are missing or infrequently occurring and attempt to teach or stimulate the growth of these specific behaviors and their corresponding linguistic rules. Thus, for SLI toddlers, goal 2 will be the predominant focus of treatment. It is hoped that the future development of our scientific knowledge base and the creation of clinical tools will increase our efforts to strive for and achieve goals 1 and 3, but until that time, the primary intervention objective will be to teach linguistic rules by treating missing or infrequently occurring behaviors.

## THE ROLE OF INTERVENTION IN ALTERING LANGUAGE ACQUISITION

With this expectation in mind for SLI toddlers, the clinician must consider how intervention can stimulate the growth of particular behaviors reflecting language rules. Specifically, the issue of greatest significance with this population is in regard to the ways in which intervention interacts with maturation in modifying children's language. For intervention to be effective, as well as ethical, it must alter growth for a particular aspect of language at a faster rate than would naturally occur (American Speech-Language-Hearing Association, 1990). This means that intervention, defined earlier as an extensive and intensive form of stimulation, will need to change children more effectively than change occurring without intervention, that is, change due to maturation alone. Maturation describes the changing physiological organism as stimulated by natural experiences in the environment. To decide whether to recommend intervention, clinicians must be aware of how it interfaces with maturation, and fully understand how it can alter the children's language acquisition process. To explore these issues, a theoretical framework adapted from the works of Gottlieb (1976, 1981) and Aslin (1981), who have examined ways in which environmental experiences can alter the natural maturational process, will be presented.

Gottlieb's research has concentrated on attempting to identify "innate" or "instinctive" species-specific behaviors, and as such, he has been interested in the ways behaviors are altered by experience. Gottlieb and Aslin have formulated a theoretical framework for describing the various ways experience fosters the development of behavior. These researchers use the term "experience" to mean any type of environmental stimulation. The authors adapted their model by interpreting "experience" as "intensive experience," or "focused stimulation," that is, "intervention," and the role intervention plays in altering language behaviors over and above maturation associated with natural environmental influences.

What are the various ways, then, that experience/intervention can change behaviors? Gottlieb (1976, 1981) has described three roles experience can play in altering behavioral development: (1) facilitation, (2) induction, and (3) maintenance. See Figure 1.

## Facilitation

According to Gottlieb, facilitation describes the role of experience in altering the rate of change for an ability, but not the endpoint of development. "Facilitative experiences regulate maturation, hasten development, improve performance, increase perceptual differentiation, etc." (Gottlieb, 1976, p. 31). In language intervention, a facilitative treatment would be one that "got the system going," as in assisting a child to learn single words (Olswang, Bain, Rosendahl, Oblak, & Smith, 1986). As illustrated in Figure 1, a facilitative experience can have an effect on an undeveloped or partially developed behavior, but the experience does not alter the eventual level of functioning; rather it serves to accelerate learning. The data reviewed by Whitehurst et al. (this issue) reflect a facilitative effect of therapy. The toddlers they studied increased their expressive vocabularies faster than did untreated peers, although the long-term endpoint (at age 5) was similar for both groups. In the Olswang et al. (1986) study, two language-impaired children were taught

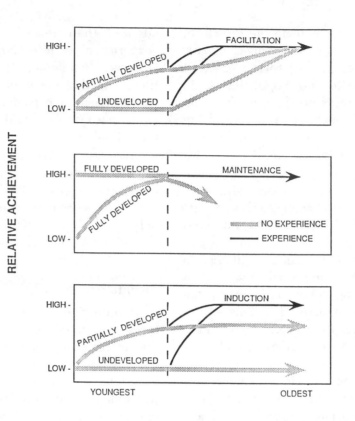

**Figure 1.** Framework for interpreting the effects of experience on behavioral development. Vertical dashed line indicates when experience starts. Fully developed, partially developed, and undeveloped refer to the state of the system prior to experience. Reprinted with permission from Gottlieb, G. (1981). Roles of early experience in species-specific perceptual development. In R. Aslin & J. Alberts (Eds.), *Development of Perception Vol 1*. Copyright 1981, Academic Press, Orlando, Fla.

single-word utterances. Both children ended up with increased single-word utterances, but for only one of the children did direct treatment appear to be the cause of the improvement. For this child, direct treatment had a facilitative effect, helping the language-impaired child acquire single words earlier than would have occurred naturally. This phenomenon was documented by monitoring the child's acquisition of vocabulary that was not targeted in treatment.

Facilitation raises several important clin-

ical issues. First, why should facilitative therapy be initiated, if the child will eventually reach the same endpoint without intervention? Whitehurst et al. (this issue) raise this question explicitly. There are several points to be made in this regard. In the first place, although the child may eventually achieve the same endpoint in the skill being targeted, other skills that build on or coordinate with that skill may be delayed by its slow rate of growth. For example, expressive vocabulary size may achieve normal levels by age 5 if untreated in preschoolers with small expressive vocabularies. However, metalinguistic skills involving knowledge of what a word is, and phonological segmentation abilities, which allow children to understand that words are made up of sounds—both skills central to the acquisition of literacy—may not develop if the child has spent the preschool period in a very slow process of acquiring new words without facilitative intervention. Second, social skill, self-esteem, and other psychosocial attitudes may be affected during the period in which communication skills are delayed, even if children do eventually "catch up" in the language area. Facilitative therapy may be important for giving the child a sense of mastery and avoiding psychosocial problems. Third, facilitative therapy may be important for improving parent–child interactions. Finally, the long-term effects of facilitative therapy must be judged in light of the limitations on our measurement ability. That is, some forms of intervention may appear to be "merely" facilitative because our standard tools for measuring language status are too crude. For example, Whitehurst et al. (this issue) claim that language therapy for young children is "merely" facilitative because both treated and untreated groups of SLI toddlers scored within the normal range of expressive vocabulary and general verbal fluency by age 5. However, language skills that are more difficult to measure, such as modulation of verb meaning through the use of auxiliary verbs, elaboration of sentences through the use of prepositional phrases, and metalinguistic awareness may have distinguished the groups. Several other issues about facilitation are important for clinical consideration. For exam-

ple, can clinicians be sure intervention is responsible for change? How does intervention interface with maturation? We will return to several of these issues later in our discussion.

## Maintenance

A maintaining experience serves "to preserve an already developed state or end point, regardless of how the state or end point itself was achieved" (Gottlieb, 1976, p. 28). The maintenance role of experience is necessary for sustaining a behavior; without such an experience, the behavior will decrease or possibly disappear. "Maintenance can also be required to keep an immature system intact, going, and functional so that it is able to reach its full development at a later stage" (Gottlieb, 1976, p. 28). Gottlieb has most recently argued that maintenance applies only when a behavior exists before the experience, so that the experience itself does not create or enhance the behavior but only preserves that which is already present (Gottlieb, 1981, p. 41). In language intervention, this would describe the necessity of treatment to maintain a behavior that was already in a child's repertoire. An example of this would be the need for intervention in the case of a child with a degenerative disease or with sudden onset of a sensory impairment. For the SLI toddler, maintenance seems to be less of a problem than acquisition. If the teaching is adequate, behaviors are learned and maintained. Once these children learn new language behaviors and their underlying linguistic rules, they seldom lose them. Behaviors do not deteriorate, but rather become the foundation for the next set of behaviors to be acquired. Indeed, this is what helps define the population; once these children learn a language behavior or rule, they are ready to move ahead in the developmental hierarchy of acquisition.

## Induction

The final role of experience described by Gottlieb is induction. His current model includes two aspects of induction. (See Figures 1 and 2). Aslin (1981) elected to call one of the aspects "attunement," thereby creating a fourth, separate role for experience to play in altering a behavior. According to Gottlieb (1981), "induction refers to the role of experience when it completely determines whether a particular endpoint, level of achievement, degree of specificity, fine tuning, and so on, will or will not be reached. These endpoints are not reached in the absence of experience

as they are in the case where experience merely accelerates the appearance of an endpoint [facilitation]" (p. 38). This would be seen as the most dramatic effect of experience. The presence or absence of a particular experience completely determines if a behavior will manifest itself later in development (Gottlieb, 1976). "When level of achievement requires an extra boost by experience (i.e., the behavior won't get to the endpoint without the experience), this would be considered induction" (Gottlieb, 1981, p. 38). One aspect of induction is the role experience plays in creating the existence of a new behavior. That is, experience is responsible for the emergence of a behavior and its continued development. If the experience is absent, the behavior will not emerge. In language treatment, this would be analo-

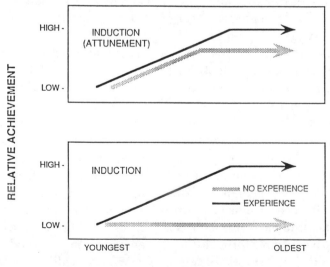

**Figure 2.** Induction is defined by the role of experience in bringing a behavior to an elevated terminal level. Experience may increase the occurrence of an already existing behavior (top) or may be required to initiate the onset of a behavior (bottom). Reprinted with permission from Gottlieb, G. (1981). Roles of early experience in species-specific perceptual development. In R. Aslin & J. Alberts (Eds.), *Development of Perception Vol 1.* Copyright 1981, Academic Press, Orlando, Fla.

gous to teaching a child a linguistic form that was not in his or her repertoire or teaching a nonverbal child to produce signs.

The second aspect of induction, which Aslin and Pisoni (1980) have termed "attunement," addresses the role experience plays in increasing an already existing behavior. A behavior may already be present in some rudimentary form, but the ability will remain only partially developed unless specific experiences are encountered by the organism (Aslin, 1981). Increasing an SLI child's initiations (for example, requestives) in different environmental contexts is an example of attunement (Olswang, Kriegsmann, & Mastergeorge, 1982). The behavior exists but is not being performed to its fullest capacity.

Thus, induction defines the role of specific experiences that are necessary for the onset and continued development of an ability. If intervention is provided, the ability will emerge and eventually reach a mature adult endpoint. If intervention is not provided, the ability will not emerge or will not reach the most advanced level of performance possible. For the SLI toddler, induction may be a way in which treatment alters acquisition. If language behaviors are totally missing from a child's repertoire, and the child seems to demonstrate the apparent prerequisites for these behaviors, then intervention would seem warranted. However, at issue is whether intervention would bring the language behavior to a level of performance that would not otherwise be achieved. Further, the ultimate level of performance and the amount of intervention necessary to achieve that level may not be known. These issues add an additional level of complexity to the clinician's decision making.

This theoretical model proposed by Gottlieb and Aslin provides a useful framework to help clinicians in their decision making. It allows us to examine the different ways we might expect to change the language development of the SLI toddler, which in turn will help in planning and implementing accountable intervention. A significant question that must be addressed when considering intervention for the SLI toddler is, when will intervention alter growth for a particular aspect of language at a rate greater than maturation? The literature supports that the timing of intervention for SLI toddlers is a valid issue for consideration (Gibson & Ingram, 1983; Olswang, Bain, Dunn, & Cooper, 1983; Olswang & Coggins, 1984; Olswang, et al., 1986). We know that SLI toddlers acquire language at different rates during the therapeutic process. The data illustrate individual variation in learning across children who appear to be quite homogeneous in their language behaviors and for whom the treatment targets seem appropriate. This variation seems to reflect in part how intervention interacts with the maturation process.

In normally developing children, emergence to mastery of a new behavior is an uneven process, sometimes proceeding slowly and other times moving more rapidly. The rapid rate of change has been referred to as a "growth spurt" and reflects a readiness to learn a particular behavior. As previously discussed, intervention can differentially affect learning, depending on when it occurs in the acquisition process (Aslin, 1981; Feuerstein, 1979; Gottlieb, 1976, 1981; Lenneberg, 1967; Vygotsky, 1978). The results of research conducted by these authors suggest the existence of critical learning periods in acquisition, that is, optimal learning times when change can be produced and the organizational process is more easily altered. Evidence supporting the nonlinearity of language learning, as defined by readiness and growth spurts, has emerged in the language-impairment intervention literature (Gibson & Ingram, 1983; Olswang & Coggins, 1984; Olswang, et al., 1982, 1983, 1986). Readiness for treatment sets the stage for the remainder of this article, where we will discuss particular ways to change the SLI toddlers' behaviors.

## WAYS TO CHANGE LANGUAGE BEHAVIORS

When planning intervention, clinicians must decide how they will go about facilitating an SLI toddler's communicative behaviors. This decision involves determining whether the toddler or the environment will be the primary focus of intervention and selecting a service delivery system and teaching strategies to match the toddler's needs.

### Service delivery options

When treating the SLI toddler, the clinician has at least two service delivery options from which to choose: (1) direct treatment in which the clinician is the primary agent for change, and (2) indirect or consultative treatment in which the clinician instructs others, usually parents and/or day-care providers, to be the primary agent for change. The framework of direct and indirect treatment is based on the American Speech-Language-Hearing Association's Guidelines for Caseload Size for Speech-Language Services in the Schools (committee on Language, Speech, and Hearing Services in the Schools, 1984). Service delivery options should be viewed on a continuum, especially with the mandates of PL 99-457 that specify parents must be involved in the intervention process. Furthermore, parents are valuable resources for the clinician to employ during intervention. The question is not should the parent be involved in the intervention process, but how. Service delivery selection should be based on toddler needs and not caseload demands or other extraneous factors.

When implementing direct treatment for intervention, the clinician assumes the primary responsibility as the service provider. The clinician becomes the "agent for change," planning and implementing the intervention and monitoring the toddler's change. The planning of intervention may be done primarily by the clinician or in collaboration with the parent and other professionals (Wilcox, 1989). Within the rubric of direct treatment, the clinician may manipulate the setting (i.e., home-based or clinic-based, Rossetti, 1986), frequency of contact, and whether the toddler is seen individually or with other children (i.e., group therapy). For example, the clinician may be the primary agent for change and see the toddler individually or in a group in the clinic, home, or preschool or day care setting. The toddler may be seen intermittently, such as once a week, or intensively, such as daily, for therapy. Furthermore, the clinician may employ the parents and day-care providers during the intervention process, but the clinician retains the role as the primary agent for change.

In providing indirect treatment, the clinician plans the intervention usually in conjunction with the parents and monitors the child's progress over time, but a parent or some other person actually implements the intervention. The clinician's role is to assist the primary interventionist. This form of service is also called the "consultative model" (Damico, 1987; Marvin, 1987). When an indirect service option is selected, the interaction between the clinician and the primary agent for change must be a collaborative one, with the clinician employing a variety of strategies including informing, instructing, modeling, demonstrating, cognitive restructuring, mediating, coordinating, reinforcing, confronting, and providing feedback. As Damico (1987) states, "the selection depends on aims of the interaction, degree of rapport, type of intervention used, and consultant's own effectiveness." (p. 29) Indirect treatment for SLI toddlers is chosen when the clinician decides that the most appropriate agent for change is the parent, teacher, or day-care provider. When considering this model, the skills and abilities of the parents and caretakers need to be assessed to ensure that the interaction will be a facilitative one. Indirect treatment is frequently employed with toddlers because they spend much of their time with the parent and/or day-care provider.

Identifying the purpose of the intervention can provide direction for the clinician in deciding which service delivery option would be most appropriate to employ. Direct treatment by the clinician may be most appropriate when the SLI toddler needs to establish a language behavior, and indirect treatment may be appropriate when the toddler needs to extend or generalize a language behavior or have a communicative behavior become more automatic.

Establishing a targeted form, content, or use behavior in an SLI toddler frequently requires the expertise of the clinician because his or her knowledge of language and its rule system, in combination with what is required to teach a new behavior, may necessitate direct treatment. The clinician's task is to manipulate the environment so that the salient linguistic or communicative features are emphasized for a specific toddler, or so that the child can more easily map meaning onto the sounds in words. This may include selecting the best exemplars of the target behavior and arranging the context so the toddler is focusing on the pertinent features of a linguistic structure. Further, the clinician may need to structure the environment so that distracting stimuli are removed while the toddler is learning the target behavior. Thus, direct treatment by the clinician may be necessary when initiating the language acquisition process for an SLI toddler.

After the toddler demonstrates the targeted language or communicative behavior, she or he often needs to practice the behavior so that the linguistic rule becomes automatic or generalized. This is an example of when indirect treatment may be most effectively used. The parent or teacher can be instructed by the clinician as to how best to structure the environment for allowing the toddler to use the behavior that recently has been established. Thus, indirect treatment provides the toddler with frequent stimulation throughout the day, giving an opportunity to practice the newly emerging behaviors in a variety of contexts that are natural and communicatively useful. Indirect treatment provides the toddler with natural antecedents and consequences for the new behavior. Toddlers may move in and out of both direct and indirect treatment, and both services may be used concurrently in order to provide the most effective and efficient intervention.

### Teaching strategies

Along with selecting the most appropriate treatment delivery option, the clinician must select treatment goals and teaching strategies to obtain these goals. The selection is influenced by the clinician's theoretical perspective regarding how language is acquired, what appropriate treatment goals are and what appropriate means for increasing communicative abilities are. Classifying teaching strategies is a difficult task because they can be viewed from a variety of perspectives and classified in diverse and arbitrary ways (Fey, 1986; Leonard, 1981; Olswang & Bain, in press). Also, some strategies use the same or similar procedures but have different names, for example, script therapy and joint action routines. Moreover, some strategies are based on a single procedure, such as modeling or expanding, whereas other strategies are a composite of procedures, such as milieu teaching. Furthermore, the same procedure may be used in several different strategies. For example, modeling is employed in inductive teaching (Connell, 1986, 1989), milieu teaching (Hart & Rogers-Warren, 1978), and script

therapy (Constable, 1986; Oblak, 1989; Snyder-McLean, Salomonson, McLean, & Sack, 1984).

Three general strategies appropriate to toddlers and illustrative of the different ways the environment can be structured are noted below. These strategies were selected because of their empirical support, which has included SLI toddlers and older preschool children, and because they represent the continuum of high structure to low structure, an important variable when selecting appropriate strategies. The strategies described are milieu teaching (Hart & Rogers-Warren, 1978; Warren, McQuarter, & Rogers-Warren, 1984; Warren & Kaiser, 1986), joint action routines (Constable, 1986; Oblak, 1989; Snyder-McLean, et al., 1984), and induction teaching (Connell, 1986, 1989). Note that induction teaching is the terminology employed by Connell and is different in meaning from the term as employed by Gottlieb and referenced earlier in the article. Other strategies are available, such as teaching through discourse structure (Schwartz, 1988; Schwartz, Chapman, Terrell, Prelock, & Rowan, 1985) and modeling plus evoked training (Weismer & Murray-Branch, 1989), but these use some of the same specific procedures employed within the three general strategies. Although these three strategies share a certain degree of similarity, they also have important differences.

#### Milieu teaching

In milieu teaching, the adult can take advantage of unstructured situations or may deliberately arrange the setting to construct events designed to shape or cue behaviors (Hart & Rogers-Warren, 1978).

Warren and Kaiser (1986) have identified the following basic ingredients of milieu training:

- teaching language and communication skills in the toddler's natural environment,
- teaching in conversational contexts,
- using a dispersed-trials training approach as opposed to a massed-trial approach,
- following the toddler's attentional lead, and
- using functional reinforcers indicated by toddler requests and attention.

The milieu strategy employs three procedures that may be emphasized or employed simultaneously.

The first procedure is mand-model, in which the adult performs the following behaviors: directs the toddler's attention to materials; mands or requests a response from the toddler; provides a model for the toddler to imitate, or prompts for a more complex response; praises the toddler for responding appropriately to the mand or for imitating; and gives the toddler the topic (material, activity, etc.) of interest. The second procedure is the use of delay, which involves the adult being in proximity and looking at the toddler questioningly or expectantly for 15 seconds. The delay provides the toddler with time to respond before the adult provides a model of the appropriate verbalization. The adult may repeat the model twice, each time waiting 15 seconds for the toddler to speak before giving the toddler what he or she seems to want regardless of whether the toddler has verbalized. Incidental teaching is the third procedure of milieu teaching, and it requires that the toddler select

a topic (activity, material, etc.) and that the adult respond relative to this topic. The adult follows the toddler's lead and only stays with an activity as long as it is reinforcing to the toddler.

The three procedures differ primarily in aspects of adult behavior. In the mand-model procedure, the adult initiates the interaction with the toddler, directs the toddler's attention, and mands verbalization. The delay procedure is directed to bring the toddler's verbalization under the control of environmental stimuli rather than the adult. The toddler's verbalization gradually comes under the control of nonsocial aspects of the context. Incidental teaching is directed to help toddlers elaborate language as a means of communicating.

### Joint action routines or script therapy

Joint action routine (JAR) is based on event models that assume young children gain knowledge from direct experiences not only alone but also in a social and cultural context (Nelson, 1986). A JAR is defined as "a ritualized interaction pattern, involving joint action, unified by a specific theme or goal, which follows a logical sequence, including a clear beginning point and in which each participant plays a recognized role, with specific response expectancies, that is essential to the successful completion of that sequence." (Snyder-McLean et al., 1984).

The rationale for employing JAR is that it provides guidelines for the structure and content of the nonlinguistic and linguistic features of intervention events. The scripted events presumably reduce cognitive workloads, thus increasing the resources that toddlers can apply to the language-learning task. The main idea is to develop routines with which the toddler becomes familiar. This, in turn, decreases the cognitive demands on the toddler, and the toddler can focus on attaining more advanced linguistic forms. The routines, events, or scripts are socially based and include the need to communicate. The event is the theme or topic of the activity. The routine is an activity that occurs frequently and in which the toddler participates. The script has to do with the dialogue that occurs within the event. The critical elements for the JAR include the following:

- having an obvious theme or purpose for the JAR;
- having a joint focus between the adult and toddler;
- following a predictable, nonarbitrary sequence;
- structuring turn-taking;
- planning repetition;
- planning controlled variations; and
- clearly delineating roles within the routine (Constable, 1986; Goldstein, Wickstrom, Hoyson, Jamieson, & Odom, 1988; Snyder-McLean et al., 1984).

### Inductive teaching

Inductive teaching is a strategy in which the clinician carefully structures the language input given to a toddler during meaningful interactions (Connell, 1989). The input (stimuli) must provide sufficient information for the SLI toddler to identify patterns, explain them, and consequently hypothesize a rule. The inductive teaching approach involves three steps designed to

teach language rules. First, the stimuli must allow the toddler to recognize that there is a pattern to the stimuli. The clinician carefully arranges or organizes the stimuli into pairs so that the items can be compared. Thus, the clinician has simplified the context and highlighted the salient features of linguistic rules for the learner, and has eliminated distractors. The toddler finds differences between each member of the pair, thus leading to the identification of a pattern across the stimuli. For example, if the therapy target was plurals, the toddler would be exposed to pairs of stimuli contrasting singular versus plural, as in dog–dogs, cat–cats, ball–balls, rattle–rattles, and so forth. Second, the pattern must be explained by understanding the meaningful context of the stimuli. The toddler searches for a solution to the problem posed by the stimulus pairs. In the present example of plurality versus singularity, it is hoped that the toddlers would note that plurals are marked with a fricative. Regardless of the target, the contrast in stimuli must represent a change in meaning. Pairing the stimuli simplifies the task for the toddler. In real life, the number of times the contrasts are adjacent to one another is rare. The preconstruction of the stimuli into contrasting pairs highlights the rule to be learned and simplifies the task for the learner by reducing the memory load. The structure of the task minimizes other communicative demands so that the language target is the focus. The third step involves the toddler hypothesizing the rule that captures the nature of the correspondence between the observed pairs of stimuli. The assumption of this procedure is that the induction process is an innate one so that by this step, if the preceding ones have been arranged correctly, hypothesizing the rule will occur automatically.

In summary, these three strategies, which vary in structure, have been successfully employed with SLI toddlers. Clinicians should select such strategies based on the needs of each SLI toddler.

## Intervention issues related to strategies

Given our profession's advances in identifying useful and effective treatment delivery options and specific teaching strategies, one cannot help but wonder why intervention remains so elusive and difficult. We would argue that several major issues influence the success of our intervention with SLI toddlers.

First, speech-language pathologists apply the "normal process" model to language-impaired children, and this may not be appropriate (Connell, 1987; Wade & Haynes, 1989). Much of the intervention provided to SLI toddlers is based on what is known about the normal acquisition of language, with treatment targets based on the sequence of normal acquisition. Evidence exists indicating normal children learn language more effectively through modeling procedures than through elicited imitation procedures. The assumption was made that this would also apply to language-impaired youngsters. Recently, Connell (1987) investigated modeling versus imitation strategies in normal and language-impaired children. He found that although normal preschoolers learned language more effectively through modeling than through elicited imitation, such was not the case for children with language impairment, who learned language more

effectively through elicited imitation procedures. The three strategies previously described allow for adult modeling and for elicited imitation. Induction teaching probably relies most on elicited imitation as a means to obtain responses from the SLI toddler. JAR and milieu teaching strategies are flexible approaches that allow the clinician to vary the amount of modeling and elicited imitation based on the needs of a specific SLI toddler. The adult may emphasize either modeling or elicited imitation procedures or use both. Obviously, the extent to which we can effectively apply normal processes to intervention with the language impaired population is a topic for future investigation.

Second, we assume the intervention strategies or techniques are strong enough to override the central organismic variables, that is, the toddler's language learning deficit; again, this may be inappropriate. Clinicians employ teaching strategies in order to facilitate the toddler's communication. The risks of applying the normal model to SLI toddlers are similar to the risk of assuming that a specific strategy will overcome the adverse language learning conditions for all toddlers. Clinicians must consider whether a specific strategy is best suited for particular toddlers at particular points in the learning process or particular toddlers with various characteristics. Although conclusive evidence supporting the interaction of child characteristics and treatment strategies is not available, trends of such a relationship emerge from the research (Cole & Dale, 1986; Friedman & Friedman, 1980). Friedman and Friedman (1980) investigated the interaction of two different treatment approaches with specific child characteristics. In general, children who had minimum verbal skills responded better to a structured teaching approach than did children with more advanced language abilities. The latter group of children responded more positively to a more natural or interactional approach. Children with lower intelligence quotients (IQs) seemed to respond more favorably to a structured approach, whereas children with higher IQs responded more favorably to an interactional approach. Clinicians need to recognize the extent to which a specific treatment strategy might interact with the characteristics and abilities of a toddler at a particular time. For example, the induction teaching strategy is an approach that is highly structured and requires an attentive toddler in order for the strategy to be implemented. Both induction teaching and JAR strategies reduce the cognitive workload for the toddlers through careful selection of salient stimuli and predictability of the routine, respectively; thus, the toddler presumably has more resources to attend to the linguistic target. Conversely, the milieu teaching strategy requires that the toddler be able to handle distracting elements in the environment as well as attend to the target stimuli. In addition, the JAR strategy can be employed in such a way as to allow or minimize distracting stimuli to be present in the environment. The complicating factor is that toddler characteristics change over time. Thus, a structured approach, for example, may be most beneficial early in the language acquisition process for particular toddlers, but may be inappropriate at a later time. Clinicians must constantly assess whether or not a particular approach is appropriate at a specific time for a specific toddler.

Third, treatment strategies also interact with treatment targets. For example, Connell (1989) found that semantic targets responded to an inductive teaching approach whereas a syntactic target (pronoun case) responded to a deductive approach. The clinical implication of this finding is that clinicians must analyze the treatment target and determine if a particular strategy would be appropriate to facilitate the acquisition of that target. Given that the inductive teaching approach is high in structure and not conducted in a social setting, it is probably not appropriate for pragmatic targets. On the other hand, milieu teaching and JAR strategies are conducted in social settings and could be appropriate for pragmatic in addition to semantic and syntatic targets. To assume that a particular strategy is effective with a wide variety of different treatment targets may be shortsighted, and the clinician must give considerable thought to ensuring that the environmental context is supportive of the selected target.

Fourth, teaching strategies may be employed differentially in service delivery options. For example, the induction teaching strategy requires the expertise of the clinician in selecting the stimuli that will highlight and make salient the linguistic rule to be learned by the toddler. The toddler's parents might implement the strategy after the initial stages of treatment. Similarly, devising an appropriate JAR may initially require the expertise of the clinician, followed by implementation by the parent or caretaker who can more readily identify routines in the natural environment that would be supportive of the target. Milieu teaching could be taught to parents to employ in the toddler's natural environment. Thus, the three strategies can be employed in direct and indirect service delivery options, although with varying degrees of ease. Additional research is needed to investigate these types of interaction between stages of treatment, treatment delivery models, and teaching strategies.

Selection of the appropriate treatment delivery model and teaching strategy is an incredibly complex task for the clinician. Although guidelines are available, these are general at best. Consequently, providing effective intervention is a difficult goal to obtain. Given that few answers are available, clinicians must repeatedly and periodically evaluate their clinical decisions. They must determine the effectiveness of their intervention and be prepared to make modifications when necessary.

## CLINICAL DECISION MAKING

Deciding if intervention is effective is a challenging and difficult task because the clinician must be able to measure accurately change in communication that is reflective of the intervention process. This requires that clinicians make some major decisions. First, they must decide what behaviors to measure. This involves identifying behaviors that will change due to intervention versus those that will change due to maturation or other factors. Second, clinicians need to decide how to measure such behaviors. The task is to determine which measurement procedures, standardized or nonstandardized, appropriately will sample the behaviors of interest. This task is made difficult because of validity and reliability issues. Finally, clinicians must decide how frequently to measure the behaviors of interest. Many clinicians eval-

uate the effectiveness of intervention by comparing pre- and posttherapy results. Changes in standard deviation units (Bain & Dollaghan, in press) and the "proportional change index" (Wolery, 1983) are two procedures to aid the clinician in determining the effectiveness of intervention when using pre- and posttherapy comparisons. If, however, the goal of measurement is to determine if intervention is being effective, then clinicians must monitor the ongoing language acquisition process, not just make pre- and posttherapy evaluations. Repeated, periodic monitoring is essential, particularly with toddlers, for their language changes can occur rapidly. Clinicians may find single-subject designs, such as a multiple-baseline design, useful tools for assessing the ongoing effectiveness of the intervention process, as described by Bain and Dollaghan (in press).

The use of data for deciding when intervention should be initiated, if intervention is being effective, and when intervention can be terminated is critical for accountable service delivery. Deciding what behaviors to measure, how to measure them, and how frequently, will provide clinicians with tools for making informed decisions regarding the effectiveness of intervention. The complexity of the process requires that clinicians be well informed about data collection procedures and interpretation. The task of determining whether intervention is being effective in changing a toddler's language acquisition is at the core of the philosophy espoused in this article. Intervention is recommended to teach SLI toddlers specific language behaviors and underlying rules. Intervention is viewed as facilitating or inducing the language acquisition process. The benefits of intervention must be weighed against the benefits of maturation alone, and the decision to intervene based on an informed judgment about the toddler's readiness to learn. Selection of the most appropriate treatment delivery option and treatment strategy is based on numerous variables regarding the toddler's language skills and needs. Although research has provided some guidelines to aid the clinician in making these selections, unfortunately, few hard facts exist. Thus, the clinician is left to make the best choices and to evaluate those choices continually. The process is dynamic. The therapeutic process is seen as one in which

a toddler moves in and out of intervention, using different treatment delivery models and treatment strategies as deemed appropriate at particular points in time. The clinician's data are used to monitor growth that is attributable to intervention versus maturation, and to support the need to revise intervention plans. Treating the SLI toddler is a process of accelerating development and enhancing learning that is occurring by maturation alone. A mixture of intervention and monitoring seems to be the most accountable approach to employ, and one that requires ongoing data collection for evaluating clinical decisions.

## REFERENCES

American Speech-Language-Hearing Association. (1990). Code of Ethics. *Asha, 32*, 91.

Aram, D., Ekelman, B., & Nation, J. (1984). Preschoolers with language disorders: 10 years later. *Journal of Speech and Hearing Research, 27*, 232–244.

Aram, D., & Nation, J. (1980). Preschool language disorders and subsequent language and academic difficulties. *Journal of Communication Disorders, 13*, 159–170.

Aslin, R. (1981, November). Effects of experience in sensory and perceptual development: Implications for infant cognition. Paper presented at a conference entitled "Neonate and infant cognition: Learning and development," sponsored by the Harry Frank Guggenheim Foundation, Rockefeller University, New York, NY.

Aslin, R., & Pisoni, D. (1980). Some developmental processes in speech perception. In G. Yeni-Komshian, J. Kavanagh, & C. Ferguson (Eds.), *Child phonology: Perception* (Vol. 2). New York, NY: Academic Press.

Bain, B.A., & Dollaghan, C.A. (in press). Treatment effectiveness: The notion of clinically significant change. *Language, Speech, and Hearing Services in Schools.*

Bishop, C., & Edmundson, A. (1987). Language-impaired 4-year olds: Distinguishing transient from persistent impairment. *Journal of Speech and Hearing Disorders, 52*, 156–173.

Brown, R. (1973). *A first language.* Cambridge, MA: Harvard University Press.

Cole, K.N., & Dale, P.S. (1986). Direct language instruction and interactive language instruction with language

delayed preschool children: A comparison study. *Journal of Speech and Hearing Research, 29*, 206–217.

Committee on Language, Speech, and Hearing Services in the Schools. (1984, July). Guidelines for caseload size for speech-language services in the schools. *Asha, 26*, 53–58.

Connell, P. (1986). Acquisition of semantic role by language-disordered children: Differences between production and comprehension. *Journal of Speech and Hearing Research, 29*, 366–374.

Connell, P. (1987). An effect of modeling and imitation teaching procedures on children with and without specific language impairment. *Journal of Speech and Hearing Research, 30*, 105–113.

Connell, P. (1989). Facilitating generalization through induction teaching. In L. McReynolds & J. Spradlin (Eds.), *Generalization strategies in the treatment of communication disorders.* Philadelphia, PA: B.C. Decker.

Constable, C. (1986). The application of scripts in the organization of language intervention contexts. In K. Nelson (Ed.), *Event knowledge: Structure and function in development.* Hillsdale, NJ: Erlbaum.

Damico, J. (1987). Addressing language concerns in the schools: The SLP as consultant. *Journal of Childhood Communication Disorders, 11*, 17–41.

Feuerstein, R. (1979). *The dynamic assessment of retarded performers.* Baltimore, MD: University Park Press.

Fey, M. (1986). *Language intervention with young children.* San Diego, CA: College-Hill Press.

Friedman, P., & Friedman, K. (1980). Accounting for individual differences when comparing the effectiveness of remedial language teaching methods. *Applied Psycholinguistics, 1,* 151–170.

Gibson, D., & Ingram, D. (1983). The onset of comprehension and production in a language delayed child. *Applied Psycholinguistics, 4,* 359–376.

Goldstein, H., Wickstrom, S., Hoyson, M., Jamieson, B., & Odom, S. (1988). Effects of sociodramatic script training on social and communicative interaction. *Education and Treatment of Children, 11,* 97–117.

Gottlieb, G. (1976). The roles of experience in the development of behavior and the nervous system. *Studies on the development of behavior and the nervous system: Neural and behavioral specificity.* New York, NY: Academic Press.

Gottlieb, C. (1981). Roles of early experience in species-specific perceptual development. *Development of Perception (Vol. 1).* New York, NY: Academic Press.

Hall, P., & Tomblin, J. (1978). A followup study of children with articulation and language disorders. *Journal of Speech and Hearing Disorders, 43,* 227–241.

Hart, B., & Rogers-Warren, A. (1978). A milieu approach to teaching language. In R. Schiefelbusch (Ed.), *Language intervention strategies.* Baltimore: University Park Press.

Johnston, J. (1983). What is language intervention? The role of theory. In J. Miller, D. Yoder, & R. Schiefelbusch (Eds.), *ASHA Reports: (Vol. 12). Contemporary issues in language intervention.* Rockville, MD: The American Speech-Language-Hearing Association.

Kamhi, A., & Catts, H. (1989). *Reading disabilities: A developmental language perspective.* Boston, MA: Little, Brown.

Lenneberg, E. (1967). *Biological foundations of language.* New York, NY: Wiley.

Leonard, L. (1981). An invited article: Facilitating linguistic skills in children with specific language impairment. *Applied Psycholinguistics, 2,* 89–118.

Marvin, C. (1987). Consultation services: Changing roles for SLPs. *Journal of Childhood Communication Disorders, 11,* 1–16.

Nelson, K. (1986). *Event knowledge: Structure and function in development.* Hillsdale, NJ: Lawrence Erlbaum.

Oblak, S.B. (1989). *Scripts: A strategy for facilitating communication.* Paper presented at the Washington Speech and Hearing Association Convention, Spokane, Washington.

Olswang, L., & Bain, B. (in press). Language intervention research applied to clinical decision-making. In P. Tallal (Ed.), *The neural basis of developmental language disorders.* New York, NY: Oxford University Press.

Olswang, L., Bain, B., Dunn, C., & Cooper, J. (1983). The effects of stimulus variation on lexical learning. *Journal of Speech and Hearing Disorders, 48,* 192–201.

Olswang, L., Bain, B., Rosendahl, P., Oblak, S., & Smith,

A. (1986). Language learning: Moving performance from a context-dependent to -independent state. *Child Language Teaching and Therapy, 2,* 180–210.

Olswang, L., & Coggins, T. (1984). The effects of adult behaviors on increasing language delayed children's production of early relational meanings. *British Journal of Disorders of Communication, 19,* 15–34.

Olswang, L., Kriegsmann, E., & Mastergeorge, A. (1982). Facilitating functional requesting in pragmatically impaired children. *Language, Speech, and Hearing Services in Schools, 13,* 202–220.

Rossetti, L. (1986). *High-risk infants: Identification, assessment, and intervention.* Boston, MA: College-Hill.

Schwartz, R. (1988). Early action word acquisition in normal and language-impaired children *Applied Psycholinguistics, 9,* 111–122.

Schwartz, R., Chapman, K., Terrell, B., Prelock, P., & Rowan, L. (1985). Facilitating word combination in language-impaired children through discourse structure. *Journal of Speech and Hearing Disorders, 50,* 31–39.

Snyder-McLean, L., Salomonson, B., McLean, J., & Sack, S. (1984). Structuring joint action routines: A strategy for facilitating communication and language development in the classroom. *Seminars in Speech and Language, 5,* 213–228.

Vygotsky, L. (1978). *Mind in society: The development of higher psychological processes.* Cambridge, MA: Harvard University Press.

Wade, K., & Haynes, W. (1989). Dynamic assessment of spontaneous language and cue responses in adult-directed and child-directed play: A statistical and descriptive analysis. *Child Language Teaching and Therapy, 5,* 157–173.

Wallach, G., & Butler, K. (1984). *Language learning disabilities in school-age children.* Baltimore, MD: Williams & Wilkins.

Warren, S., & Kaiser, A. (1986). Incidental language teaching: A critical review. *Journal of Speech and Hearing Disorders, 51,* 191–199.

Warren, S., McQuarter, R., & Rogers-Warren, A. (1984). The effects of mands and models on the speech of unresponsive language-delayed preschool children. *Journal of Speech and Hearing Disorders, 49,* 43–52.

Weismer, S., & Murray-Branch, J. (1989). Modeling versus modeling plus evoked production training: A comparison of two language intervention methods. *Journal of Speech and Hearing Disorders, 54,* 269–281.

Wilcox, M. (1989). Delivering communication-based services to infants, toddlers, and their families: Approaches and models. *Topics in Language Disorders, 10*(1) 68–79.

Wolery, M. (1983). Proportional change index: An alternative for comparing child change data. *Exceptional Children, 50,* 167–170.

# Providing services to children with autism (ages 0 to 2 years) and their families

**Barry M. Prizant, PhD**
*Director*
*Communication Disorders Department*
*Emma Pendleton Bradley Hospital*

*Assistant Professor*
*Division of Child and Adolescent*
  *Psychiatry*
*Department of Psychiatry and Human*
  *Behavior*
*Brown University Program in Medicine*
*Providence, Rhode Island*

**Amy M. Wetherby, PhD**
*Associate Professor*
*Department of Communication*
  *Disorders*
*Florida State University*
*Tallahassee, Florida*

OVER THE PAST two decades, major advances have been made in our knowledge of the syndrome of autism. These advances have resulted in improvements in the provision of education and treatment to children with autism and their families. In the 1960s, applied researchers using behavioral approaches demonstrated that autistic children can learn and be educated. Work in the 1970s refined behavioral techniques, provided preliminary evidence for the neurological bases of the disorder, and laid the groundwork for exploring the developmental relationship between cognitive, social, and language impairments in autism. Achievements of the 1980s have provided preliminary evidence of neurological impairment involving subcortical structures with secondary impairment of cortical development. Additionally, recent emphasis has been placed on the application of developmental information to explain the various social, cognitive, and communicative symptoms of autism. Impending goals for

*Top Lang Disord*, 1988, 9(1), 1–23
© 1988 Aspen Publishers, Inc.

the next decade are to improve early identification efforts, to further increase our understanding of etiological factors, to demonstrate the efficacy of different treatment and educational approaches, and to integrate educational contributions from various approaches (e.g., behavioral and developmental approaches).

The language specialist plays a key role in the education and treatment of autistic children since the core symptoms of autism include impairments in speech, language, and communication, and in language-related cognitive and social skills (Prizant, 1982). The current definition of autism proposed by the American Psychiatric Association includes the following three diagnostic criteria: "qualitative impairment in reciprocal social interaction," "qualitative impairment in verbal and nonverbal communication, and in imaginative activity," and a "markedly restricted repertoire of activities and interests" (American Psychiatric Association, 1987, p. 38–39). This definition reflects the recent emphasis on impairments of social interaction, communication, and symbolic activities.

The majority of children identified as having the autistic syndrome are reported to demonstrate symptomatology within the first 2 years of life, but in practice, may not be diagnosed until 3 to 5 years of age at the earliest, with many diagnosed at a later age. Early identification of autism should improve considerably due to the expansion of child find services and increased sophistication in psychosocial and communication evaluations for infants and toddlers. The passage of the Education of the Handicapped Act Amendments of 1986 (P.L. 99-457) establishes the availability of federal funds to states choosing to implement early intervention programs for handicapped/high risk children from birth to 2 years (i.e., during the first 3 years of life until the third birthday). The downward extension of early intervention programs serving children from birth to 2 years will become more prevalent in the coming years. Thus, there is an urgent need for professionals to sharpen their clinical skills in all aspects of service provision for this young age level.

## EARLY SYMPTOMATOLOGY AND EARLY IDENTIFICATION

### Early diagnosis a difficult task

Identification and diagnosis of autism during the first 18 months of life have been extremely rare occurrences. Factors precluding early identification are many and varied, and include the variability of behavior in children, the lack of appropriate referrals by professionals to whom parents express concern, and/or the family's lack of knowledge of services or access to services. Currently, retrospective accounts of parents whose children have been diagnosed as having autism are the primary source of information about behavioral symptomatology in the first 18 months of life (for example, see DeMyer, 1979). Validity of such accounts is problematic due to limitations on recall (parents may "tell their story" many years later), and the need for parents to have a standard of comparison for what "normal" behavior is during this period of development, especially when the affected child is the first born.

Further complicating the picture is the

variability of behavioral profiles of infants later diagnosed as autistic. A consistent early profile predictive of autism could help to reliably distinguish these children from other children with developmental disorders or even from normally developing children. However, research findings suggest that there may not be a single early behavioral profile characterizing this population. For example, Coleman and Gillberg (1985) noted that in the first year of life, there are at least two general "modes of presentation" for children later diagnosed as autistic: the "model" infant who not only presents few demands, but who also may be somewhat lethargic and appears to prefer to be left alone, and the "terrible" or highly irritable infant who has sleeping problems, is frequently screaming or crying, and is difficult to console.

In addition to these two extreme profiles, it is now widely accepted that there are at least two different subgroups of autistic children distinguished on the basis of clinical onset (Freeman & Ritvo, 1984). Most autistic children demonstrate developmental delays and observable symptoms early in life, while as many as 20% have a history of normal development in the first year or two of life with subsequent developmental arrest or regression accompanied by the onset of specific symptomatology. For the latter group, parents often report that problems were first noted following an illness accompanied by a high fever. In some cases, no identifiable precipitant is reported. Until recently, an additional criterion of the diagnosis of autism was an onset prior to 30 months. This criterion was eliminated due to the difficulty in confirming age of onset for some children, as well as increased recognition that others may demonstrate the full symptom picture of autism, but have an onset up to 5 or 6 years of age, and in rare cases later in childhood (APA, 1987).

Ornitz, Guthrie, and Farley (1977) identified nonspecific and specific symptomatology observed in those infants who are symptomatic in the first year. Nonspecific symptoms are those that may be observed in children with other disabilities or even in children whose development is essentially normal in other ways, for example, hyperactivity, lethargy, sleep problems, and/or feeding difficulties. Specific symptoms entail those more closely related to social and communicative functioning and other characteristics associated with autism and include peculiarities of gaze behavior (i.e., frequent gaze aversion or empty staring), lack of a social smile, lack of responsiveness to sounds, and lack of anticipation of others' social approaches. In addition, vocalization may be minimal or babbling may stop, and imitation of sound or gestures and responsiveness to early social games may be absent or limited (Freeman & Ritvo, 1984). Some parents also report the presence of stereotypic motility patterns such as rocking behaviors or repetitive hand movements. As with nonspecific symptoms, many of these so-called specific symptoms also may be observed in normally developing children. For example, infants use gaze aversion to regulate social interaction and control the amount of stimulation they receive (Stern, 1977). However, it is the frequency and clustering of these symptoms that result in a picture of severely impaired social relatedness early in development—the hallmark of the autistic syndrome.

The early identification of autistic children is further complicated by some aspects of development that proceed normally. Most children diagnosed as autistic do not present with significant medical problems early in development even though there tends to be an increased incidence of prenatal and postnatal problems when compared to normal controls (Coleman & Gillberg, 1985). Many children also do not demonstrate significant delays in gross motor milestones, may be physically attractive, and even appear to be extremely alert at times, resulting in an inconsistent and spurious picture of normalcy. Without obvious medical problems, further referrals may not be made, giving parents an implicit message that nothing is terribly wrong. Without early diagnosis, the child's condition remains somewhat ambiguous, which may lead to disagreements between family members as to whether there is cause for concern and what the appropriate course of action should be (Bristol, 1985).

Social and communicative impairment is one of the most stressful aspects of a young child's behavior for the family (Bristol, 1988). In addition to delayed language development, children may actively avoid social contact with others. Conventional nonverbal communication (e.g., pointing, requesting, showing gestures, head shakes, and nods) may be virtually absent. Some children who had been developing language may become mute. Kurita (1985) reported that 37.2% of a sample of 261 Japanese autistic children lost meaningful speech prior to 30 months of age. Others may become echolalic during the later part of this period

raising the hopes of parents because of the development of speech, yet causing distress to parents at the typically noncommunicative nature and strange quality of early echolalic patterns.

During the period between 18 and 36 months, problems that become more pronounced may include the development of temper tantrums, more frequent repetitive movements (whirling, hand flapping) and ritualistic play (e.g., lining up objects), extreme reactions to specific sensory stimuli, and hyperactivity (Freeman & Ritvo, 1984; Ornitz, Guthrie, & Farley, 1977). Social and symbolic play may be strikingly absent and difficulties in language comprehension may become evident. Interactions have a one-sided quality, with adults or other children having to take the major responsibility for initiating and maintaining social contact. The stereotype of the autistic child being in a world of his or her own is probably more true between 18 to 36 months than during any other time period.

### Refining early identification efforts

Over the past decade major advances have been made in early identification and diagnosis due to increased professional and social awareness of autism and

---

*Over the past decade major advances have been made in early identification and diagnosis due to increased professional and social awareness of autism and more comprehensive multidisciplinary services available in both urban and rural areas.*

---

more comprehensive multidisciplinary services available in both urban and rural areas. A greater understanding of the variability of behavior within the autistic syndrome and increased recognition of the positive impact of early intervention have resulted in attitudinal changes leading many professionals to abandon "wait and see" attitudes in favor of making referrals to obtain further information or to rule out problems. Unfortunately, ignorance of and misinformation about autism still abounds, leaving parents frustrated and even bitter about their experience with professionals, while precluding early identification and service provision.

Since autistic children may not show significant medical problems or delays in gross motor development early in life, they typically are not identified as at-risk for developmental problems. The first obvious indicator to parents or physicians that the child is not developing normally may be the absence of, delay in, or regression in, language acquisition. Children normally begin using words between 12 and 18 months of age. Therefore, a child may not be referred for a delay in language development until 18 to 24 months at the earliest, allowing for a normal range of variation when the point of reference is the emergence of words. Some autistic children may use first words before 18 months, further obscuring early identification. Thus, the time of language emergence may not be a sensitive indicator for the early identification of autism. However, recent research in communicative intent has provided a valuable framework to improve early assessment efforts (Prizant & Wetherby, 1987).

The importance of prelinguistic communicative, cognitive, and social develop-

ment for the acquisition of language has been emphasized in the child language literature during the past decade (Bates, 1979; Bruner, 1981). This information holds important implications for the early identification of children with communication impairments. The range of symptoms that characterize autism suggests that impairments of social interaction, communication, and symbolic activities should be evident in young autistic children, even prior to the emergence of words. Thus, the child's profile of communicative and symbolic behavior likely will be a sensitive measure for the early identification and differential diagnosis of children with autistic characteristics.

## EARLY INTERVENTION AS PREVENTION

A major premise underlying the provision of early intervention is that the facilitative effects of intervention on development are greater earlier in life than later (Wetherby, 1985). The effects of early intervention may involve both neurological and behavioral changes, as well as positive influences on a family's ability to deal with this perplexing disorder.

The formation of neural connections is dependent on stimulation from the environment during critical periods of development (e.g., Rutledge, 1976; Schapiro & Vulkovich, 1970). The influence of the environment on brain structure and function is greatest during the first few years of life when the brain is relatively immature and growing rapidly, to take advantage of neural plasticity (Lenneberg, 1967). Neural plasticity, the capacity of the structure and function of the nervous system to be modified, diminishes with maturation.

Since autism is presumed to be caused by brain dysfunction with primary involvement of subcortical systems (see Schopler & Mesibov, 1987), early intervention offers a better chance of stimulating new connections or compensatory pathways for these impaired systems (see Lund, 1978).

The young autistic child is impaired in the ability to engage in social interaction, to process social stimuli, and to use flexible, exploratory action schemes to foster cognitive development. These impairments in social interaction, communication, and symbolic activities may result in an environment that is inadequate for neural maturation, that is, the child may not be able to elicit and/or process necessary social and environmental stimulation during critical periods. This inability may have a detrimental impact on neurological development, and thus, may compound the underlying brain dysfunction. While further research clearly is needed to provide support for this argument, some indirect evidence can be found in Sameroff and Chandler's (1975) review of the literature on early development of children. They indicated that developmental outcomes are influenced more by a family's socioeconomic status, and conceivably, quality of the environment and caregiving, than by early neurological status. This notion should underscore the importance of early intervention and help families develop an optimistic rather than a pessimistic view on the potential for neurodevelopmental change.

Early intervention also may prevent the development of maladaptive behaviors. Due to the nature of the severe social and communication impairment, children with autism are at high risk for the development of significant behavior problems. Recent research and clinical literature have emphasized the social–communicative basis of maladaptive behavior (e.g., temper tantrums being used to protest rather than more conventional symbolic signals). One obvious implication is that early communication intervention may serve to preclude the development of potentially dangerous and disruptive behavior. Current literature in child psychiatry is also emphasizing early communication intervention as a strategy for prevention of emotional and behavioral problems in communicatively impaired children (Beitchman, 1985; Baker & Cantwell, 1984). Clearly, issues of communication development and behavior management can no longer be viewed as mutually exclusive for children with communication impairments (Prizant & Wetherby, in press).

Finally, early communication intervention may impact positively on social development. Communication problems exacerbate problems of social relatedness for autistic children (Garfin & Lord, 1986). As children with autism become more motivated to engage others in social exchange, breakdowns may occur primarily due to linguistic and communicative limitations. Thus, early communication intervention has the potential to prevent increased social isolation and withdrawal. When the focus of intervention is on enhancing interaction between the child and others, improvement in both communication and social ability is mutually interdependent. This should allow a child to benefit from increased social stimulation, and help family members to experience some enjoyment from the resulting social inter-action.

To date, there is virtually no empirical evidence of the effectiveness of interven-tion with autistic children from birth to 2 years, since in practice children have not been identified by this age. However, there is now accumulating evidence on the effectiveness of early intervention with 3- to 5-year-old autistic children. Simeons-son, Olley, and Rosenthal (1987) reviewed empirical studies of treatment of autistic children 5 years of age and younger. Although the number of studies with ade-quate research designs was small, the find-ings of the three most comprehensive studies (Fenske, Zalenski, Krantz, & McClannahan, in press; Hoyson, Jamie-son, & Strain, 1984; Lovaas, 1987) were impressive, with a substantial number of children achieving normal levels of social and intellectual functioning by kinder-garten. Simeonsson, Olley, and Rosenthal (1987) identified the following common features that may have contributed to the success of these programs: (1) use of struc-tured behavioral approaches that targeted specific skills and employed positive con-sequences; (2) training of parents to implement the program at home; (3) implementation of the program before the age of 5; (4) use of an intensive program that involved many hours a day, 5 days a week, year-round, with parents carrying over at home; and (5) emphasis on gener-alization by using natural settings and involving parents and peers.

The studies reviewed by Simeonsson, Olley, and Rosenthal (1987), for the most part, used behavioral approaches. The lack of a significant literature reporting outcome with other than "behavioral approaches" does not necessarily imply that only behavioral approaches are effec-tive. Furthermore, behavioral approaches are highly heterogeneous in reference to methodology and content. Certainly, aspects of developmental as well as behav-ioral approaches are being integrated in current programs (see Prizant & Wether-by, in press, for further discussion). Indeed, it has been suggested that devel-opmental approaches are more appropri-ate with young children but have limita-tions with adolescents and adults (Dawson & Galpert, 1986). Further research is needed to explore the relationship be-tween educational approach and age as well as developmental level of the child. However, during the interim it seems pru-dent to use developmental strategies with very young autistic children.

While there is evidence of the greater effectiveness of intervention before the age of 5 than after age 5 (Fenske, Zalenski, Krantz, & McClannahan, in press), it seems reasonable to assume that the impact of intervention for the child and the family would be even greater before age 3. In designing programs for young autistic children, special consideration should be given to using developmentally sound approaches, with an emphasis on addressing the core symptoms of autism, that is, social interaction and social relatedness, communication, and symbolic behavior. Early intervention has the potential to make a substantial impact on the child, and in some cases may prevent the need for special education by school age (Lovaas, 1987). It may also provide support for families and thus lessen the significant stress parents and siblings may experience (Bristol, 1985).

## APPROACHES TO EARLY ASSESSMENT

The purpose of assessing the communication skills of a young child with autistic characteristics may range from identifying a problem to determining a child's developmental level across domains in order to target intervention goals. The communication assessment may also contribute information toward the differential diagnosis of autism from other developmental disorders. For children from birth to 2 years of age, however, the major emphasis should be on identifying and understanding the nature of a social communicative impairment and providing preliminary directions for intervention, rather than establishing a diagnosis. The assessment plan should be guided by normal developmental information and theories explaining the nature of the communication impairment of autistic children (Prizant & Wetherby, in press). Since autistic children's speech, language, and communication impairments are most apparent in the social use of language (i.e., pragmatics), traditional formal assessment instruments have limited utility. Therefore, clinicians must rely on the systematic use of informal procedures to assess communication. In designing an assessment plan, the clinician first needs to determine the key content areas to be addressed, and then can select strategies to explore these areas. This section will provide a framework for a clinician-designed assessment of communication with young children diagnosed as, or suspected of having, autism. This framework also is relevant for all young children who have or are suspected of having developmental delays.

### Content of assessment

In the first 2 years, a child's behavior becomes increasingly more deliberate and goal directed, showing increased evidence of foresight, and culminating with the ability to plan behavior through symbolic thought. The development of intentional communication lies at the interface of emerging intentionality within cognitive, social, and affective domains. In normal development, preverbal intentional communication provides a foundation for the emergence of symbolic, referential language. The autistic child experiences cognitive, social, and affective impairments, which disrupt the normal development of language. In order to address underlying impairments in social cognition, a communication assessment needs to focus on two major content areas: (1) the child's profile of communicative behaviors, and (2) the child's symbolic level across cognitive–social and language domains.

Table 1 identifies the major content areas that need to be examined to develop a communicative profile. If a child is at a preintentional level, assessment should identify any behavior that serves a communicative function based on the adult's interpretation of the act. Assessment should identify what a child attempts to accomplish (intents expressed) and actu-

---

*Assessment should identify what a child attempts to accomplish (intents expressed) and actually accomplishes (functions of communication) in his or her communicative behavior.*

**Table 1.** Assessment dimensions of a communication profile

---

**Repertoire of communicative functions**
- regulate another's behavior
- engage in social interaction
- reference joint attention

**Degree of intentionality for each function**
- awareness of a desired goal
- simple plan designed to achieve the goal
- coordinated plan designed to achieve a goal
- alternative plans used if met with failure
- metapragmatic awareness of the success or failure of the plan

**Variety and sophistication of communicative means for each function**
- reenactive to symbolic representation
- idiosyncratic to conventional act
- aberrant to socially acceptable behavior
- echolalic to creative speech
- gestural and/or vocal modality
- prelinguistic to complex linguistic rules

**Reciprocity of communication**
- ability to participate in turn-taking interactions
- ability to repeat or revise message as needed to repair communication breakdowns
- ability to assume shared knowledge and encode information needed by the listener to understand the message
- ability to collaborate on topics based on conventional meanings

---

ally accomplishes (functions of communication) in his or her communicative behavior. Normally developing children use prelinguistic gestures and vocalizations for the following functions prior to the emergence of speech: to regulate others' behavior, to engage in social interaction, and to reference joint attention (Bruner, 1981; Wetherby, Cain, Yonclas, & Walker, in press). Autistic children in the early stages of communication and language development have been found to show deficiencies in the range of communicative functions expressed (Wetherby & Prutting, 1984). Wetherby (1986) suggested that the easiest and first emerging category of functions for autistic children is regulating others' behavior, while the most difficult is referencing joint atten-

tion, presumably because of the differing social underpinnings of these abilities.

Autistic children may show discrepancies in the degree of intentionality, conventionality, and sophistication of communicative means for these different functions. For example, a young autistic child may use creative speech to regulate others' behavior, echolalic speech or gestural reenactment strategies to engage in social interaction, and show no intentional communication to reference joint attention. In assessment it is critical to determine the level of intentionality for each communicative function. That is, does the individual use a behavior for preplanned or intentional effects on others, and does the degree of intentionality vary with different communicative functions? Recent research has demonstrated that unconventional, idiosyncratic, and aberrant behavior may be used intentionally to communicate for a variety of functions (Carr & Durand, 1986; Donnellan, Mirenda, Mesaros, & Fassbender, 1984; Wetherby & Prutting, 1984); therefore, a lack of conventionality or social acceptability should not preclude the possibility that a behavior is used purposefully to communicate. Similarly, the sophistication of communicative means should be evaluated for each function. A developmental continuum of intentionality and dimensions of communicative means to be assessed are listed in Table 1.

Autistic children also show difficulties with the reciprocity of communication, ranging from impairments in synchronizing and regulating turn-taking interactions to making poor judgments about what the listener needs to know to interpret their message (Dawson & Galpert, 1986). Higher functioning autistic children who reach a discourse level show difficulties with conversational contingency. They may initiate topics without identifying the referent and have difficulties revising a message to clarify what the listener needs to know. Maintaining a topic of joint focus is problematic when conversing with autistic children. For example, they may engage in a particular dialogue to complete a ritual rather than to share information. They may group words or follow topics by clanging, that is, by the way words sound rather than by their meaning (e.g., associating words that rhyme or have the same initial phoneme), making it hard for the listener to identify or maintain the topic. The dimensions of

reciprocity that need to be evaluated are listed in Table 1.

Numerous studies of autistic children have found impairments in cognitive–social correlates of language (e.g., Dawson & Adams, 1984; Sigman & Ungerer, 1984; Wetherby & Prutting, 1984). Therefore, a communication assessment must compare the autistic child's ability to use symbols across cognitive–social and language domains. Determining autistic children's symbolic levels may be difficult because of their propensity for using reenactment strategies. That is, they may replicate an entire event or aspects of it as a means to achieve a goal (e.g., manipulating an adult's hand to open a door; or repeating a memorized portion of a book to request that book). Reenactment is indexical representation, rather than symbolic, in that the original event or part of the event is being used to stand for the whole event, and it precedes symbolic thought in normal development (Bruner, 1978; Piaget, 1954). Symbolic representation entails the use of one scheme as a symbol to stand for or represent a different scheme, and the relationship between the symbol and the referent may range from iconic to arbitrary. Paradoxically, a verbal autistic child, whose speech consists exclusively of immediate or delayed echolalia, may be functioning at a presymbolic level (Prizant & Rydell, 1984).

Autistic children's expressive language must be compared with their symbolic level in other domains to obtain an accurate picture of symbolic functioning. Domains that should be included in the assessment and general developmental progressions of symbolic representation

**Table 2.** Assessment dimensions of cognitive, social, and language correlates with developmental progressions from presymbolic to symbolic behavior

**Means–end/tool use**
- uses a tool that is contiguous with the goal as a means to obtain the goal (e.g., pulls string tied to object; pulls cloth under object)
- uses a tool that is noncontiguous with the goal as a means to obtain the goal (e.g., rakes in object with stick; moves chair in position and climbs on chair to obtain object on shelf)

**Causality/communicative intent**
- touches adult's hand or object to recreate spectacle
- uses gestural or vocal signal to regulate adult's behavior or to direct adult's attention
- discovers the source of an action (e.g., how to activate a mechanical toy; looks for the source of a thrown object)

**Gestural/vocal imitation**
- takes turns after adult imitates child's behavior or in familiar social routines
- imitates vocal or gestural behavior initiated by adult
- imitates a behavior at a much later time in the absence of the original model

**Schemes for relating to objects/symbolic play**
- explores the physical properties of objects
- uses recognitory gestures on realistic objects (e.g., combs own hair; brushes own teeth; eats from spoon)
- uses pretend schemes with miniature objects toward self (e.g., rolls toy car; drinks from doll's cup; pounds toy hammer)
- uses pretend schemes toward others (e.g., feeds doll with bottle; combs mother's hair)
- uses multiple pretend schemes in sequence (e.g., stirs pretend food in pan; pours food onto dish; and feeds doll)

**Social relatedness/expression of emotion**
- expresses emotions of joy, fear, and anger in appropriate situations or in response to adult's emotional expression
- responds differentially to strangers and caregivers
- uses gestural or vocal signals to establish closeness (e.g., pulls on adult's leg and reaches up to be picked up)
- knows how to get adult to react (e.g., to make adult laugh and make adult angry)
- expresses emotions of empathy, shame, guilt, affection, and defiance

**Language comprehension**
- uses nonlinguistic response strategies, including situational routines, contextual clues, intonation, gestures, and facial expression
- comprehends the meaning of single words (e.g., person names, object names, actions)
- comprehends multiword utterances based on semantic relations (e.g., action + object; agent + action; attribute + object)

**Language production**
- uses consistent preverbal forms tied to the context
- uses single word approximations or intoned jargon to encode dynamic, changing states, or objects that can be acted upon by the child
- uses multiword utterances to encode semantic relations (e.g., action + object; attribute + object)

*Note:* Adapted from Greenspan, & Lieberman (1980); McCune-Nicolich (1981); Miller, Chapman, Branston, & Reichle (1980); Uzgiris, & Hunt (1975); and Wetherby, & Prutting (1984).

within each of these domains are presented in Table 2. Again, these domains are relevant for all young children referred for assessment.

## Assessment strategies

Due to the difficulty in assessing communicative behavior of autistic children, a combination of assessment strategies is recommended (Wetherby & Prizant, in press). A useful initial method for gathering information about the child's communicative behavior and symbolic level is to interview caregivers. The interview should include questions about, and solicit examples of, communicative behaviors outlined in Table 1 and symbolic skills in the domains outlined in Table 2. Peck and Schuler (1987) and Lapidus (1985) have developed interviews addressing communicative means and functions that may be referred to for this purpose. The use of caregivers as informants ensures that the assessment will address the communicative needs of the child and of people interacting with the child in everyday situations.

Based on the information obtained from the interview, a checklist or inventory of possible communicative behaviors and the functions they serve can be developed to measure communicative behavior observed in natural contexts. Observation of the child during daily activities is necessary to determine communicative needs and to evaluate the adequacy of natural opportunities for the child to communicate. Checklists, such as those developed by Donnellan, Mirenda, Mesaros, and Fassbender (1984) and Lapidus (1985), are particularly useful to establish which

communicative means are used to express each communicative function in different settings with various partners. Similarly, checklists can be devised for observation of symbolic behaviors used spontaneously by the child in natural environments. While observation checklists provide critical information about the child's spontaneous use of communicative and symbolic behavior, it may be rather time consuming to wait for behaviors to occur naturally, and some of the child's abilities may not be demonstrated during the observation period.

Thus, a third method to supplement the observation checklist is behavior sampling. The purpose is to collect a representative sample of communicative and symbolic behavior typical of a child's range of functioning in a relatively short period of time, preferably on videotape for later analysis. Structured communicative situations may be staged to entice the child to interact and use a variety of communicative functions (see Schuler & Prizant, 1987; Wetherby & Prutting, 1984). Opportunities can also be set up for the child to use toys or objects instrumentally and symbolically to evaluate the child's level of symbolic representation. Some formal developmental scales for young children include items that may be useful for sampling symbolic skills. Consideration must be given to deciding who will interact with the child during behavior sampling. While it may be less time consuming for the clinician to serve as interactant, a more valid sample may be collected by having a caregiver interact with the child with the clinician demonstrating the procedures to the caregiver. With the birth to 2 years population, emphasis should be on child interactions with a familiar adult.

During the interview, observation, and behavior sampling, the clinician can formulate hypotheses about the child's communicative profile and symbolic level across domains. The next step in assessment is hypothesis testing. Donnellan, Mirenda, Mesaros, and Fassbender (1984) described a procedure for testing hypotheses about the functions of aberrant behavior, which may be extended to other communicative behavior and symbolic abilities. The procedure entails manipulating antecedent and consequent events surrounding the occurrence of the behavior. For example, if a child persistently screams or displays self-injurious behavior when presented with a certain activity, one hypothesis is that the child is protesting. The adult can alternate between presenting that activity and a desirable one. If the child's behavior does not occur with the desired activity and ceases to occur once the undesired activity has been removed, this hypothesis has received support.

Hypothesis testing should be done on a continual basis over an extended period of time, not during only a single assessment session. This is especially pertinent when testing unconventional and primitive communicative acts. Furthermore, to ensure representativeness, the behaviors of concern should be tested in different environments with a variety of interactants. Thus, assessment should be considered an exploratory process that is ongoing rather than episodic.

These guidelines for assessment have been made with the assumption that the evaluation team or clinician will have access to a child and family members on an ongoing basis. In cases where a child is identified as requiring services, and services are available for the ages birth to 2 population, parents should be urged to take advantage of this support, and ongoing assessment can then become part of the services offered. However, a family may not live in a region with birth to 2 years services, may not have access to such services due to fiscal and geographical constraints, or the child may not demonstrate sufficient developmental delay or behavioral symptomatology at the time of evaluation to justify services. In such cases where questions remain, periodic follow-up assessments should be scheduled in order to monitor a child's development. At these times, parents should continue to be the primary source of information about their child's language and communicative development.

## APPROACHES TO INTERVENTION

A thorough multidisciplinary evaluation should determine the need for early intervention services. When this need is indicated, the initiation of services for a child younger than 3 years of age may be both a relief as well as a great stress for families. Parents may be relieved that they are finally getting some professional support and guidance that should result in their child reaching his or her potential. On the other hand, a determination of the need for services confirms the significance of the child's disability. At this point families face the arduous task of coming to grips with the reality of their child's limitations. It is this acceptance that allows parents to begin to move forward and become actively involved in intervention efforts (see Featherstone, 1980, for further consideration of the complex issue of accepting a child's disability). However, acceptance and understanding of autism may be particularly difficult due to the ambiguity of the disability (Bristol, 1988) and the uneven profile of abilities and disabilities (Prizant & Schuler, 1987a).

In this discussion of approaches to intervention, the emphasis will be on a family systems approach (Bristol, 1985) in designing appropriate intervention strategies for enhancing language and communication abilities. Within this framework, parents are viewed as partners in the process rather than as patients that need to be treated or dictated to (Bristol, 1985). Furthermore, this approach recognizes the impact that a severe disability such as autism can have on the day-to-day functioning of the family unit. Thus, intervention planning must include family members as active participants as well as addressing the needs of both the affected child and the family. In advocating for this approach, Bristol (1985) noted that

"Intervention that affects only the child or even the child and one parent is not considered appropriate. The entire family is seen as one of an interactive, interdependent set of systems "nested" within each other. The child affects and is affected by the entire family system" (p.49).

Thus, success of an early intervention program cannot be measured solely in terms of child progress. Family involvement and family adaptation to the child must also be taken into account. A carefully coordinated multidisciplinary approach to early intervention is crucial to the goal of meeting a broad range of needs for the child and the family (see Rossetti, 1986, for further discussion of multidisciplinary team approaches).

These principles are especially relevant for efforts to enhance language and communication, for it is limitations in these skills that create the *most significant barriers* between the child and other family members. Conversely, progress in language and communication development may have a positive impact on a child's social, emotional, and adaptive functioning and foster more successful and mutually satisfying interactions between the child and significant others.

## Home vs. center-based approaches

The two general models of service delivery in early intervention are distinguished on the basis of whether early intervention efforts occur in the child's home environment (i.e., home based) or at a professional or educational agency (center based). Each approach has specific strengths for language and communication enhancement.

Home-based approaches may be directed to the child and/or to the parents in enhancing the child's social communication and cognitive–social abilities, and helping the parents to develop an interactive style conducive to communicative growth. In addition to the convenience for the family, the provision of services within the home allows the early interventionist to observe, and take advantage of, regular family routines as a vehicle for communication enhancement. Modifications of the physical environment can be suggested in order to help create natural opportunities

---

*In addition to the convenience for the family, the provision of services within the home allows the early interventionist to observe, and take advantage of, regular family routines as a vehicle for communication enhancement.*

---

and needs for communication. Finally, other family members, including siblings and grandparents, can become involved in a setting that is familiar and comfortable to them. The major advantage of these approaches is their ecological soundness; that is, the services that are being provided directly to the family and the child are more likely to meet their needs, and acquired abilities are more likely to be used in daily routines. This is especially crucial for autistic children whose situation-specific learning style often results in generalization problems. Professionals also are able to get a more accurate picture of the child's abilities and the challenges parents face.

Center-based approaches also may be directed to the child, parents, or both. Going to a center for services can help to combat the feeling of isolation experienced by many families with handicapped children. Many centers run parent and sibling groups to provide an emotionally supportive forum to express concerns and share experiences. In specific reference to understanding communication problems and enhancing communication abilities, parents can compare notes and share "home-made" strategies. They also learn to understand their role as advocate

for their child, an important skill considering the coming years of potential frustration in finding appropriate services.

Center-based approaches also provide an opportunity for the child to have varied experiences with many different people. Half-day or full-day programs can provide contact with other children in regularly scheduled activities or routines, providing opportunities for targeting specific language and social communicative goals. When such programs are available, parents are afforded much needed time to attend to other obligations or to get a "breather" from the demands of caring for their child. Some centers also offer respite services enabling families to live a more normal life. For more demanding children, these indirect support services often result in the family being able to maintain a child in the home setting rather than resorting to residential placement. Furthermore, family members have more energy for working with the affected child when it is not a full-time occurrence (Bristol, 1988).

Home- and center-based approaches are not mutually exclusive strategies. Benefits of both can be realized when agencies have the financial support and flexibility to provide both kinds of services. However, the effectiveness of either approach depends largely on the degree of active involvement and cooperation on the part of the family (Rossetti, 1986). As noted, approaches focusing solely on the child are episodic, and do not address life-span issues for the family. On the other hand, approaches that empower families by including them as partners in the early intervention process, and when requested, by educating them and providing them with needed skills, have a much greater chance of having an immediate as well as a lasting impact (National Center for Clinical Infant Programs, 1985). For a more in-depth consideration of these issues, see Guralnick and Bennett (1987).

### Content of intervention

The content of communication intervention may be derived from the assessment framework presented in Tables 1 and 2. Goals may be conceptualized bidimensionally along a horizontal and vertical axis (McLean, Snyder-McLean, Jacobs, & Rowland, 1991), borrowing from Piaget's (1954) concept of horizontal and vertical decalage. On the horizontal axis, goals involve expanding the child's repertoire of behaviors at the same developmental level. An example of a horizontal goal is to expand the child's range of communicative functions that emerge during the prelinguistic stage. Wetherby (1986) suggested an ontogeny of communicative functions to be used in intervention with autistic children. The first specific target should be the function of regulating others' behavior to achieve an environmental end through requests for objects and actions, and protests, if the child does not communicate for these functions. As the child progresses toward this goal, the adult can introduce social routines or games that involve adult–child turn-taking interactions with exchangeable roles, such as peek-a-boo (see McLean & Snyder-McLean, 1984). These games or routines form the bases for facilitating communication for the social end of attracting attention to oneself. After the child begins using communication to engage in social interaction, the adult can devise turn-taking interactions that introduce or manipulate objects systematically to facilitate the child's use of communication to direct attention to an object or event.

Other horizontal communication goals include expanding the child's repertoire of means to express intentions and to repair breakdowns. For example, at a prelanguage level, goals may include increasing the variety of vocalizations or gestures. At a language level, horizontal goals might include expanding vocabulary, semantic relations, or grammatical morphemes to enhance the variety of meanings and intents expressed. Horizontal goals should also target deficient cognitive–social skills. For example, for a child functioning in Stage IV of symbolic play, a horizontal goal would be to increase the variety of different action schemes used on objects and the number of different objects with which an action scheme can be used.

On the vertical axis, goals involve increasing the developmental complexity of behavior within the child's repertoire. In enhancing communicative knowledge and behavior, a primary goal is to help the child understand that signals can be used to affect people and to control the environment. For the very young or more severely impaired children, this vertical goal involves shaping noncommunicative exploratory behavior into deliberate and intentional use of the same or similar forms to effect specific outcomes. This may be achieved by constructing predictable interactive routines. Once knowledge of routine structure has been established, delay or discontinuance of an anticipated event often becomes a strong motivator for communication (Schuler & Prizant, 1987).

Communicative persistence and repair reflect higher degrees of intentionality. Autistic children may not persist in expressing intent if initial communicative efforts are unsuccessful. While horizontal goals involve expanding the child's repertoire of communicative behavior, vertical movement entails teaching the child to persist in using these means, and if necessary, to repair unsuccessful communicative attempts by using alternative means. For children at preverbal levels or with poor speech intelligibility, communicative effectiveness may depend on a child's ability to combine communicative means (e.g., use vocalizations plus gestures) or shift to alternative communicative means. The recent movement to nonspeech systems for communicating (e.g., picture boards, sign language, sight–word boards, computerized devices) is providing subjects who have limited communicative ability with more conventional and more efficient means of communicating to repair breakdowns. At verbal levels, children may need to learn that there are alternative ways to express intent through language. The ability to develop strategies for repairing communicative breakdowns is essential in ensuring that the child's communicative act functions as intended.

Secondarily, more sophisticated, and more easily interpretable or conventional means should be targeted to express intent. Due to the idiosyncratic forms often used by autistic individuals, intervention goals must address conventionality of form. At nonverbal levels, partial reenactments may be comprehensible as an expression of intent only to those who are familiar with those situations. At verbal levels, echolalia and metaphorical language may be used with clear intent but limited effectiveness if their origin or referent is not shared by the listener. Another vertical goal related to conventionalization is the social acceptability of the expression of intent. However, social acceptability is not isomorphic with conventionality. Aberrant means such as aggression may be easily understood by others as a form of protest, and therefore may be relatively conventional. Other aberrant means such as self-injury may not be as easily understood as intentional communicative behavior. Short-term considerations include the subject's immediate safety and the safety of others. Long-term considerations involve the acceptability of an individual's behavior in social contexts. The primary goal when dealing with socially unacceptable expression of intent is to replace the aberrant behavior with more socially acceptable forms for expressing that intent (e.g., more acceptable ways to express protest, rejection, and frustration), rather than simply attempting to eradicate or extinguish such behavior (Donnellan, Mirenda, Mesaros, & Fassbender, 1984; Schuler & Prizant; 1987). Research has demonstrated that these problem behaviors may be reduced significantly when children and even adults learn to use more acceptable means to serve the same functions (e.g., protest or requesting assistance) (Carr & Durand, 1986; Smith, 1985).

Success in communication is also dependent on the explicitness of the signals used in expressing meanings and intents. More generalized prelinguistic means for expressing intent (such as the use of undifferentiated gestures or vocalizations) do not communicate explicit content, but shift the burden of interpretation to the listener's ability to use contextual and other nonlinguistic cues in inferring intent. In the dimension of vertical programming, the rule of thumb is to target forms slightly beyond the child's current language level. As indicated, however, some intents may be expressed in far more sophisticated form than others (Wetherby, 1986). Therefore, for a particular child, an appropriate goal for one function might be the use of single- or multi-word utterances while an appropriate goal for another function might be the use of a reenactment gesture to replace disruptive behavior.

It must be kept in mind that the frequent use of memorized language forms may present a spurious picture of linguistic sophistication. Problems in understanding and assessing echolalia have been discussed elsewhere (Prizant, 1983; Schuler & Prizant, 1985). Suffice it to say, sophistication of form is not simply a matter of grammatical complexity. It is also a matter of creativity and generativity. Thus, even simple two- to three-word utterances reflecting generative productive processes should be considered more sophisticated in linguistic form than longer memorized language "chunks."

The concept of horizontal and vertical programming emphasizes the developmental interaction of communicative functions and means. New communicative functions should be taught initially through simple means within the child's repertoire. More conventional, acceptable, and sophisticated means should be mapped onto established communicative functions. Both horizontal and vertical goals may be targeted simultaneously; however, too much emphasis on vertical goals should be avoided. Autistic individuals with limited repertoires of conventional communicative behaviors may display volatile maladaptive behaviors when they cannot successfully communicate, for example, to express that they are frustrated or bored with an activity, or to indicate distress over a routine being disrupted. To circumvent this developmental progression, horizontal goals should be emphasized in young autistic children to give them a variety of appropriate alternative means to express their intentions.

In addition to vertical communication goals, vertical goals should also be targeted in deficient cognitive–social domains. For the example of the child functioning in Stage IV of symbolic play, vertical movement would be to teach conventional uses of realistic objects. Several cognitive–social goals may be targeted simultaneously. However, because the autistic child may show discrepancies across domains, it is likely that goals will be targeted at different developmental levels for different domains.

Thus, early communication intervention is not merely teaching verbal and nonverbal behavior to the child; it entails facilitating the communicative, cognitive, and social foundations of language as well as enhancing linguistic knowledge and use.

### Intervention strategies

In order to address intervention goals that target communicative and symbolic behavior, special consideration must be given to the learning context and the interaction strategies used in intervention. The design of the learning context for autistic children should be guided by the following principles.

### Work at the level of the dyad, rather than the individual child

Successful communicative interactions involve the cooperative effort of two people. Therefore, changes in both members of the dyad are necessary to enhance communication development (MacDonald, 1985). For young children, the emphasis should be on adult–child interactions involving caregivers.

### Structure the environment to scaffold ample opportunity for learning

For young children, the environment needs to provide a consistent and predictable schedule to encourage the child to develop a sense of anticipation and to initiate communicative behavior (see Bruner, 1978; McLean & Snyder-McLean, 1984). A variety of objects and experiences should be available to develop flexible exploratory and problem-solving strategies. Natural or contrived opportunities should be available for the child to initiate communication for a variety of reasons.

### Expect the child to communicate

Wait and look expectantly at the child to signal the child's turn (MacDonald, 1985). To preclude learned helplessness, do not anticipate the child's needs; rather, encourage the child to use active signaling. Avoid verbal cues that the child may become dependent on, because the child will learn to wait for these cues and may not initiate without them.

### Work on communicative acts that are either informative or collaborative

The child should be communicating, whether preverbally or verbally, either to provide information that the listener needs to know or to draw the listener's attention to something for the purpose of sharing. The physical environment can be easily modified to ensure informativeness. For example, to teach a child to say or point to a cookie to request it is not informative when the cookie is the only object of choice, but is informative when the cookie is among several choices of objects. Questions that the adult obviously already knows the answer to should be avoided. If the child's communicative behavior is not providing needed information, then it should be serving an affiliative purpose, for example, to share an interaction or a topic.

### Use natural reinforcers that are consistent with the child's intent

Consider whether the child's act serves to regulate another's behavior, to engage in social interaction, or to reference joint attention, and then respond naturally to that function (Wetherby, 1986). If the child is requesting or protesting an object, the natural reinforcer is to offer or remove the object. If the child is greeting or calling, the natural reinforcer is to attend to the child. If the child is labeling or commenting, the natural reinforcer is to attend to the object or event.

### Attune to the child

Adults should adjust their interaction style and level of language input to the child. For the very young child, the emphasis should be on synchronizing interactions with the child. One effective way to do this is by imitating the child to establish a smooth flow of turn taking (see Dawson & Adams, 1984). The complexity of the adult's speech should be matched to the child's level of language comprehension (see Prizant & Schuler, 1987b). Contextual cues and gestures should be used with speech to develop verbal comprehension.

Current developmental language intervention approaches caution against adult-directed interactions. Fey (1986) described three steps in child-oriented approaches designed to follow the child's lead: (1) wait for the child to initiate some behavior; (2) interpret that behavior as communicative and meaningful; and (3) respond to that behavior in a manner that

will facilitate further communicative interaction and language learning. This issue is even more critical in early intervention programs since research has shown that the vast majority of parent–child interactions involving children from birth to age 3 are child initiated (Hart, 1985). Current behavioral approaches to language treatment emphasize using incidental teaching procedures, which involve waiting for the child to initiate an interaction and then following the child's lead. Because autistic children's major problem is with communication and the use of language, a child-oriented approach may be advantageous (Prizant & Wetherby, in press). Specific antecedent strategies that encourage the child to initiate communication using minimal verbal stimuli are presented in Table 3. Consequential strat-

**Table 3.** Intervention strategies to entice communication

| Antecedent strategies to entice child-initiated communicative acts |
|---|
| 1. Place desired objects so that they are visible to the child but out of the child's reach or in containers that the child needs help opening. |
| 2. Offer the child items that the child does not like or that the child does not need for an activity he or she is engaged in. |
| 3. Engage the child in an activity that necessitates a utensil, then withhold the utensil or "sabotage" the function of the utensil. |
| 4. Set up a turn-taking routine for three or more turns until the child anticipates the steps and then violate a step in the routine. |
| 5. Do or say something that is unexpected or obviously absurd for the situation. |
| **Consequential strategies to facilitate further communicative attempts** |
| 1. Interpret the child's preintentional communicative behaviors as if they were intentional. |
| 2. Translate the child's unconventional act by coding the intent with conventional means. |
| 3. Repeat all or a portion of the child's act to acknowledge or confirm the message. |
| 4. Use obvious back-channel responses (i.e., verbal or nonverbal acknowledgments) to maintain the topic. |
| 5. Provide a simplified model to encode the intent of the child's echolalic utterance. |
| 6. Expand the child's creative utterance by making it more grammatically complete. |
| 7. Extend the child's utterance by adding new information. |
| 8. Ask for a clarification of the child's utterance or for further information about the topic of the child's utterance. |

*Note:* Adapted from Constable (1983); Lucas (1980); MacDonald (1895); Prizant (1983); and Wetherby (1986).

egies to facilitate continued communicative interactions are also presented. A key component when implementing these antecedent and consequential strategies is to wait and to look expectantly at the child.

•   •   •

The benefits of early intervention with autistic children are now becoming apparent in improved outcome for the children receiving these services (Simeonsson, Olley, & Rosenthal, 1987). As early intervention services increase with the impetus of

P.L. 99-457, children displaying characteristics of autism will no doubt be identified earlier. With early provision of services for these children and their families, the potential for growth in communication and related abilities may be realized. Professionals providing these services may take pride in the fact such progress is truly for the whole family, and not for the child alone. With more sensitive tools for early identification and the provision of services for the birth to age 2 population, the next decade will bring opportunities for impacting the outcome of autism that have not been possible in the past.

## REFERENCES

American Psychiatric Association. (1987). *Diagnostic and statistical manual of mental disorders* (3rd ed., rev.). Washington, DC: American Psychiatric Association.

Baker, L., & Cantwell, D. (1984). Primary prevention of the psychiatric consequences of childhood communication disorders. *Journal of Preventive Psychiatry, 2*(1), 75–97.

Bates, E. (1979). *The emergence of symbols: Cognition and communication in infancy.* New York: Academic Press.

Beitchman, J.H. (1985). Speech and language impairment and psychiatric risk: Toward a model of neurodevelopmental immaturity. *Psychiatric Clinics of North America, 8,* 721–735.

Bristol, M. (1985). Designing programs for young developmentally disabled children: A family systems approach to autism. *Remedial and Special Education, 6*(4), 46–53.

Bristol, M. (1988). Impact of autistic children on families. In B. Prizant & B. Schaechter (Eds.), *Autism: The emotional and social dimensions.* Boston: The Exceptional Parent.

Bruner, J. (1978). From communication to language: A psychological perspective. In I. Markova (Ed.), *The social context of language* (pp. 17–48). New York: Wiley.

Bruner, J. (1981). The social context of language acquisition. *Language and Communication, 1,* 155–178.

Carr, E., & Durand, V. (1986). Reducing behavior problems through functional communication training. *Journal of Applied Behavior Analysis, 18,* 111–126.

Coleman, M., & Gillberg, C. (1985). *The biology of the autistic syndrome.* New York: Praeger.

Constable, C.M. (1983). Creating communicative context. In H. Winitz (Ed.), *Treating language disorders: For clinicians by clinicians.* Baltimore: University Park Press.

Dawson, G., & Adams, A. (1984). Imitation and social responsiveness in autistic children. *Journal of Abnormal Child Psychology, 12,* 209–226.

Dawson, G., & Galpert, L. (1986). A developmental model for facilitating the social behavior of autistic children. In E. Schopler & G.B. Mesibov (Eds.), *Social behavior in autism.* New York: Plenum Press.

DeMyer, M. (1979). *Parents and children in autism.* New York: Wiley.

Donnellan, A., Mirenda, P., Mesaros, R., & Fassbender, L. (1984). Analyzing the communicative functions of aberrant behavior. *Journal of the Association for Persons with Severe Handicaps, 9,* 201–212.

Featherstone, H. (1980). *A difference in the family.* New York: Basic Books.

Fenske, E.C., Zalenski, S., Krantz, P.J., & McClannahan, L.E. (in press). Age at intervention and treatment outcome for autistic children in a comprehensive intervention program. *Analysis and Intervention in Developmental Disabilities.*

Fey, M. (1986). *Language intervention with young children.* San Diego: College-Hill Press.

Freeman, B.J., & Ritvo, E.R. (1984). The syndrome of autism: Establishing the diagnosis and principles of management. *Pediatric Annals, 13,* 284–296.

Garfin, D., & Lord, C. (1986). Communication as a social problem in autism. In E. Schopler & G. Mesibov (Eds.), *Social behavior in autism*. New York: Plenum Press.

Greenspan, S., & Lieberman, A. (1980). Infants, mothers, and their interaction: A quantitative clinical approach to developmental assessment. In S. Greenspan & G. Pollack (Eds.), *The course of life, Volume I, Infancy and childhood*. (DHHS Pub. # 80-999). Washington, DC: U.S. Government Printing Office.

Guralnick, M.J., & Bennett, F.C. (Eds.) (1987). *The effectiveness of early intervention for at-risk and handicapped children*. New York: Academic Press.

Hart, B. (1985). Naturalistic language training techniques. In S. Warren & A. Rogers-Warren (Eds.), *Teaching functional language: Generalization and maintenance of language skills*. Baltimore: University Park Press.

Hoyson, F.M., Jamieson, B., & Strain, P.S. (1984). Individualized group instruction of normally developing and autistic-like children: The LEAP curriculum model. *Journal of the Division for Early Childhood, 8*, 157–109.

Kurita, H. (1985). Infantile autism with speech loss before the age of thirty months. *Journal of the American Academy of Child Psychiatry, 24*, 191–196.

Lapidus, D.C. (1985). *Developing communication and language skills in autism*. Unpublished manuscript.

Lenneberg, E. (1967). *Biological foundations of language*. New York: Wiley.

Lovaas, I. (1987). Behavioral treatment and normal educational/intellectual functioning in young autistic children. *Journal of Clinical and Consulting Psychology, 55*(1), 3–9.

Lucas, E. (1980). *Semantic and pragmatic language disorders: Assessment and remediation*. Rockville, MD: Aspen Publishers.

Lund, R.D. (1978). *Development and plasticity of the brain: An introduction*. New York: Oxford University Press.

MacDonald, J.D. (1985). Language through conversation: A model for intervention with language-delayed persons. In S. Warren & A. Rogers-Warren (Eds.), *Teaching functional language: Generalization and maintenance of language skills*. Baltimore: University Park Press.

McCune-Nicolich, L. (1981). Toward symbolic functioning: Structure of early pretend games and potential parallels with language. *Child Development, 52*, 785–797.

McLean, J., & Snyder-McLean, L. (Eds.) (1984). Strategies of facilitating language development in clinics, schools, and homes. *Seminars in Speech and Language, 5*(3), 159–266.

McLean, J., Snyder-McLean, L., Jacobs, P., & Rowland, C.M. (1981). *Process oriented educational programming for the severely-profoundly handicapped adolescent*. Parsons: University of Kansas, Bureau of Research.

Miller, J., Chapman, R., Branston, M., & Reichle, J. (1980). Language comprehension in sensorimotor stages V and VI. *Journal of Speech and Hearing Research, 23*, 284–311.

National Center for Clinical Infant Programs. (1985). *Equals in this partnership: Parents of disabled and at-risk infants and toddlers speak to professionals*. Washington, DC: National Maternal and Child Health Clearinghouse.

Ornitz, E., Guthrie, D., & Farley, A. (1977). The early development of autistic children. *Journal of Autism and Childhood Schizophrenia, 7*, 207–229.

Peck, C., & Schuler, A. (1987). Assessment of social/communicative behavior for students with autism and severe handicaps: The importance of asking the right question. In T. Layton (Ed.), *Language and treatment of autistic and developmentally disordered children*. Springfield, IL: Charles C Thomas.

Piaget, J. (1954). *The construction of reality in the child*. New York: Basic Books.

Prizant, B. (1982). Part II. Speech–language pathologists and autistic children: What is our role? *ASHA, 24*, 531–537.

Prizant, B. (1983). Echolalia in autism: Assessment and intervention. *Seminars in Speech and Language, 4*(1), 63–78.

Prizant, B., & Rydell, P. (1984). An analysis of the functions of delayed echolalia in autistic children. *Journal of Speech and Hearing Disorders, 27*, 183–192.

Prizant, B., & Schuler, A. (1987a). Facilitating communication: Theoretical foundations. In D. Cohen & A. Donnellan (Eds.), *Handbook of Autism and Pervasive Developmental Disorders*. New York: Wiley.

Prizant, B., & Schuler, A. (1987b). Facilitating communication: Language approaches. In D. Cohen & A. Donnellan (Eds.), *Handbook of Autism and Pervasive Developmental Disorders*. New York: Wiley.

Prizant, B., & Wetherby, A. (1987). Communicative intent: A framework for understanding social–communicative behavior in autism. *Journal of the American Academy of Child Psychiatry, 26*, 472–479.

Prizant, B., & Wetherby, A. (in press). Enhancing language and communication in autism: From theory to practice. In G. Dawson (Ed.), *Autism: New perspectives on diagnosis, nature, and treatment*. New York: Guilford Press.

Rossetti, L. (1986). *High-risk infants: Identification, assessment, and intervention*. San Diego: College-Hill Press.

Rutledge, L.T. (1976). Synaptogenesis: Effects of synaptic use. In M.R. Rosenzweig & E.L. Bennett (Eds.), *Neural mechanisms of learning and memory.* Cambridge, MA: The M.I.T. Press.

Sameroff, A., & Chandler, M. (1975). Reproductive risk and the continuum of caretaking causality. In F. Horowitz, M. Hetherington, F. Scarr-Salapatek, & G. Siegel (Eds.), *Review of child development research* (Vol. 4). Chicago: University of Chicago Press.

Schapiro, S., & Vulkovich, K.R. (1970). Early experience effects upon cortical dendrites: A proposed model for development. *Science, 167,* 292–294.

Schopler, E., & Mesibov, G. (Eds.) (1987). *Neurobiological issues in autism.* New York: Plenum Press.

Schuler, A., & Prizant, B. (1985). Echolalia in autism. In E. Schopler & G. Mesibov (Eds.), *Communication problems in autism.* New York: Plenum Press.

Schuler, A., & Prizant, B. (1987). Facilitating communication: Pre-language approaches. In D. Cohen & A. Donnellan (Eds.), *Handbook of autism and pervasive developmental disorders.* New York: Wiley.

Sigman, M., & Ungerer, J. (1984). Cognitive and language skills in autistic, mentally retarded and normal children. *Developmental Psychology, 20,* 293–302.

Simeonsson, R.J., Olley, J.G., & Rosenthal, S.L. (1987). Early intervention for children with autism. In M. Guralnick & F. Bennett (Eds.), *The effectiveness of early intervention for at-risk and handicapped children.* New York: Academic Press.

Smith, M. (1985). Managing the aggressive and self-injurious behavior of adults disabled by autism. *Journal of the Association for Persons with Severe Handicaps, 4,* 228–232.

Stern, D. (1977). *The first relationship: Infant and mother.* Cambridge, MA: Harvard University Press.

Uzgiris, I., & Hunt, J. (1975). *Assessment in infancy: Ordinal scales of psychological development.* Champaign: University of Illinois Press.

Wetherby, A. (1985). Speech and language disorders in children—An overview. In J. Darby (Ed.), *Speech and language evaluation in neurology: Childhood disorders.* Orlando, FL: Grune & Stratton.

Wetherby, A (1986). Ontogeny of communicative functions in autism. *Journal of Autism and Developmental Disorders, 16,* 295–316.

Wetherby, A., Cain, D., Yonclas, D., & Walker, V. (in press). Analysis of intentional communication of normal children from the prelinguistic to the multi-word stage. *Journal of Speech and Hearing Research.*

Wetherby, A., & Prizant, B. (in press). The expression of communicative intent: Assessment guidelines. *Seminars in Speech and Language.*

Wetherby, A., & Prutting, C. (1984). Profiles of communicative and cognitive–social abilities in autistic children. *Journal of Speech and Hearing Research, 27,* 364–377.

# "Verb-alizing": Facilitating action word usage in young language-impaired children

**Kathy L. Chapman, PhD**
Assistant Professor

**Brenda Y. Terrell, PhD**
Assistant Professor
Department of Communication Sciences
Case Western Reserve University
Cleveland, Ohio

OVER THE PAST decade, much new information has been gained about the lexical development of normal children (e.g., Benedict, 1979; Chapman, Leonard, & Mervis, 1986; Gentner, 1978; Leonard, Schwartz, Chapman, & Morris, 1981; Schwartz & Leonard, 1982). Recently, the lexical acquisition of children with specific language disorders has also been the focus of attention (e.g., Leonard, Camarata, Rowan, & Chapman, 1982a; Leonard, Schwartz, Chapman, Rowan, Prelock, Terrell, Weiss, & Messick, 1982b; Schwartz, Leonard, Messick, & Chapman, 1987. Together, these two bodies of research show that early lexicons are composed of both object and action words. This consideration would appear to be important in facilitating lexical acquisition in language-impaired children. Both types of words should be trained. However, while clinicians rountinely train object words, less attention has been given to the training of action words. Guidelines

*Top Lang Disord*, 1988, 8(2), 1–13
© 1988 Aspen Publishers, Inc.

are needed for the incorporation of action words into early lexical training. Early development of action words will be explored here, along with a strong rationale and basis for the choice of action forms to include in an early lexicon. Strategies that seem appropriate for facilitating action word development are then proposed.

## EARLY DEVELOPMENT OF ACTION WORDS

During the single-word-utterance period, although object words predominate, children also acquire a number of other word types (Benedict, 1979; Nelson, 1973; Rescorla, 1976). Among these types are action words and action-related words. Action words are terms that eventually become true verbs. Action-related words are words that are not categorized as verbs in an adult lexicon but are used by children during the single-word period to accompany actions. Examples include *in*, used to accompany putting one object inside another; *off*, used to describe separation of objects; and *there*, used to accompany placement of an object in some location. Because the earliest action terms used by children are often not adult verbs, "action-related" seems a more appropriate nomenclature for this lexical category.

The first category of action-related words encoded in the single-word-utterance period is *protoverbs* (e.g., *up, in, off*) (Barrett, 1983; Clark, 1979). These are productions that children use in verblike contexts. Consistent with other protoforms, these productions do not have all the characteristics of pure verbs. They are transitional lexical phenomena that are often used to express "the state of something or the outcome of an action" (Clark, 1979, p. 153). Furthermore, their usage is often "highly ritualistic" and strongly tied to the accompanying action scheme (Barrett, 1983, p. 199). Examples of protoverbs found in the early vocabularies of normal children include *up, down, off* (Clark, 1979); *no, on-here, inside, there* (Barrett, 1983); and *get-down, bye-bye, nite-nite,* and *out* (Benedict, 1979).

Following the appearance of protoverbs, several other categories of action-related words appear. These include general-purpose words (e.g., *do*), deictic words (e.g., *see*), object-related action-specific words (e.g., *drink*, Clark, 1979), and intransitive action-specific words (e.g., *run*, Huttenlocher, Smiley, & Charney, 1983). General-purpose action-related words are a category of words that do not define a specific action. The meaning of words in this group can be determined only by reference to the context. For example, *do it* (e.g., as the mother is putting on the child's coat) can be understood only with respect to actions that are ongoing or appropriate to the context in which the phrase is produced. Action-related deictic words are words used for calling attention to something. Such use of these words is much like the use of *here* in similar contexts. For example, a child might say *see* to call his mother's attention to some object or event he has noticed.

A child's use of *push*, while moving a toy car across the floor, is an example of the category of object-related action-specific words. The words in this category have precise meanings; they can be used only in reference to a specific action or set of actions. Also, all the actions in this category are actions that are performed on objects. The word *push* in this context means using some body part to move an object away from the body. Were the child not encoding this specific action, some other lexical item would have been chosen. Similarly, intransitive action-specific words have precise meanings. However, these actions are not object related. An example would be the child's production of *walk* to describe the action he was making a doll perform.

It is unclear whether object-related action-specific or intransitive action-specific terms are more easily acquired during the single-word period. If relational complexity influences the ease of acquisition (Gentner, 1982), intransitive action-specific terms should be easier to learn. However, an examination of the action-related words present in young normally developing children's early lexicons suggests that more object-related action-specific terms are acquired (Barrett, 1983; Benedict, 1979; Braunwald, 1978; Goldin-Meadow, Seligman, & Gelman, 1976; Gruendel, 1977). A listing of action-related words acquired by normally developing children during the single-word and early two-word utterance period appears as Appendix.

In addition to the developmental ordering of these action-related categories, changes occur in the range of extension and use of action-related terms. Children first produce action words to describe their own actions as opposed to actions that they observe being performed by others (Barrett, 1983; Bowerman, 1976; Greenfield & Smith, 1976; Huttenlocher, Smiley, & Charney, 1983; Leonard, 1976; Nelson & Lucariello, 1983).

Barrett (1983) has suggested that children's early action word usage is underextended in application. Initially, extension is limited to performative usage. That is, children use their earliest action-related words to specify particular action schemes (the actions performed together with the objects and actors involved) for actions performed exclusively by the child (Barrett, 1983). An example is when a child says *off* only while undressing. Such performative use of action-related words in many cases may overlap with the child's use of protoverbs.

In the next stage of development of action-related terms, even though usage remains primarily nonreferential, generalization and elaboration of meaning occur. During this stage the child's meaning of the term may be generalized to include other actors or objects affected by the action. Further elaboration of the action leads to a more appropriate range of extension for the action concept. During the third stage, decontextualization occurs, and the word is used referentially (e.g., *off* used appropriately to describe any separation of objects).

Children's acquisition of action concepts, like object concepts, can best be explained in terms of a prototype model of category structure. Within a prototype model, category membership is internally structured in terms of a "core" or prototype that represents the clearest or best example of a concept (Rosch, 1973, 1975; Rosch, Mervis, Gray, Johnson, & Boyes-Braem, 1976). Each exemplar to which the term is extended generally has some characteristic in common with the proto-

typical exemplar. Bowerman (1978) provides a clear illustration of an action concept structured and extended in terms of a
prototype. The prototypical action for her
daughter's use of *kick* was "kicking a ball
with the foot so that it propelled forward"
(p. 274). Other examples to which she
extended the term all contained one or
more of the critical features of the prototype: waving limb, sudden sharp contact,
and object propelled. Examples of these
extensions were kicking a floor fan with
her foot, a picture of a kitten with a ball
near its paw, and, in a television cartoon, a
row of turtles doing the cancan. Understanding the course of development of
action-related words can serve as a basis
for selecting specific words to incorporate
into early lexical training.

## STRUCTURING THE ACTION LEXICON

Regardless of the type of word being
trained, there are some general considerations in choosing those words for early
lexical training. Holland (1975) and
Lahey and Bloom (1977) have provided
guidelines for the content and context of
early lexical training. Both emphasized
that training should extend beyond simple
referential meanings. In addition, they
stressed that the lexical items chosen for
training should be communicatively useful and have the potential for being combined with other words. Lahey and Bloom
also suggested that training should focus
on items that can serve a number of
communicative functions (e.g., request,
comment on action, comment on object)
and that can be used in reference to a
variety of actions and objects.

In addition, choosing action words for
training requires consideration of the
child's developmental level with regard to
action word usage. The child's present
level of usage will determine the form of
the action-related terms chosen. For the
child who demonstrates no previous use of
action-related terms, protoverbs would
appear to be the appropriate form for
training. For a child further along in the
sequence, general-purpose or object-
related action-specific terms should be

---

*For the child who demonstrates no
previous use of action-related terms,
protoverbs would appear to be the
appropriate form for training.*

---

targeted. When choosing a specific word
within a category (protoverbs, general-
purpose terms, etc.), priority might be
given to lexical items that occur more
frequently in the speech of normally
developing children (see Appendix), together with actions with the greatest
potential of occurring, given the child's
environment.

A final consideration in choosing words
to be included in the training lexicon is
phonological characteristics (Fey, 1986;
Leonard & Fey, 1979; Leonard et al.,
1982b). During the single-word-utterance
period, children have been observed to
select or avoid certain productions based
on the phonological form of the word
(Ferguson, Peizer, & Weeks, 1973; Mack-
en, 1976; Menn, 1971). The selection and
avoidance criteria are child-specific, depending on the child's own production
system. For instance, Menn (1971)

described a child who preferred to produce words containing initial velar consonants. Other investigators have described children whose early lexicons contained primarily words with initial-position fricatives (Ferguson & Farwell, 1975). In addition to such constraints, some children restrict the words attempted on the basis of syllable shape (e.g., CVCV words only, Ingram, 1974). Finally, some children use both sound and syllable-shape constraints. Ferguson, Peizer, and Weeks (1973) studied a child who produced only CVCV words with /i/ as the final vowel. Lexical training studies of normal and language impaired children functioning at the single-word stage have shown that children are more likely to acquire words and syllable shapes that are within their phonological repertoire (Leonard et al., 1982b). Therefore, a careful examination of the child's phonological system is necessary. Words chosen for training should be consistent with the constraints of the child's developing system.

## FACILITATING THE USE OF ACTION-RELATED TERMS

A number of language intervention techniques might be useful for lexical training with young language-impaired children (see Fey, 1986; Leonard, 1981, for a review). Focused stimulation is among the techniques that might be used in the context of event structuring to facilitate action-word usage in language-impaired children.

Basic to this approach is the modeling of numerous communicative uses of the target language form. Examples may be provided within the context of a story or as the accompaniment of ongoing actions in the therapy environment. Focused stimulation requires the clinician to structure the environment so that use of the target is obligatory. In one adaptation of focused stimulation, the child may be prompted to produce the target after having been shown several examples (Leonard, 1981). For example, after several pairings of the target with the action, the clinician can use a question (e.g., *What are you doing?*) to prompt the child's production. Whereas use of the prompt does not obligate the child to respond, it does provide a pragmatically appropriate context for the child's use of the target. This may represent an appropriate and often necessary intervention step for some children. However, prompts should always appear as a natural part of the communication and should not be used simply to elicit imitations.

As a procedure for training action-related words, focused stimulation has appeal for a number of reasons. First, the effectiveness of focused stimulation has been demonstrated with a broad spectrum of language-impaired children (e.g., Culatta & Horn, 1981, 1982; Leonard et al., 1982b; Schwartz & Leonard, 1982). Culatta and Horn (1981) trained mothers of young hearing-impaired children, age 18 to 26 months, to use focused stimulation to train lexical items. The mothers produced the target words (e.g., *open*) to accompany ongoing actions (e.g., opening a variety of boxes, doors, and drawers), and presented repeated exposures several times a day in naturally occurring situations, as well as planned, nonnatural contexts. Leonard et al. (1982b) used a focused stimulation approach with specific language-impaired and normal children to train intransitive action-specific verbs (e.g., *dip, bow, spin*), as well as object words. In training the verbs, an experimenter produced an action word while manipulating a doll to perform the associated action (e.g., *Watch the baby bow*). These exposures occurred in a play context. During each training session, the exposures (i.e., action word + doll performance) were repeated five times.

Second, focused stimulation is useful for training a variety of levels of action terms. For example, Leonard et al. (1982b) used focused stimulation to train intransitive action-specific terms. Culatta and Horn (1981) have illustrated the use of focused stimulation to train protoverbs.

Third, focused stimulation can be used to facilitate both lexical comprehension and production. Culatta and Horn (1981) and Leonard et al. (1982b) clearly illustrated its effectiveness in facilitating productive use of training targets. Fey (1986) sees focused stimulation as particularly important for facilitating comprehension. For children with limited receptive knowledge of action concepts, focused stimulation can be used to facilitate comprehension. Leonard et al. (1982b) assessed both comprehension and production of the training targets. As a result of focused stimulation, gains in comprehension were also evidenced.

Finally, focused stimulation as a procedure for training action words has appeal because of its flexibility. Because it does not require rigid adherence to a specific protocol, it is adaptable for use by any number of people who interact with the children in their normal environment. In training lexical items for actions that occur

naturally and frequently in the environment, focused stimulation requires little more from the clinician than careful observation and the provision of model utterances. When training less commonly occurring targets, the procedures require only that activities be organized to elicit the action, or that usual activities are modified to prompt the target action. Focused stimulation is flexible as it can be continued as a training procedure beyond the stage of early lexical acquisition. Thus the child is not required to become familiar with a completely new set of rules once lexical training stops being a major focus.

A focused stimulation approach can be adapted to train each of the action-related categories described earlier. The Culatta and Horn (1981) procedure is an illustration of focused stimulation used to train protoverbs. (See previous example.) Focused stimulation to facilitate protoverb usage would be appropriate for children who show no evidence of using action words. The specific protoverb to train would be chosen on the basis of the factors delineated earlier: communicative usefulness, potential for being combined, normal developmental ordering, phonological considerations, frequency of occurrence in lexicons of normally developing children, and potential of occurrence in the child's environment.

For example, for a child whose phonological repertoire includes VC syllables with nasals, and who habitually climbs in and out of boxes, puts objects in boxes and dumps them out, *in* would be an appropriate word to train. In addition to being at the appropriate developmental level for a child who exhibits no action word usage, *in* has been observed in the early lexicons of young normally developing children (Barrett, 1983; Gruendel, 1977). Because this child performs many *in* activities, it seems appropriate to train *in* as a first extension of an action-related term. This lexical item also meets the criterion of communicative usefulness because it can be used in a variety of ways, such as to describe the child's ongoing action, to request another to perform an action, and to protest the performance of an action that is oppositional to *in*. With regard to combinations, *in* can be used with nouns (*in* + noun or noun + *in*) to perform the same communicative functions as the single word productions.

Focused stimulation might also be used to train general-purpose action-related words. During play with a variety of age-appropriate toys, the clinician can use a general-purpose action-related word to describe the child's actions as well as the actions of other participants in the play activity. For example, as the child builds a tower with blocks, rolls a ball, moves cars across the floor, or dresses a doll, the clinician says *do it*. The clinician would also use this term in reference to his or her own actions, such as helping the child build, putting toys on the shelf or rolling the ball to the child. Obviously, the various actions encoded by *do it* are all quite different. Such variety is illustrative of the nature of general-purpose action-related words, whose meaning is determined by the context of their use.

Use of focused stimulation to train higher-level action words (i.e., object-related action-specific and intransitive action-specific terms) calls for additional considerations. First, the actions must be trained using a variety of actors and with a variety of appropriate objects (for object-related actions). Second, because action concepts, like object concepts, appear to be structured around a prototypical exemplar (Bowerman, 1978), the initial training examples should include all the features of the prototype. Further extension to less prototypical, but still appropriate exemplars also should be undertaken.

In choosing questions or other prompts at any level of training, it is important to consider the variable of informativeness (Greenfield & Smith, 1976). The principle of informativeness suggests that in communication, children encode the aspects of events that are the most informative

---

*The principle of informativeness suggests that in communication, children encode the aspects of events that are the most informative.*

---

(Fey, 1986). Failure to consider informativeness leads to highly stilted, formulaic, unnatural clinician–child interactions. To illustrate, consider an activity to train a general-purpose term. If during the activity the child does not produce the action word spontaneously, the clinician could attempt to elicit the target (*do it*) by using a prompt. In response to the prompt *What do you want to do?* the child's use of the general-purpose term *do it* may be unnatural and unnecessary. In such a case, *that*, possibly accompanied by a pointing gesture, would be an appropriate and informative response. Alternatively, the target action term *do it* is more informative and pragmatically appropriate as a response to the prompt *What?* (M.E. Fey, personal communication, 1987). Because the former prompt presupposes an action context, the child's recoding of the action would be redundant. In contrast, the neutral query *What?* does not presuppose the action, and it is therefore more likely to elicit an action word.

A particularly potent context for facilitating action-related word usage involves the use of scripts. Scripts are "ordered sequences of actions appropriate to a particular spatial–temporal context and organized around a goal. Scripts specify the actors, actions and props used to carry out those goals within specified circumstances" (Nelson, 1986, p. 13). Scripts, then, are mental representations of events. The relational nature of action words makes it necessary, when training these words, to represent the action involved, the agent of the action, as well as any objects that may be affected by the action. Scripted-event structures present all of these components in a pragmatically appropriate context.

Constable (1986) has outlined some factors that may contribute to the successful application of scripted formats in language intervention. First, because the scripted events are organized and familiar, the child need not focus on extralinguistic components of the event, but rather on language use. Secondly, repetition and recurrence of the events over time help the child make appropriate associations between the language produced and the events encoded.

In using scripts as a context for training action-related words, the script should be constructed so that primary emphasis is on the actions within the event structure rather than on the actors or props. A diagram of a script for making muffins is provided in Figure 1. At the extreme left of the diagram are all the "acts" involved in making muffins. The acts are arranged in the diagram in sequential order. Subscripts for each of these acts can be developed that further delineate specific actions involved in the scripted event. For example, the diagram shows that the third general act, "mix the ingredients," is further subscripted into six sequentially ordered actions. These actions in turn can be subscripted into finer detail. The actions encoded for the script are determined by the developmental form of the action-related words being trained. In the script of Figure 1, training of *in* as a protoverb is a possible focus. For this training, *in* can be encoded at several different levels of the script. At each point where it is encoded, the protoverb should be used to accompany a consistent and highly similar set of movements. For general-purpose action word training, however, the movements associated with the term need not be highly similar, and may even differ in structure.

The script approach assumes that the child has a high degree of familiarity with the scripted event. Therefore, the actions involved and the temporal ordering of the actions are known and familiar, so that using a general-purpose word at a specific point in the event would be understood as coding the temporally appropriate action. For example, should the clinician say *do it* after putting in the mix and putting in the egg, this action-related term would refer to putting in the water, the next action in the sequence.

Within the event structure, the clinician

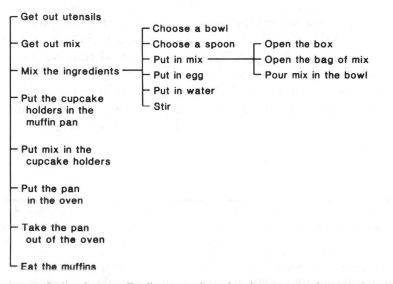

Figure 1. Components of a "making muffins" script. Adapted with permission from Neslon, K. (1982). The syntagmatics and paradigmatics of conceptual development. In S. Kuczaj II (Ed.), *Language Development* (pp. 335–365.). Hillsdale, NJ: Erlbaum.

can prompt the child's production of action words by asking *What's next?* The child may then respond with the appropriate term. What is appropriate depends on the level of action word being trained (e.g., *in* [protoverb], *do it* [general purpose] *stir* [intransitive action-specific]). The event script can be modified and elaborated to include various actors or objects to be acted on. Such adaptability is particularly important when training intransitive action-specific or object-related action-specific words.

•   •   •

These guidelines were not prepared with any specific group of language-impaired children in mind. Language-impaired children may exhibit deficits in one or all components of language. This paradigm is especially useful, however, with children for whom it has been determined that lexical acquisition is an appro-

priate target; with modifications, it should be applicable to a broad range of language-impaired children. Training for any particular child may not require progression through the full developmental sequence (i.e., beginning with protoverbs). As with any training procedure, training should begin at a level appropriate to the child's current level of functioning. For example, if working with a 3- or 4-year-old child whose cognitive skills are within normal limits, whose receptive skills appear better than expressive abilities, and who currently uses protoverbs and/or general-purpose terms, a clinician might appropriately target the child's use of action-specific verbs to encode action.

In training action-related words for children with severe handicaps, it may not be necessary for the child to actually perform the actions to be trained. Instead, the child's comprehension of the action word should be assessed. In the event that the child does not demonstrate comprehension of the action-related term, focused stimulation could be used to facilitate acquisition of the action concept. For these children, it also seems reasonable to include more action-specific terms (e.g., *drink*) during early stages of training. This adaptation ensures a maximal communicative effect with minimal communicative effort. Including action-related words in the initial training lexicons of all language-impaired children increases the communicative precision of single-word speech and may facilitate transition to later stages of language.

## REFERENCES

Barrett, M.D. (1983). The early acquisition and development of the meanings of action-related words. In T.B. Seiler & W. Wannenmacher (Eds.), *Concept development and the development of word meaning* (pp. 191–209). Berlin, Germany: Springer-Verlag.

Benedict, H. (1979). Early lexical development: Comprehension and production. *Journal of Child Language, 6,* 183–199.

Bowerman, M. (1976). Semantic factors in the acquisition of rules for word use and sentence construction. In D. Morehead & P. Morehead (Eds.), *Normal and deficient child language* (pp. 99–179). Baltimore, MD: University Park Press.

Bowerman, M. (1978). The acquisition of word meaning: An investigation into some current conflicts. In N. Waterson & C. Snow (Eds.), *The development of communication* (pp. 263–287). New York: Wiley.

Braunwald, S. (1978). Context, word and meaning: Toward a communicational analysis of lexical acquisition. In A. Lock (Ed.), *Action, gesture and symbol* (pp. 486–525). New York: Academic Press.

Chapman, K., Leonard, L.B., & Mervis, C.B. (1986). The effects of feedback on young children's inappropriate word usage. *Journal of Child Language, 13,* 101–117.

Clark, E.V. (1979). Building a vocabulary: Words for objects, actions, and relations. In P. Fletcher and M. Garman (Eds.), *Language acquisition: Studies in first language development* (pp. 149–161). Cambridge: Cambridge University Press.

Constable, C.M. (1986). The application of scripts in the organization of language intervention contexts. In K. Nelson (Ed.), *First knowledge: Structure and function in development* (pp. 97–121). Hillsdale, NJ: Erlbaum.

Culatta, B, & Horn, D. (1981). Systematic modification of parental input to train language symbols. *Language, Speech and Hearing Services in Schools, 12,* 4–13.

Culatta, B., & Horn, D. (1982). A program for achieving generalization of grammatical rules to spontaneous discourse. *Journal of Speech and Hearing Disorders, 47,* 174–180.

Ferguson, C., & Farwell, C. (1975). Words and sounds in early language acquisition: English initial consonants in the first 50 words. *Language, 51,* 419–439.

Ferguson, C., Peizer, D., & Weeks, T. (1973). Model and replica: Phonological grammar of a child's first words. *Lingua, 31,* 35–65.

Fey, M.E. (1986). *Language intervention with young children.* San Diego: College-Hill.

Gentner, D. (1978). On relational meaning: The acquisition of verb meaning. *Child Development, 48,* 988–998.

Gentner, D. (1982). Why nouns are learned before verbs: Linguistic relativity versus natural partitioning. In S.A. Kuczaj II (Ed.), *Language development* (pp. 301–334). Hillsdale, NJ: Erlbaum.

Goldin-Meadow, S., Seligman, M., & Gelman, R. (1976). Language in the two-year-old. *Cognition, 4,* 189–202.

Greenfield, P., & Smith, J. (1976). *The structure of communication in early language development.* New York: Academic Press.

Gruendel, J. (1977). Referential extension in early language development. *Child Development, 48,* 1567–1576.

Holland, A. (1975). Language therapy for children: Some thoughts on context and content. *Journal of Speech and Hearing Disorders, 40, 183–199.*

Huttenlocher, J., Smiley, P., & Charney, R. (1983). The emergence of action categories in the child: Evidence from verb meanings. *Psychological Review, 90,* 72–93.

Ingram, D. (1974). Phonological rules in young children. *Journal of Child Language 1,* 97–106.

Lahey, M., & Bloom L. (1977). Planning a first lexicon: Which words to teach first. *Journal of Speech and Hearing Disorders, 42,* 340–349.

Leonard, L. (1976). *Meaning in child language.* New York: Grune & Stratton.

Leonard, L.B. (1981). An invited article: Facilitating linguistic skills in children with specific language impairment. *Applied Psycholinguistics, 2,* 89–118.

Leonard, L.B., & Fey, M. (1979). The early lexicons of

normal and language-disordered children: Development and training considerations. In N. Lass (Ed.), *Speech and language advances in basic research and practice.* (pp. 113–147). New York: Academic Press.

Leonard, L.B., Schwartz, R., Chapman, K., & Morris, B. (1981). Factors influencing early lexical acquisition: Lexical orientation and phonological orientation. *Child Development, 52,* 882–887.

Leonard, L.B., Camarata, S., Rowan, L.E., & Chapman, K. (1982a). The communicative functions of lexical usage by language-impaired children. *Applied Psycholinguistics, 3,* 109–125.

Leonard, L.B., Schwartz, R., Chapman, K., Rowan, L., Prelock, P., Terrell, B., Weiss, A., & Messick, C. (1982b). Early lexical acquisition in children with specific language impairment. *Journal of Speech and Hearing Research, 25,* 554–564.

Macken, M. (1976). Permitted complexity in phonological development: One child's acquisition of Spanish consonants. *Papers and Reports on Child Language Development, 11,* 28–60.

Menn, L. (1971). Phonotactic rules in beginning speech. *Lingua, 26,* 225–251.

Nelson, K. (1973). Structure and strategy in learning to talk. *Monographs of the Society for Research in Child Development, 38,* (1–2, Serial No. 149).

Nelson, K. (1982). The syntagmatics and paradigmatics of conceptual development. In S. Kuczaj II (Ed.), Language Development (pp. 335–365). Hillsdale, NJ: Erlbaum.

Nelson, K. (1986). Event knowledge and cognitive. In K. Nelson (Ed.), *Event knowledge: Structure and function in development* (pp. 1–18). Hillsdale, NJ: Erlbaum.

Nelson, K., & Lucariello, J. (1983). The development of meaning in first words. In M.D. Barrett (Ed.), *Children's single-word speech* (pp. 149–181). Chichester, England: Wiley.

Rescorla, L. (1976). *Concept formation in word learning.* Unpublished doctoral dissertation, Yale University, New Haven.

Rosch, E. (1973). On the internal representation of perceptual and semantic categories. In T. Moore (Ed.), *Cognitive development and the acquisition of language* (pp. 111–144). New York: Academic Press.

Rosch, E. (1975). Universals and cultural specifics in human categorization. In R. Brislin, S. Boschner, & W. Lonner (Eds.), *Cross-cultural perspectives in learning.* New York: Halsted Press.

Rosch, E., Mervis, C.B., Gray, W.D., Johnson, D.M., & Boyes-Braem, P. (1976). Basic objects in natural categories. *Cognitive Psychology, 8,* 382–349.

Schwartz, R.G., & Leonard, L.B. (1982). Do children pick and choose? Phonological selection and avoidance in early lexical acquisition. *Journal of Child Language, 9,* 319–336.

Schwartz, R.G., Leonard, L.B., Messick, C.K., & Chapman, K. (1987). The acquisition of object names in children with specific language impairment: Action, context and word extension. *Applied Psycholinguistics, 8,* 233–244.

# Appendix

# Action-related words during the single-word- and early two-word-utterance period

**Barrett (1983)** (two subjects studied longitudinally from 1;4 to 2;6)

| | | | | | |
|---|---|---|---|---|---|
| there | (1)[a] | 1;5[b] | off | (1) | |
| no | (2) | 1;7 | wash | (1) | |
| catch | (1) | 1;7 | dance | (1) | |
| in | (1) | 1;8 | hold | (1) | |
| on | (1) | 1;10 | clap | (1) | |

**Benedict (1979)** (eight subjects studied longitudinally from 0;9 to 1;8)

| | | | |
|---|---|---|---|
| no | (6) | tickle | (2) |
| see | (5) | get | (2) |
| bye-bye | (5) | read | (1) |
| nite-nite | (4) | sit | (1) |
| go | (3) | walk | (1) |
| out | (3) | eat | (1) |
| get-down | (3) | close | (1) |
| rock-rock | (2) | stop-it | (1) |

**Bowerman (1978)** (two subjects studied longitudinally)

| | | | |
|---|---|---|---|
| off | 1;2 | close | 1;3 |
| giddiup | 1;2 | open | 1;5 |
| night-night | 1;3 | kick | 1;5 |

**Braunwald (1978)** (one subject studied longitudinally from 0;8 to 1;8)

| | | | |
|---|---|---|---|
| bye-bye | 0;9 | ring | 1;1 |
| down | 1;0 | swing | 1;2 |
| off | 1;1 | again | 1;2 |
| up | 1;1 | out | 1;3 |

**Goldin-Meadow, Seligman, & Gelman (1976)** (twelve subjects studied longitudinally from 1;2 to 2;2)

| | | | |
|---|---|---|---|
| eat | (7) | kick | (2) |
| open | (7) | stand | (2) |
| close | (6) | fly | (2) |
| sit | (6) | cry | (2) |
| jump | (5) | blow | (1) |
| fall | (5) | hug | (1) |
| wash | (4) | pick-up | (1) |
| kiss | (4) | touch | (1) |
| drink | (3) | push | (1) |
| throw | (3) | pull | (1) |
| run | (3) | lie down | (1) |
| drop | (2) | turn around | (1) |
| shake | (2) | dance | (1) |

*(continues)*

# Appendix (continued)

**Gruendel (1977)** (two subjects studied longitudinally from 1;0 to 1;6)

|  | (in first 1–10 words) |  |  |
|---|---|---|---|
| giggle-giggle | (1) | see | (1) |
| up | (1) |  |  |

|  | (in first 11–50 words) |  |  |
|---|---|---|---|
| go-go or go | (2) | down | (1) |
| tickle-tickle | (1) | off | (1) |
| sing | (1) | on | (1) |
| up | (1) | no | (1) |

|  | (in first 51–100 words) |  |  |
|---|---|---|---|
| night-night | (2) | come | (1) |
| bye-bye | (2) | in | (1) |
| out | (2) | down | (1) |
| wipe | (1) | feed | (1) |
| find | (1) | hide | (1) |
| help | (1) | open | (1) |
| on | (1) | write | (1) |
| count | (1) | wind-up | (1) |

**Messick (personal communication, 1986)** (nine subjects studied longitudinally from 0;11 to 1;3)

| bye-bye | (3) | walk | (1) |
|---|---|---|---|
| see | (2) | bite | (1) |
| down | (2) | open | (1) |
| up | (2) | boo | (1) |
| out | (2) | keep | (1) |
| nite-nite | (2) | roll | (1) |
| peek | (2) | bang-bang | (1) |
| touch | (1) | off | (1) |
| sit | (1) | tick-tock | (1) |
| all done | (1) | meep | (1) |
| go | (1) | bing | (1) |
| catch | (1) | smell | (1) |
| ride | (1) |  |  |

[a]number of subjects using the action-related term
[b]age at which usage was first observed

# Index

## A

Abstract relational concepts, in spatial term
   acquisition, 68
Acquired immunodeficiency syndrome (AIDS), 4
Action lexicon, structuring, 208–209
Action-related words
   early development of, 206–208
   facilitation of usage, 209–214
   performative usage, 207
   during single-word period, 216–217
   in two-word utterance period, 216–217
Adjectives, spatial, 67, 71
Affective signaling, 38
Affricates, 118
   developmental sequence, 117
   lack of, in toddler speech, 115–116
Aggression, 123
Alcohol, maternal consumption, intrauterine
   exposure to, 20
Antibiotics, ototoxic, 24, 25
Apgar scoring system, 23
APR (auropalpebral reflex), 25
Asphyxia, birth, 23, 56–57
Assessment
   of children's ability, 124–126
   of communication disorders with emotional/
     behavioral symptoms, 124–127
   content, for autistic children, 189–193
   influence of context on, 145–146

of spatial term knowledge, 73–75
   strategies, for autism, 193–194
   taxonomies, 141
   for temporally displaced speech, 91–92
At-risk children, 37
   development of, 49–50
   early communication, 38
   efficacy of preventive intervention and, 58–59
   infant service delivery models, 3–4
   preventive intervention, 56
   remedial approach eligibility and, 54
Attunement, 170–172
Audiological evaluation, indications, 26
Auropalpebral reflex (APR), 25
Autism
   assessment
     content of, 189–193
     early approaches, 189–194
     strategies, 193–194
   behavioral approaches, 182, 188
   cognitive-social impairments, 191
   communicative intentions, 139–141
   communicative persistence/repair, 198
   definition of, 183
   diagnosis, early, 183–185
   early identification efforts, refining, 185–186
   education in, language specialist and, 183
   efficacy of interventions, 188
   future goals, 182–183

interventions
    approaches, 194–202
    content, 197–199
    early, as prevention, 186–188
    horizontal communication goals, 197, 199
    for social interaction impairment, 187–188
    strategies, 199–202
    success of, program characteristics for, 188
    vertical communication goals, 197–198, 199
neurologic impairment, 182
neurological development, 187
social interaction impairments, 185, 187–88
symptomatology
    early, identification of, 183–186
    specific, 184

**B**

Babbling, 110
Back consonants, 117, 119
Barrier games, 156–157
Bayley Scales, 31, 32
Behavior
    experience and, 167–172
    problem prevention, in autism, 187
    regulation, communicative intentions during
        infancy and, 43
    sampling, in autism assessment, 193–194
Behavior state communication, 38, 125
Bilirubin, 24
Biological risk factors, 56
Birth asphyxia, 23, 56–57
Box-like stimuli, comprehension of spatial terms, 70
Brain structure, environment and, 186

**C**

Cadmium, prenatal exposure, 20
Caregiver(s)
    child-centered response style, 128
    consistent and contingent responses, 57
    depression, 133
    of developmentally delayed infants, 124
    disengagement, 133
    educational support programs, 134
    intrusive behavior, 127
    language adjustments of, 127
    providing services for, 129–132
    redefinition strategies for, 131
    response strategies, 131
Caregiver-child interactions, 124

assessment, 126–127
disturbances, treatment of, 132–133
during infancy, 42–45
positive experiences, development of, 128–129
shared knowledge about scripted events and, 80
transactional nature of, 40–41
Caregiver-child therapy, for emotional/behavioral
    communication disorders, 133–134
Caregiver-toddler groups, for emotional/behavioral
    communication disorders, 134
CDI. See Communicative Development Inventory
    (CDI)
Center-based approach, for autism, 195–197
Child-oriented intervention, for autism, 200–202
Chromosomal abnormalities, hearing loss and, 17–
    20
CLAMS (Clinical Linguistic and Auditory Milestone
    Scale), 30
Cleft palate, 12
Clinical Linguistic and Auditory Milestone Scale
    (CLAMS), 30
Clinician
    in consultative model, 172–173
    role in JAR procedure, 101
    temporally displaced speech implications
        for assessment, 91–92
        for intervention/training, 92–93
Clubbed foot, 12
Cluster reduction, 115
CMV (congenital cytomegalovirus), 21
Cockayne syndrome, 19
Cognition
    contribution to temporally displaced speech, 82–
        87
    in language acquisition, 81
Cognitive signals, 37–38
Cohen's Kappa, 103
Collaborative consultation
    discipline-specific competencies of speech-
        language pathologist and, 14–15
    interpersonal skills, for speech-language patholo-
        gist, 15
    in service delivery models, 6–14, 60–61
    services, examples of, 11–13
    team members, 16
Communication
    context-dependent nature of, 142
    primary level, classification of, 125
Communication development, 37

in at-risk children, 49–50
in developmentally disabled children, 49–50
mutual/self-regulatory capacities and, 39–40
nonverbal, 38
socioemotional development and, 39–49
stage-specific considerations, 41
  in early childhood, 47–49
  in infancy, 42–45
  in toddlerhood, 45–47
transactional model of, 40–41
Communication disorders, with emotional/behavior
  symptoms. *See* Emotional/behavioral disorders
Communication interactions, speaker knowledge
  and, 158–159
Communicative breakdown repairs, remediation
  strategies, 130–131
Communicative Development Inventory (CDI)
  research, 30–32
  validity, 31
  vs. Language Development Survey, 34
Communicative intentions
  in clinical populations, 139–141
  context and, 145–146, 146
  development, 138
  diversity of use, 139
  elicitation procedures, 142–143
  importance, 138–139
  in infancy, 43
  maintaining joint attentional episodes and, 144
  mode of expression, 140
  opportunities, 142–143
  rate of, 140–141
  situational structure and, 97
  task characteristics and, 142
Communicative interaction, responsivity and, 144–
  145
Communicative persistence/repair, autism and, 198
Communicative signaling
  during infancy, 44–45
  remediation strategies, 130
Compensatory strategies, 59, 166
Comprehension
  assessment, 125
  decoding model of, 152
  development, 158
  event experience and, 161–162
  of irony, 157–158
  of spatial terms, 74
  speaker knowledge and, 157

world-knowledge driven model, 153–154
Concept extension, 69
Conditional/hypothetical language, temporally
  displaced speech and, 88
Congenital anomalies/disorders, 12, 17, 20–21
Consonant(s)
  back, 117, 119
  correct pronunciation, by toddlers, 114
  final, deletion of, 119
  glottal, 119
  initial, widespread deletion of, 119
  inventories, 113
    of toddlers, 117–118
Consonant-vowel syllable (CV syllable), 118–119
Consultative model, 172–173
Context
  for assessment, 12
  influence on assessment, 145–146
  language and, 137
  language learning and, 138
  language sampling and, 96
  linguistic, of world knowledge, 154–155
  linguistic/cognitive skills and, 91–92
  logical ability and, 91
  physical, of world knowledge, 155–157
  sensitivity, of maternal language, 93
  in sentence decoding, 152
  in spatial-term acquisition, 69–70
  variables, 141–142
    communicative use of language and, 142–145
    manipulating, performance and, 145–146
Contrastive stimuli, for spatial-term intervention, 76
Conversational language-sampling measurement, 97
Conversational routines, temporally displaced
  speech and, 88–89
Conversational samples, general accuracy, toddler
  assessment and, 114
Craniofacial development, 17
Craniofacial malformations, 17
Cumulative risk model, 124
CV words, 113
CVCV words, 134, 209
CVCVC words, 113
Cytomegalovirus, congenital, 21

**D**

Data reduction and coding, in language sampling
  procedure, 102–103
Deafness. *See* Hearing loss

Decontextualization, of action-related terms, 207
Deictic words, 155, 206
Delay procedure, in milieu teaching, 175
Denver Developmental Screening Test, 73
Development. *See also specific types of development*
  alterable factors, 55
  instruction and, 92
  normal processes, 37
  unalterable factors, 55
Developmental care
  continuity of, 9–10
  team structure, 4–6
Developmental delays/disorders, 37
  communicative intention usage, 139
  development of, 49–50
  diagnosis, 53–54
Developmental disabilities, mandated services for, 4
Developmental psychopathology, 37
Discipline-specific competencies, of speech-
  language pathologists, 14–15
Displaced events, 80–81
Displaced reference, 79–80, 83
Diuretics, ototoxic, 24–25
Down syndrome
  associated malformations, 18
  communicative intentions, 139–141
  incidence, 18
  preventive intervention, 56, 58–59
  problem-focused therapy, 12
Dramatic play, language learning and, 160

**E**

Early childhood development
  of communication, 47–49
  communication delays/disorders, later disabilities
    and, 52
  of language, 47–49
  of socioemotional functions, 47–49
Early intervention. *See* Intervention, early
Early Intervention Program for Infants and Toddlers
  with Handicaps, 122
Early Language Inventory (ELI), 31. *See also*
  Communicative Development Inventory (CDI)
Early Language Milestone Scale (ELM Scale), 26–
  27, 30
Education of the Handicapped Act Amendments of
  1986. *See* Public Law 99–457
Educational support programs, 134

18q-syndrome, 18
ELM (Early Language Milestone Scale), 26–27, 30
Emotional attachments
  building, 48, 128
  in infancy, 42
Emotional/behavioral disorders, 39, 122–123
  assessment, 37
  assessment considerations, 124–127
  communication disorders and, 39
  redefinition strategies, 131–132
  remediation strategies, 130–131
  risk factors, 123–124
  service delivery options, 133–135
  service provision, 129–132
  transactional intervention, 127–129
Emotional conflict resolution, caregiver language
  for, 127
Emotional development. *See* Socioemotional
  development
Emotional difficulties, 123
Emotional involvement, memory for exact wording
  and, 160
Emotional state, expression, assessment of, 125
Environment
  developmentally shaped, 9
  manipulation, for SLI toddler, 173
  risk factors of, 56
  structuring, for autism intervention, 200
Environmental noise, hearing loss and, 25
Environmental risk factors, 124
Environmental toxins, fetal development and, 20
Environmentally at-risk children, providing services
  for, 132–133
Epstein-Barr virus, 22
Eradication, remediation and, 53
Error patterns
  in atypical phonological development, 119
  in phonological assessment of toddlers, 114–115
Established risk factors, 56
Event context, communicative intents and, 143–144
Event knowledge
  comprehension and, 161–162
  temporal displacement and, 80–83
Event representations, temporally displaced speech
  and, 79–80
Experience
  behavior and, 167–172
  comprehension and, 161–162

Expressive language delay, in toddlers, 29–30
Extensional approach, spatial-term concepts and, 68

**F**

Facial expression, 125
Facilitative therapy, for altered language acquisition, 167–169
Families
  dysfunctional
    interactional disturbances, treatment of, 132–133
    reeducation strategies for, 132
  intervention role of, 4
Family-focused intervention
  defined, 124
  for environmentally at-risk children, 132–133
  goals, 124
Family systems approach, for autism, 195–197
Feature approach, spatial-term concepts and, 68–69
Feeding
  development, 14
  problems, 14
    interventions, 14
Fetal alcohol syndrome, 12
Fetal development, environmental toxins and, 21
Fetal rubella syndrome, 20–21
Final consonants, deletion of, 119
Flexibility
  of focused stimulation, 210
  in language learning interventions, 160–161
Focused stimulation
  for altered language acquisition, 167
  for facilitation of action-related words, 209–211, 214
  informativeness principle and, 211
Free-play situations
  in communications assessment, 126
  context, 82, 141
  of early vs. late word learners, 38
  for language sampling, 99
    procedure, 100–101
    results, 106–107
  misassessment of linguistic ability and, 91
  physical contexts of, 156
  structured, 108
  transactional intervention and, 128
Fricatives, 117, 118
  developmental sequence, 113
  lack of, in toddler speech, 115–116

Front consonants, 117
Frustration, 123

**G**

General-purpose action related words
  early development of, 206, 208
  training
    focused stimulation for, 211
    scripted approach for, 211
General scaffolding techniques, in temporally displaced speech, 88–89
Generalization behaviors, 96
Gestural communicative means, 125
Gestures
  in encoding communicative intent, 140
  during infancy, 43
  intentional nonverbal, 145
Glides, 113, 117, 118
Goldenhar syndrome, 19
Grammar development, in early childhood, 47
Gricean cooperative principle, 137
Group B streptococcus, 22
Growth spurt, 171

**H**

Handicaps, prevention of, 58
Hansen Early Language Parent Program, 134
Hearing impairments, preventive interventions, 55
Hearing loss
  congenital, 17
  environmental noise and, 25
  environmental toxins and, 20
  perinatal infections and, 22–23
  postnatal infections and, 22–23
  in utero fetal infections and, 20–23
Hearing screening, 25–27
Heavy metals, prenatal exposure, 20
Hemorrhage, intracranial, 23–24
Hepatitis B, 22
Here-and-now physical activity, 80
Herpes, 22
HIV (human immunodeficiency virus), 4, 22
Home-based approach, for autism, 195–197
Hospitalization
  developmental routines in, 6–8
  discharge, developmentalist role and, 10
Human immunodeficiency virus (HIV), 4, 22
Hunter syndrome (mucopolysaccharidosis type II), 18

Hurler syndrome (mucopolysaccharidosis type I), 18
Hypothesis testing
    acquisition of spatial terms and, 69
    in autism assessment, 194

## I

Imaginative language, 156
Impulsivity, 123
Inborn errors of metabolism, 18
Incidental teaching, in milieu teaching, 175
Independent analysis, of normal phonological
    development, 112–113, 115–116
Individual Family Service Plan, 127
Individuals with Disabilities Education Act, 4
Induction teaching, 174
    for altered language acquisition, 170–172
    cognitive workload and, 178
    elicited imitation and, 177
    for SLI toddlers, 176–177
Inductive teaching, 174. *See also* Induction teaching
Infant development, 3
    of communication, 42–45
    of language, 42–45
    of socioemotional function, 42–45
Infant-family care continuum, between hospital and
    home/community, 6–8
Infections
    perinatal, 22–23
    postnatal, 22–23
    in utero fetal, 20–22
Informativeness principle, 211
Instruction, development and, 92
Intensional approach, spatial-term concepts and, 68
Inter/psychological learning score, 92
Interactional approach, intelligence quotients and, 178
Interactional disturbances, treatment, 132–133
Interactive capacities. *See* Mutual capacities
Intercoder reliability, 84
Interdisciplinary model, 60–61
Interpersonal skills, for collaborative consultation, 15
Intersubjective relatedness, 44
Intervention. *See also specific intervention
approaches*
    in altering language acquisition, 166–172
    definition of, 165
    determining toddler's need for, 165
    early
        approaches, 53–59
        changing issues in, 3–4

compensatory approaches, 59
    effectiveness, 55
    importance, 52
    preventive approaches, 55–59
    remediation approaches, 53–55
    selection of approach, 59
    team structure, 4–6
    transactional approach, 127–129
efficacy evaluation, 96
focus, 165
goals, 165–166
maturation and, 167
planning, 172
for spatial-term acquisition, 75–77
for specific language impaired toddlers, 164–165
for temporally displaced speech, 92–93
Interview, in autism assessment, 193, 194
Intracranial hemorrhage, 23–24
Intransitive action-specific words
    early development of, 206, 207
    training, focused stimulation and, 210, 211
Irony comprehension, 157–158

## J

JAR. *See* Joint action routine (JAR)
Jaundice, 24
Joint action routine (JAR)
    cognitive workload and, 178
    definition of, 96–97, 175
    for language sampling, 99
    procedure for language sampling, 101–102
    rationale for using, 175–176
    segment from, 102
    for specific language impairment, 177
    for specific language impairments, 107, 174
    variability in children's involvement and, 107
Joint attention
    communicative intentions during infancy and, 42
    maintaining, 144

## K

Kartagener syndrome, 19

## L

Language, emotional bonding and, 48
Language acquisition
    altered, intervention for, 166–172
    cognitive, temporal displaced speech acquisition
        and, 79

delay
  in autism, 186
  in preschool children, 29
  social-interactive, temporally displaced speech
    and, 79, 80
Language acquisition support system (LASS), 80
Language behaviors, changing, 172–179
Language development
  in at-risk children, 49–50
  in developmentally disabled children, 49–50
  emotional factors and, 38
  mutual/self-regulatory capacities and, 39–40
  social factors and, 38
  stage-specific considerations, 41
    in early childhood, 47–49
    in infancy, 42–45
    in toddlerhood, 45–47
  transactional model of, 40–41
Language Development Survey (LDS), 30, 32–34
Language-impaired children
  behavioral disorders and, 29
  communicative intention usage, 139
  familiarity of routines and, 161–162
  normal process model, 177
  pragmatic theory, 155
  psychiatric disorders and, 29
Language learning, world knowledge and, 151–152
Language-measurement task, 96
Language processing
  models, background knowledge and, 153
  theory, world knowledge and, 152
Language sampling, 95–96
  contexts, 96, 146
  data analysis, 103
  data reduction and coding, 102–103
  differences in procedures, 107
  free-play procedure, 100–101
  goal, 96
  pragmatic differences in contexts, 107–108
  predictability, 96, 97
  reliability, 103
  results, 106–108
    group analysis, 103–104
    individual analysis, 104–106
  setting and, 96
  situation and, 96
  situational structure and, 97
  for specific language-impairment, 97–98
  structure and, 96

LASS (language acquisition support system), 80
Late talkers, 111, 120, 139
LDS (Language Development Survey), 30, 32–34
Lead, prenatal exposure, 20
Learned helplessness, 200
Lexicon
  acquisition and usage, 54, 57–58
  action, structuring, 208–209
  comprehension, focused stimulation and, 210
  size, 117–1118
Lexicon-phonology interface, in atypical phonologi-
    cal development, 119–120
Linguistic/cognitive skills, context and, 91–92
Linguistic development, 110
Liquids, 117, 118
  developmental sequence, 113
  deviation of, 115
Listeria, 22
Logical ability, context and, 91

**M**

MacArthur Communicative Development Inventory:
    Toddlers (CDI). *See* Communicative Develop-
    ment Inventory (CDI)
Maintenance therapy, for altered language acquisi-
    tion, 169–170
Maladaptive response strategies, 130
Maltreated children
  affective expressions of, 45
  early communication, 38
  socioemotional development, in early childhood,
    48
Mand-model, in milieu teaching, 175
Matching strategies, 128
Maternal language, context-sensitivity of, 93
Maternal scaffolding, temporally displaced speech
    and, 81, 85–87, 92–93
Mean length of utterance (MLU)
  in CDI: Toddlers, 31
  in normal phonological development, 112
Medical/developmental approach, to developmental
    intervention, 6–8
Medically Fragile Children's Program, 12–14
Medically ill infants, developmental needs of, 7
Melnick-Fraser syndrome, 19
Mercury, prenatal exposure, 20
Milieu teaching, 174–175, 177
Mitigation, 53, 57
Mohr syndrome, 19

Mononucleosis, 22

Mood of reader, narrative processing and, 159–160

Morquio syndrome (mucopolysaccharidosis type IV), 18

Mother-child talk, shared knowledge about scripted events and, 80

Mucopolysaccharidoses, 18

Multidisciplinary model, 60

Multiple synostosis, 19

Mutual capacities
 development during infancy, 43–44
 language, communication and, 39–40

Mutual regulatory skills, 13

Myelomeningocele, 12

**N**

Narrative processing, mood of reader and, 159–160

Nasals, 113, 117, 18

Natural reinforcers, 200

Negative affective states, expression of, 126

Neonatal intensive care unit (NICU), 15

Neural plasticity, 186

Nipple feeding, 14

Nondirective responding, 128

Nonoral feeders, 14

Nonsubstantive contributions, to temporally displaced speech, 85

Normal process model, for language-impaired children, 177

Nouns, as spatial terms, 67

**O**

Object manipulation, in spatial-term knowledge assessment, 74

Object-related action-specific words
 early development of, 206–207, 208
 training, focused stimulation for, 211

Object stimuli, for spatial-term intervention, 76

Observation checklist, in autism assessment, 193, 194

Observation of Communicative Interactions Scale (OCI Scale), 126

Opportunities, for communicative intents, 142–143

Otitis media, in newborn, 22–23

Oto-palato-digital syndrome, 19

Ototoxic drugs, 24–25

Overactivity, 123

**P**

Parent Infant Interaction Scale, 126–127

Parent involvement, in service delivery, 172–173

Parental cuing, 144

Parenting education, 132

Partnership, with child, 128

Peabody Picture Vocabulary Test-Revised (PPVT), 98

Perceived difficulties, 57

Perinatal infections, 22–23

Phoneme-by-phoneme analysis, 114

Phonemes, individual accuracy assessment, 114

Phonetic inventories/repertoires, correct production and, 116

Phonological development
 acquisition patterns, 11
 atypical, 11, 118–120
  error patterns, 119
  lexicon-phonology interface, 119–120
  order of acquisition and, 118–119
  rate of acquisition, 120
 commonalities, 111
 course, 111
 general patterns of, 112
 individual differences, 111, 116–118
 normal
  analyses summary, 115–116
  independent analysis, 112–113, 115–116
  relational analysis, 114–115
  variations in, 116–118
  vowel acquisition and, 116
 rate, 111

Phonological processes, classification of, 115

Phonology, 110

Play. See Free-play situations

Postnatal infections, 2–23

PPVT (Peabody Picture Vocabulary Test-Revised), 98

Pragmatic theory, 155

Pre- and posttherapy comparisons, 179

Preintentional communicative behavior, 43

Prelinguistic development, 110

Premature infants, 7, 23, 41

Prenatal risk factors, 17–20

Prepositions, spatial, 67, 71–73

Prespeech capacity, 14

Presymbolic behavior, autistic children and, 191–193

Pretense activity, in temporally displaced speech, 84
Preventive intervention
  effectiveness, 58
  goals, 57–58
  selection, 59
  service eligibility, 55–56
Primary developmentalist, 5
Problem-focused therapy, 10–14
Production
  correct, phonetic inventories/repertoires and, 116
  focused stimulation and, 210
  limitations, of spatial terms, 74
Prompts, in focused stimulation, 209
Pronunciation, correct, in normal phonological
  development, 114
Proportional change index, 179
Prototype approach, spatial-term concepts and, 69
Protoverbs
  early development of, 206, 208
  training
    focused stimulation for, 210
    scripted approach for, 212
Public Law 99-457, 4
  assessment and, 29–30
  federal funding and, 183
  Individual Family Service Plan, 127
  interdisciplinary approach and, 39
  interdisciplinary model and, 61
  service delivery options and, 172
  speech-language pathologists and, 33, 53, 122
Puppet task, for spatial-term intervention, 77

**Q**

Quantity, 97

**R**

Receptive Expressive Emergent Language Scale, 73
Reciprocity, 125, 128, 191
Redefinition
  strategies, 131–132
  in transactional intervention, 129
Reeducation strategies
  for environmentally at-risk children, 132
  in transactional intervention, 129
Referential communication, 38, 155–156
Referential speech, 142
Relational analysis, of normal phonological
  development, 114–115
Relevant knowledge. *See* World knowledge

Remediation, 53
  effectiveness, 55
  intervention selection, 59
  for skills in functional areas, 54
  strategies, for communication disorder with
    emotional/behavioral symptoms, 130–131
  in transactional intervention, 129
Responding
  nondirective, 128
  sensitively, 128
Responsivity, communicative interaction and, 144–
  145
Reynell Expressive Language Scale, 32
Risk factors, 9, 123
  categories, 56
  in each family situation, 127
Routines, 80
  familiarity with , 161–162
  natural, transactional intervention and, 128
  predictable and consistent, 131
  signalling, transitional objects for, 131–132
  substantive contributions to temporally displaced
    speech and, 85–86
  in temporally displaced speech, 84
Rubella, congenital, 20–21

**S**

SALT (Systematic Analysis of Language Transcript), 102–103
Scaffolding
  general, 88–89
  language acquisition and, 80
  maternal, 81, 85–87, 92–93
Screening
  for hearing loss, 25–27
  pediatric instruments, 30
Scripted context, 81, 82, 83
Scripts. *See also* Joint action routines (JAR);
  Routines
  for facilitating action-related words, 212–213
  situational variables and, 144
Self-directed behavior, 44, 130
Self-efficacy, 48
Self-esteem, 48
Self-image, 48
Self-regulatory capacities
  development during infancy, 43–44
  language, communication and, 39–40
Semantic development, in early childhood, 47

Semantic devices, 92
Semantic relations, for language sampling technique, 97, 99–100
Sentence decoding, 153
Sequenced Inventory of Communication Development (SICD), 98
Service delivery
  collaborative approaches, 6–14
  developmental care continuum and, 9–10
  developmentally shaped environment and, 9
  models, 60–61
    for at-risk infants, 3–4
    collaborative, 60–61
    independent, 60
  options
    for emotional/behavioral disorders, 133–135
    employment of different teaching strategies and, 178–179
    for specific language impaired toddlers, 172–174
  problem-focused therapy and, 10–14
Setting, language sampling and, 96
Shared knowledge, temporal displaced speech and, 82–83
SICK (Sequenced Inventory of Communication Development), 98
Single-word utterance period, action-related words and, 206, 208, 216–217
Situational variables, scripts and, 144
SLI. See Specific language impairment (SLI)
Small-for-gestational age infants, 23
Social-action games, adult structure and, 143–144
Social-affective functioning, assessment, 125
Social-communicative functioning, assessment, 126
Social context. See Context
Social-effective exchange, 127
Social interaction
  communicative intentions during infancy and, 43
  contribution, in temporally displaced speech, 85–87
  temporally displaced speech and, 80
Socially unacceptable behavior, 130
Socioemotional development
  achievements, 44, 46
  in at-risk children, 49–50
  communication development and, 39–49
  definition of. 36–37
  in developmentally disabled children, 49–50
  stage-specific considerations, 41
    in early childhood, 47–49

in infancy, 42–45
  in toddlerhood, 45–47
Spatial-term acquisition, 67–68
  assessment, 73–75
    context and, 74
    developmental order, 74–75
    of front/back orientation, 74
  conceptual knowledge, 67
  contextual influences, 68, 69–70
  developmental order, 70–73, 76
  developmental progression, 69–73
  interventions, 75–77
    developmental order and, 76
    training stimuli for, 76–77
  relationships of terms, 67–68
  theoretical background, 68–69
  types of terms, 67
Speaker knowledge, 157–159
Specific activity, in temporally displaced speech, 83–84
Specific language impairments (SLI), 106–107
  clinical decision making, 179–180
  communicative intentions, 139
  indirect treatment, 173–174
  interventions, 164–165
    benefits, 180
    effectiveness, measurement of, 179–180
    goals, 165–166
    purpose, 173
    teaching strategies and, 177–179
  language sampling technique comparison, 97–98
    procedures, 98–100
    subjects, 98
  lexical acquisition, 205–206
  rate of communicative intentions, 140–141
  service delivery options, 172–174
  teaching strategies, 174–179
Speech-language pathologists (SLPs), 5–6, 97
  delivery of communication-based services, 53
  integrative approach and, 38–39
  Public Law 99-457 and, 33, 53, 122
  in reeducation process, 132
  role in caregiver-child therapy, 134–135
  specialized competencies, 14–15
  in treatment of interactional disturbances, 132–133
Standardized assessment procedures, 95
Stanford-Binet Test of Intelligence-Fourth Edition, 98

Stimuli
box-like, for comprehension of spatial terms, 70
contrastive, for spatial-term intervention, 76
object, for spatial-term intervention, 76
pairs, in inductive teaching, 176
for spatial-term intervention, 76–77
Stops, 113, 117, 118
Stressors, of families with preschoolers, 130
Stridency deletion, 115, 116
Structured teaching, for minimum verbal skills, 178
Subscripts, 212
Substantive contributions, to temporally displaced
speech, 85
6-Sulfo-N-acetylhexosominide sulfatase, 18
Swallowing problems, 14–15
Syllables, 113
Symbolic behavior, autistic children and, 191–193
Syntactic devices, 92
Syphilis, 21–22
Systematic Analysis of Language Transcript
(SALT), 102–103

**T**

Target behaviors
intervention goals and, 166
performance differences, 96
for SLI toddler, 173–174
treatment strategies and, 178
Task characteristics, communicative use of language
and, 142
Teaching strategies, for specific language impaired
toddlers, 174–177
Team membership, 61
Team structure, two-tiered, 4–6
Temporal language, temporally displaced speech
and, 87–88
Temporally displaced speech, 79
analysis
procedure, 81–82
results/discussion, 82–93
subjects, 81
child contributions, 85–87, 90
conditional/hypothetical language and, 88
conversational routines and, 88–89
definition, 82
event representations and, 79–80
general scaffolding techniques, 88–89
implications for clinician, assessment and, 91–92

knowledge base in, 83–84
maternal contributions, 87
situational variation, 83
social-interactive contribution, 85–87
temporal language and, 87–88
time-frame of episodes, 84–85
WH-questions and, 87, 89–90
Teratogens, environmental exposure, 4
Therapy stimuli or targets, as world knowledge, 154
Time-displaced talk, 161–162
Toddlers
communication development, 45–47
language-delayed
identification of, 29–30
multistep screening for, 33–34
language development, 45–47
phonological development, subjects, 111
socioemotional development, 45–47
Toxoplasmosis, 21
Transactional development model, 40–41
Transactional intervention
principles, 127–129
strategies, 129
Transactional risk factors, 123–124
Transdisciplinary model, 60
Treacher-Collins syndrome, 19
Trisomy 21. *See* Down syndrome
Turner syndrome (XO syndrome), 18
Turntaking, reciprocal, 128
Two-word utterance period, action-related words,
216–217

**U**

University of New Mexico, Developmental Care
clinical team, 4–6

**V**

Velo-cardio-facial syndrome, 19
Verbal activity, in temporally displaced speech, 83
Verbal communication, 125
Videotaping
of caregiver-child therapy, 134
of educational support programs, 134
Vocabulary
CDI: Toddlers assessment, 31
development, 46, 116
recognition-format checklist, 30
size, 110

Vocalizations, 145
Vowel acquisition, in normal phonological develop-
    ment, 116
Vowel errors, numerous, 119

## W

Waardenburg syndromes, type I and II, 19
Wh-questions, in temporally displaced speech
    episodes, 87, 89–90
Within-child risk factors, 123
Words
    action-related. *See* Action-related words
    CV, 113
    CVCV, 113, 209
    CVCVC, 113
    deictic, 155, 206

possible meanings of, 153
    word history and, 162
World knowledge
    comprehension and, 152–154
    definition of, 151–152
    goals and level of involvement, 159–161
    knowledge of speaker, 157–159
    language processing theory and, 152
    linguistic context, 154–155
    physical context, 155–157

## X

XO syndrome (Turner syndrome), 18

## Z

Zone of proximal development (ZPD), 80, 91